THE BIG BOOK ᴏғ
BACKYARD
MEDICINE

The Ultimate Guide to
Home-Grown Herbal Remedies

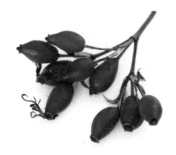

JULIE BRUTON-SEAL
MATTHEW SEAL

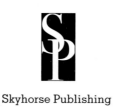

Skyhorse Publishing

To our parents:

Jen and Des Bartlett
Midge and George Seal

and in memory of inspirational herbal teachers:

Christopher Hedley (1946–2017)
Dr. James Duke (1929–2017)
Margaret Roberts (1937–2017)

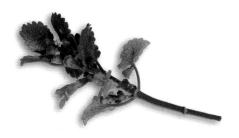

Country people heretofore did often use [ground ivy, above] to tun
it up with their drink.... But this Age forsakes all old things, though
never so good, and embraceth all kind of novelties whatsoever; but
the time will come, that the fopperies of the present time shall be
slighted, and the true and honest prescriptions of the Ancients come
in request again.
– William Coles (1656)*

Rather than dismissing items of plant lore as quaint reminders of
a more ignorant past, they should be seen as clues to an earlier, far
more comprehensive knowledge of the use of plants.
– Gabrielle Hatfield (1999)

Complete Contents

Part I: Backyard Medicine 5
Part II: Backyard Medicine for All 221

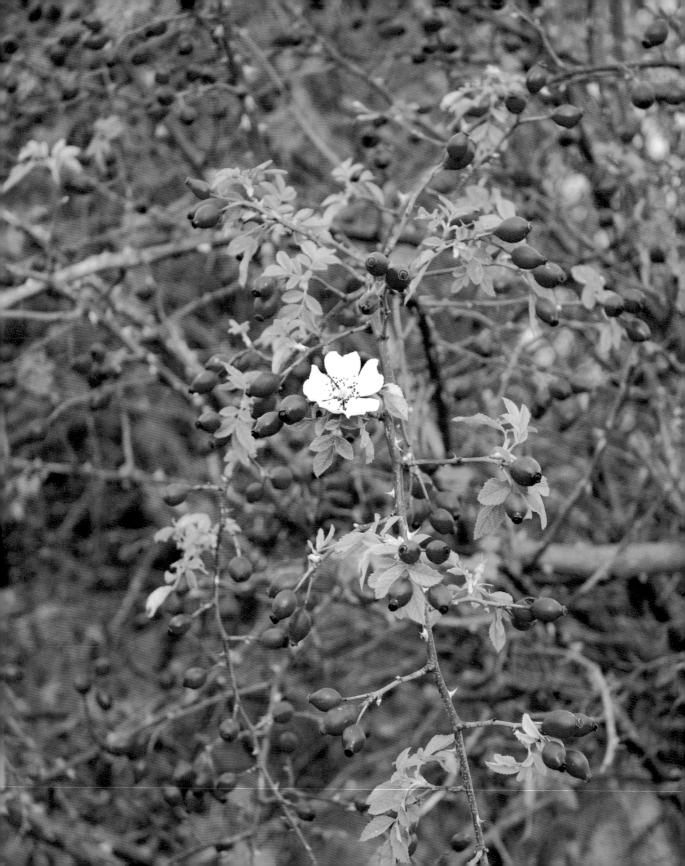

PART I: Backyard Medicine
Harvest and Make Your Own Herbal Remedies

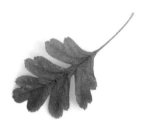

Contents

Preface to the North American edition

This is a book about wild plants and their medicinal uses. As authors we began with a list of over 100 species, which we thought was a limitation already, but our publisher wisely persuaded us to halve the number and write in greater depth. These are all wild plants, many of which are considered "weeds," which are abundant, easy to identify, cost nothing and are safe to pick.

Each of our selected plants has medicinal values – what the old herbals called the "virtues" of the plant. These are powerful, proven and significant herbs albeit they are often familiar and common. Commonness is not to be despised: it means a plant has the survival adaptations needed to accompany and thrive alongside our changing civilization.

We list our plants alphabetically by the English name, give a short description, and outline the habitat, distribution, related species and parts of the plant used. The text blends history, folklore, botany, uses of the plant and its modern medicinal benefits. We think it important to include easy-to-follow recipes too, and add bullet points of the herbal benefits. We tie ailments and benefits together in a comprehensive index.

We have made a number of changes in this latest version of the book. Two plants, figwort and sorrel, clamored for our attention, and we have made room for them by removing coltsfoot (following concerns about its pyrrolizidine alkaloid content) and shortening bilberry. We have improved some photographs, updated the "Using your Herbal Harvest" section, notes to the text, resources and recommended reading lists, simplified the page numbering and altered the index accordingly. We have added PubMed open access research information where appropriate.

Since the book was first published, on both sides of the Atlantic, more than a decade ago, it has become widely used in courses and workshops, and we hear from readers that it is often their first herb book or was their first course textbook. We thank you all, and especially for making this a bestseller in Amazon's Traditional Medicine and Remedies category. Our message to you was and remains the same: go out and find these plants for yourselves, get to know them and make your own useful medicines from them.

We cannot end without thanking a number of individuals from the herbal community for their help and support, including Andrew Chevallier, Christine Herbert, David Hoffmann, Sara James, Anna-Rósa Róbertsdóttir, Maida Silverman, Karin Uphoff, David Winston, and Matthew Wood.

Last but not least, we must thank the plants themselves. Wild medicine harvesting, like foraging for wild food, is best done with conscious respect for both habitat and individual plants, and we have received gifts from all of our plants. We understand better now why the famed Dutch herbalist Herman Boerhaave routinely lifted his hat in gratitude when we walked past 'mother elder.'

Preface to the 10th anniversary edition

This book has had a hectic life so far, with seven UK printings in ten years. The idea "hedgerow medicine" has also found its way into many courses, conferences, and workshops. In North America the book has had a parallel life as *Backyard Medicine*, and indeed that idea too seems to be spreading.

It is highly gratifying when we hear from people around the world that this was their first herb book, or it was their course textbook. Our message to you all has been and remains: go out and find these plants for yourself, get to know them, and make useful medicines from them.

Changes made in this edition of *Hedgerow Medicine / Backyard Medicine* include adding two new entries, for figwort and sorrel; we have shortened bilberry and removed coltsfoot. We have also replaced some photographs, updated the hedgerow harvest section, notes to the text, resources and recommended reading, simplified the page numbering and altered the index accordingly, and have incorporated PubMed open access research information where appropriate.

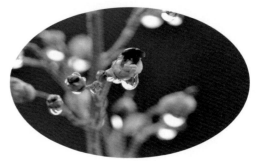

Despite these changes do be reassured that this remains essentially the book you have known, and made into a bestseller in Amazon's Traditional Medicine and Remedies category. We do appreciate this continuing support: you cannot know how grateful we are. In this new edition we particularly want to thank Andrew Chevallier and Anna Rósa Róbertsdóttir.

For more information, including details on workshops and courses, contact us on: www.hedgerowmedicine.com.

Julie Bruton-Seal & Matthew Seal
Ashwellthorpe, Norfolk   October 2018

Introduction

The British edition of this book used the title "hedgerow medicine," which we have changed to "backyard medicine" for the present edition.

Hedgerows in Britain are an integral part of the landscape, and the word conveys a sense of countryside and often-forgotten traditional harvesting and use of plants – there are miles of public footpaths with rights of access. We wanted to suggest the same sense of self-sufficiency in using the plants that "grow on your doorstep," hence our choice of the term "backyard medicine."

The plants we have selected are found in various habitats, including both cultivated and neglected land. So do not be surprised to see pictures here of plants growing on cliff scree, an abbey wall or open moorland. Quite a few of our plants are happy in cities, in waste lots, and parks, or cracks in sidewalks.

If we give ourselves some latitude in the first part of our title, what of "medicine"? Herbal medicines are traditional and effective, and we encourage you to use our chosen plants in making your own medicines. In the process you are taking responsibility for your own health. We do not intend to decry either pharmaceutical or manufactured herbal products, for clearly both have their place and many people want them. What we'd prefer to do is make a positive case for our wild plants.

Consider the following quotation from a 2004 survey of *Britain's Wild Harvest*, which is also relevant for the US. In terms of sourcing herbal medicines, this account pointed out that Britain is one of the world's major importers of herbs, but "despite this interest our own wild species play a remarkably small role in this market. Almost all of the tinctures, creams or infusions we use derive from plants that we import or cultivate."

Using native wild species for herbal remedies will save on imports and air miles; backyard medicines are not only cheap, they are free. There is also a sustainability issue: many popular imported herbal medicines have negative environmental effects in their place of origin. Our chosen plants are common, local, often invasive plants that are written off as weeds.

An excellent reason to harvest and make your own local herbal medicines is the pleasure the whole process brings. You will also have the peace of mind of knowing exactly what is in your medicines. Then again, the current regulatory environment is running against over-the-counter herbal preparations, and there is almost certain to be less choice and more control in future. All in all, the best option is to learn to make your own remedies.

Do please be aware that this book is intended to be a general guide to plant medicines and is not specific to personal circumstances or meant to replace a professional consultation. Do not self-diagnose or self-treat for serious or long-term conditions without consulting a qualified herbal or medical practitioner.

Having said that, we hope we can show you how easy it is to make your own remedies from wild plants. You will soon build up a home medicine cabinet better than anything you could buy. We support you in taking responsibility for your own health, and wish you well in seeking to benefit from the healing virtues offered by the plants all around us.

Harvesting from the wild

Harvesting wild plants for food or medicine is a great pleasure, and healing in its own right. We all need the company of plants and wild places in our lives, whether this is in an old wood, a mountainside or the seashore, just down the street or even in our own backyard. Gathering herbs for free is the beginning of a valuable and therapeutic relationship with the wild. Here are a few basic guidelines to help you get started.

Why pay others to frolic in the luscious gardens of Earth, picking flowers and enjoying themselves making herbal products? You can do all that frolicking, immersing yourself in wondrous herbal beauty, and uplifting your mind and spirit. Making your own herbal medicine both enhances your happiness and boosts your immune system.
– Green (2000)

When collecting, try to choose a place where the plant you are harvesting is abundant and vibrant. Woods, fields and minor roads are best, though many of our fifty plants are also found in the city. Avoiding heavy traffic is safer for you and for your lungs, and plants growing in quiet places will be less polluted. Plants growing next to fields may well receive crop sprays.

We usually want to harvest herbs when they are at their lushest. It's best to pick on a dry day, after the morning dew has burned off. For St. John's wort and aromatic plants the energy of the sun is important, so wait for a hot day and collect while the sun is high in the sky, ideally just before noon.

It is fundamental to ensure you have the right plant. A good field guide is essential – for North America we recommend the Peterson Field Guide series, which has regional guides including *A Field Guide to Medicinal Plants and Herbs of Eastern and Central North America*. Some herbalists and foragers offer herb walks, especially at herbal conferences – great for learning to identify plants.

For distribution maps and other information, go to the USDA PLANTS database: http://plants.usda.gov/.

Harvest only what you need and will use; leave some of the plant so that it will grow back. When picking "above-ground parts" of a plant, only take the top half to two-thirds. Never harvest a plant if it is the only one in a particular area.

We have included a few roots in our recipes. It is important not to over-harvest these, even though most of the plants we have selected are widespread and classed as weeds. The law states that you must seek the permission of the landowner before you dig up roots, if this is not on your own land (see page 216 for more on law).

Collecting equipment is simple: think carrier bags or a basket, and perhaps gloves, scissors or shears. If you are harvesting roots take a shovel or digging fork. See also page 12 below.

A quiet English country lane in May, with hawthorn flowering and a healthy undergrowth of nettles and cleavers

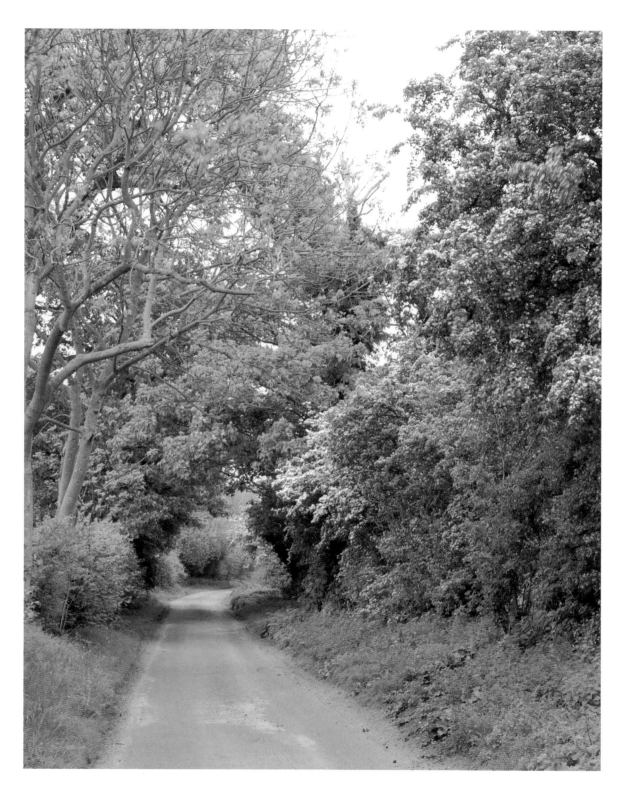

Using your herbal harvest

Herbs can be used in many different ways. Simplest of all is nibbling on the fresh plant, crushing the leaves to apply them as a poultice or perhaps boiling up some leaves as a tea. Many of the plants discussed in this book are foods as well as medicines, and incorporating them seasonally in your diet is a tasty and enjoyable way to improve your health.

But because fresh herbs aren't available year round or may not grow right on your doorstep, you may want to preserve them for later use. Follow these guidelines.

Equipment needed
You don't need any special equipment for making your own foraged medicines, and probably already have most of what you will use. Kitchen basics like a teapot, measuring jugs, saucepans and a blender are all useful, as are jam-making supplies such as a jelly bag and jam jars. A mortar and pestle are handy but not essential. You'll also need jars and bottles, and labels for these.

There is a list of suppliers at the end of the book to help you source any supplies or ingredients you may need (see p220).

It is a good idea to have a notebook to write down your experiences, so you'll have a record for yourself and can repeat successes. Who knows, it could become a future family heirloom like the stillroom books of old!

Drying herbs
The simplest way to preserve a plant is to dry it, and then use the dried part to makes teas (infusions or decoctions). Dried plant material can also go into tinctures, infused oils and other preparations, though these

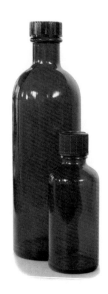

are often made directly from fresh plants.

To dry herbs, tie them in small bundles and hang these from the rafters or a laundry airer, or spread the herbs on a sheet of brown paper or a screen. (Avoid using newspaper as the inks contain toxic chemicals.)

You can easily make your own drying screen by stapling some mosquito netting or other open-weave fabric to a wooden frame. This is ideal, as the air can circulate around the plant, and yet you won't lose any small flowers or leaves through the mesh.

Generally, plants are best dried while out of the sun. An airing or warming cupboard works well, particularly in damp weather.

A dehydrator set on a low temperature setting is perfect for drying herbs as well as summer fruit.

Storing dried herbs
Once the plant is crisply dry, you can discard any larger stalks. Whole leaves and flowers will keep best, but if they are large you may want to

crumble them so they take up less space. They will be easier to measure for teas, etc. if they are crumbled before use.

Dried herbs can be stored in brown paper bags or in airtight containers such as candy jars or plastic tubs, in a cool place. If your container is made of clear glass or other transparent material, keep it in the dark as light will fade leaves and flowers quite quickly.

Dried herbs will usually keep for a year, until you can replace them with a fresh harvest. Roots and bark last longer than leaves and flowers.

In looking at medicine-making we start with the familiar teas and tinctures, then move on to often-forgotten but still valuable methods to give you a range of medicine-making options.

Teas: infusions and decoctions

The simplest way to make a plant extract is with hot water. Either fresh or dried herbs can be used. An **infusion,** where hot water is poured over the herb and left to steep for several minutes, is the usual method for a tea of leaves and flowers.

A **cold infusion** is made by steeping plants in cold water, often overnight, as in our recipe for cleavers (see p49).

A **decoction**, where the herb is simmered or boiled in water for some time, is the best process for roots and bark. Decoctions stored in sterile bottles will keep for a year or more if unopened.

Infusions and decoctions can also be used as mouthwashes, gargles, eyebaths, fomentations and douches.

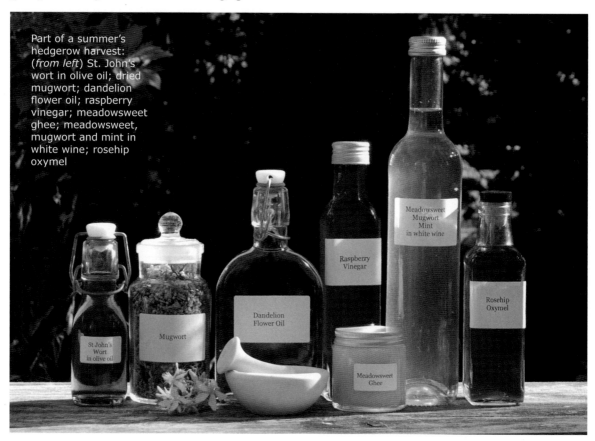

Part of a summer's hedgerow harvest: (*from left*) St. John's wort in olive oil; dried mugwort; dandelion flower oil; raspberry vinegar; meadowsweet ghee; meadowsweet, mugwort and mint in white wine; rosehip oxymel

St John's Wort in olive oil

Mugwort

Dandelion Flower Oil

Raspberry Vinegar

Meadowsweet Mugwort Mint in white wine

Meadowsweet Ghee

Rosehip Oxymel

Tinctures

While the term tincture can refer to any liquid extract of a plant, what is usually meant is an alcohol and water extract. Many plant constituents dissolve more easily in a mixture of alcohol and water than in pure water. There is the added advantage of the alcohol being a preservative, allowing the extract to be stored for several years.

The alcohol content of the finished extract needs to be at least 20% to adequately preserve it. Most commercially produced tinctures have a minimum alcohol content of 25%. A higher concentration is needed to extract more resinous substances, such as pine resin.

For making your own tinctures, vodka is the simplest alcohol as it can be used neat, has no flavor, and allows the taste of the herbs to come through. If you can get pure grain alcohol (95%) it can be diluted as needed. Whisky, brandy or rum can also be used. Herbs can also be infused in wine, but will not have as long a shelf life

To make a tincture, you simply fill a jar with the herb and top up with alcohol, or you can put the whole lot in the blender first. The mixture is then kept out of the light for anything from a day to a month to infuse before being strained and bottled. The extraction is ready when the plant material has lost most of its colour.

Tinctures are convenient to store and to take. We find amber or blue glass jars best for keeping, although clear bottles will let you enjoy the colours of your tinctures. Store them in a cool place. Kept properly, most tinctures have a shelf life of around five years. Tinctures are rapidly absorbed into the bloodstream, and alcohol makes the herbal preparation more heating and dispersing in its effect.

Wines and beers

Many herbs can be brewed into wines and beers, which will retain the medicinal virtues of the plants. Elderberry wine and nettle beer are traditional, but don't forget that ordinary beer is brewed with hops, a medicinal plant.

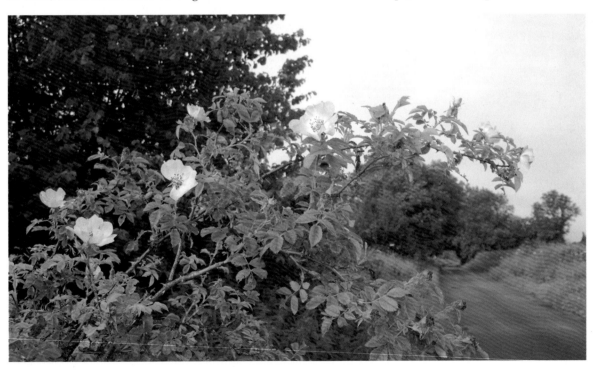

Other fermentations

Several other fermentations use a symbiotic combination of yeasts and bacteria. Sourdough bread is one example, but more relevant here are drinks such as kefir and kombucha. The starter grains are usually available on eBay. There are two kinds of kefir, one made with milk and one made with sugar and water. We find the latter a delicious and healthful drink, especially when flavoured with various herbs.

Glycerites

Vegetable glycerine (glycerol) is extracted from palm or other oil, and is a sweet, syrupy substance. It is recommended for making medicines for children, and for soothing preparations intended for the throat and digestive tract, or coughs. A glycerite will keep well if the concentration of glycerine is at least 50% to 60% in the finished product. Food-grade vegetable glycerine can be obtained online.

Glycerine does not extract most plant constituents as well as alcohol does, but preserves flavors and colors better, and is particularly good for flowers. Glycerites are made in the same way as tinctures, except the jar is kept in the sun or in a warm place to infuse.

Many herbalists like to add a small amount of alcohol to their glycerites to help preserve them, and to make them less sweet.

Glycerine is a good preservative for fresh plant juices, in which half fresh plant juice and half glycerine are mixed, as it keeps the juice green and in suspension better than alcohol. This preparation is called a succus.

Gemmotherapy extracts

Gemmotherapy is nothing to do with gem stones but rather uses the buds, shoots and sometimes root tips of trees and shrubs. The idea is that the embryonic tissue in the growing tips contains all the information of the whole plant, as well as various hormones not present elsewhere in the plant.

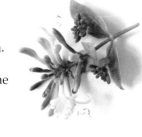

Buds are collected when they are plump but still firm, just before they open. Shoots are picked green, when they emerge from the dormant twigs. Because picking off the growth tip of a tree branch stops that part producing leaves, it needs to be done respectfully, not taking too many from any one plant.

For extracting the chemistry of buds and shoots a mixture of equal parts water, alcohol and glycerine has been found most effective. If you are using vodka or another spirit that is 50% alcohol (or more usually 40% alcohol and 60% water), simply use two parts alcohol to one part glycerine.

We have found this an effective mixture for other parts of the plant, too, and often prefer it to making a standard tincture or glycerite.

Vinegars

Another easy way to extract and preserve plant material is to use vinegar. Some plant constituents will extract better in an acidic medium, making vinegar the perfect choice.

Herbal vinegars are often made from pleasant-tasting herbs, and used in salad dressings and for cooking. They are also a good addition to the bath or for rinsing hair, as the acetic acid of the vinegar helps restore the natural protective acid pH of the body's exterior. Cider vinegar is a remedy for colds and other viruses, so it is a good solvent for herbal medicines made for these conditions.

Herbal honeys

Honey has natural antibiotic and antiseptic properties, making it an excellent vehicle for medicines to fight infection. It can be applied topically to wounds, burns and leg ulcers. Local honeys can help prevent hay-fever attacks.

Honey is naturally sweet, making it palatable in medicines for children. It is highly suited to medicines for the throat and the respiratory system as it is soothing and clears congestion. Make your herb-infused honeys as you do glycerites, or gently heat them in a bain-marie.

Oxymels

An oxymel is a preparation of honey and vinegar. Oxymels were once popular as cordials, both in Middle Eastern and European herbal traditions. They are particularly good for cold and flu remedies. Honey can be added to a herb-infused vinegar, or an infused honey used.

Electuaries

These are basically herbal pastes. Make them by stirring powdered dried herbs into honey or glycerine, or by grinding up herbs, seeds and dried fruit together. Electuaries are good as children's remedies, soothe the digestive tract and make tasty medicine balls or truffles.

Syrups

Syrups are made by boiling the herb with sugar and water. The sugar acts as a preservative, and can help extract the plant material. Syrups generally keep well, especially the thicker ones containing more sugar, as long as they are stored in sterilized bottles. They are particularly suitable for children because of their sweet taste, and are generally soothing.

Herbal sweets

While we are not recommending large amounts of sugar as being healthy, herbal sweets such as licorice and peppermints are a traditional way of taking herbs in a pleasurable way. Children enjoy making crystallized flowers, such as violets.

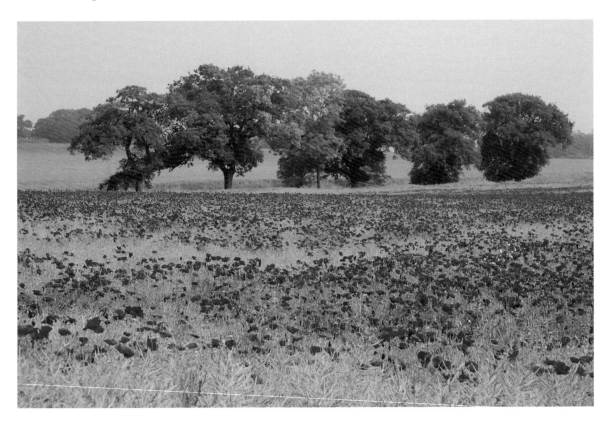

Plant essences

Plant essences, usually flower essences, differ from other herbal preparations in that they only contain the vibrational energy of the plant, and none of the plant chemistry. They have the advantage of being potent in small doses. Julie nearly always dispenses flower essences for her patients alongside other herbal preparations as they help the herbs do their job.

To make an essence, the flowers or other plant parts are usually put in water in a glass bowl and left to infuse in the sun for a couple of hours, as in the instructions for our self-heal essence on page 170. This essence is then preserved with brandy, and diluted for use.

Distilling herbs

While distilling essential oils from plants requires large plant quantities, it is simple to distill your own herbal waters (hydrolats).

Simply use a stockpot or other large saucepan with a domed lid that can be put on upside-down. A glass lid is best, as you can see what's going on inside. Put a brick into the saucepan under the center of the lid. Then put a collecting bowl on the brick, and add water plus your herbs. The idea is that the collecting bowl sits above the water level on its brick.

Heat the pot so that the water starts to become steam; this collects inside the lid and drips down into your collecting bowl. Ice cubes (or frozen peas!) put on the upturned lid speed up this condensation process. Keep going on a low heat until your collecting bowl is nearly full. Pour the distilled herbal water carefully into sterile bottles. It sounds difficult, but YouTube has many videos showing you how to do it.

If you want to make larger quantities, we recommend the traditional hand-made copper alembics still being produced in Portugal and now in the U.S.

Distilled plant waters keep quite well, but do not have any preservatives, so are often dispensed in spray bottles to keep them from getting contaminated. They are good as face washes and eyebaths, and can be taken internally. They are gentler than tinctures, but effective.

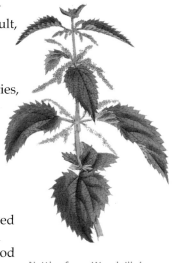

Nettle, from Woodville's *Medical Botany* (1790–3)

Infused oils

Oil is mostly used to extract plants for external use on the skin, but infused oils can equally well be taken internally. Like vinegars, they are good in salad dressings and in cooking.

We prefer extra virgin olive oil as a base, as it does not go rancid as many polyunsaturated oils do. Other oils, such as coconut and sesame, may be chosen because of their individual characteristics.

Infused oils are often called macerated oils, and should not be confused with essential oils, which are aromatic oils isolated by distilling the plant material.

Ointments or salves

Ointments or salves are rubbed onto the skin. The simplest ointments are made by adding beeswax to an infused oil and heating until the beeswax has melted. The amount of wax will vary, depending on the climate or temperature in which it will be used, with more wax needed in hotter climates or weather. Ointments made this way have a very good shelf life. They absorb well, while providing a protective layer on top of the skin.

Ointments can also be made with animal fats or hard plant fats such as cocoa butter, and with plant waxes such as candelilla.

Butters and ghees
Butter can be used instead of oil to extract herbs, and, once clarified by simmering, it keeps well without refrigeration, as a simple ointment. Clarified butter (ghee) is a staple in Indian cooking and medicine. It is soothing on the skin and absorbs well, plumping up the skin. Herbal butters and ghees can also be used as food.

Skin creams
Creams are a mixture of a water-based preparation with an oil-based one, to make an emulsion. Creams are absorbed into the skin more rapidly than ointments, but have the disadvantages of being more difficult to make and of not keeping as well. Creams are best refrigerated, and essential oils can be added to help preserve them. Creams are better than ointments for use on hot skin conditions, as they are more cooling.

Poultices
The simplest poultice is mashed fresh herb put onto the skin, as when you crush a plantain leaf and apply it to a wasp sting. Poultices can be made from fresh herb juice mixed with slippery elm powder or simply flour, or from dried herb moistened with hot water or vinegar.

Change the poultice every few hours and keep it in place with a bandage or bandaid.

Fomentations or compresses
A fomentation or compress is an infusion or a decoction applied externally. Simply soak a flannel or bandage in the warm or cold herbal liquid, and apply.

Hot fomentations are used to disperse and clear, and are good for conditions as varied as backache, joint pain, boils, and acne. Note that hot fomentations need to be refreshed frequently once they cool down. **Cold fomentations** can be used for cases of inflammation or for headaches. Alternating hot and cold fomentations works well for sprains and other injuries.

Embrocations or liniments
Embrocations or liniments are used in massage, with the herbs preserved in an oil or alcohol base, or a mixture of the two. Absorbed quickly through the skin, they can readily relieve muscle tension, pain and inflammation, and speed the healing of injuries.

Baths
Herbs can be added conveniently to bathwater by tying a sock or cloth full of dried or fresh herb to the hot tap as you run the bath, or by adding a few cups of an infusion or decoction. Herbal vinegars, tinctures, and oils can be added to bath water, as can a few drops of essential oil.

Besides full baths, hand and foot baths are very refreshing, as are sitz or hip baths where only your bottom is in the water.

Part of the therapeutic effect of any of these baths is the fact that they make you stop and be still, something we fail to do often enough.

Douches
Once they have cooled, herbal infusions or decoctions can be used as douches for vaginal infections or inflammation.

Opposite: Elder in flower in Lincolnshire, England, June

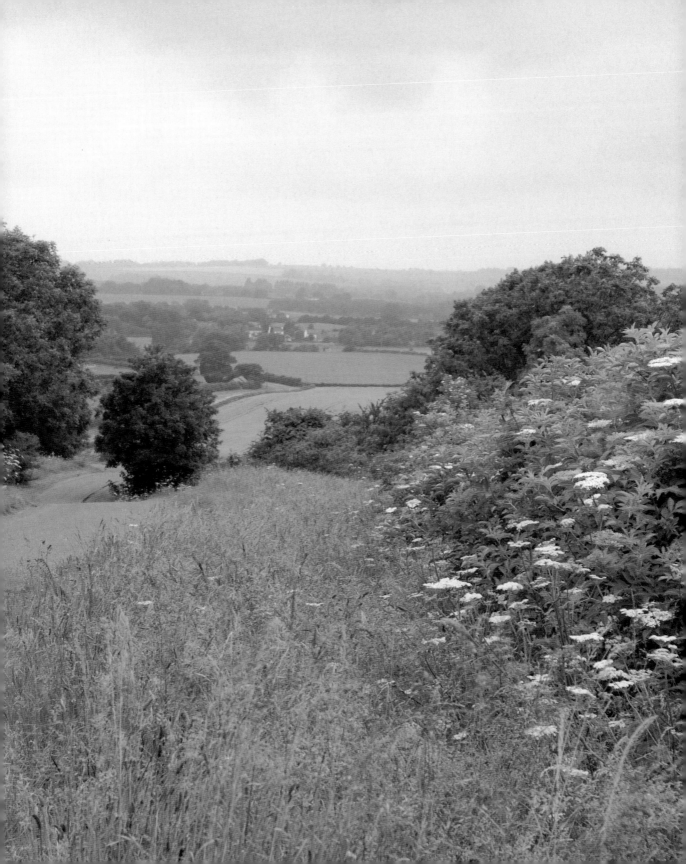

Rosaceae
Rose family

Description: Upright perennials with spikes of yellow flowers reaching up to 2 feet.

Habitat: Meadows and roadsides/grassy places.

Distribution: *A. eupatoria* is native to Europe, and introduced to North America. Tall hairy agrimony, *A. gryposepala*, is more widespread and is used interchangeably with the European species.

Related species: There are around 15 species of agrimony found in northern temperate regions and South America. In China, *xian he cao* (*A. pilosa*) is used medicinally, mainly for bleeding and diarrhea. Cinquefoil and tormentil are old medicinal herbs with very similar properties to agrimony.

Parts used: Above-ground parts, when in flower in summer.

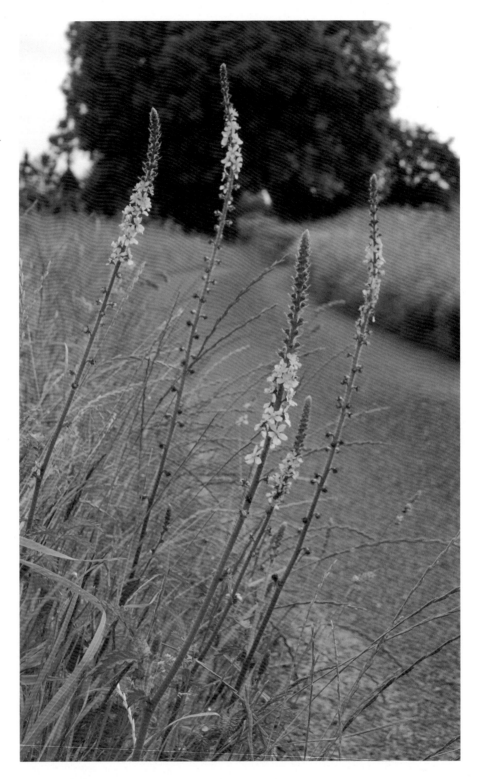

Agrimony *Agrimonia eupatoria, A. procera*

Agrimony stops bleeding of all sorts, and is used in trauma treatment and surgery in Chinese hospitals. It helps relieve pain too, and has a long tradition as a wound herb as well as for treating liver, digestive, and urinary tract problems.

Agrimony tightens and tones the tissues, and, in a seeming contradiction, will also relax tension, both physical and mental. This is the herb for when you're feeling frazzled, when stress and tension or pain are causing torment.

You can hardly miss this tall and bright summer herb, which readily earns its old name of church steeples. The sticky burrs that cling to passers-by lie behind another name, cocklebur.

Agrimony used to be a significant herb in the European tradition, being the Anglo-Saxon healing plant "garclive," but it is underused and underrated in modern western herbalism.

Agrimonia eupatoria is the "official" agrimony, but John Parkinson in *Theatrum Botanicum* (1640) preferred fragrant agrimony, *Agrimonia procera*, if available. The two can be used interchangeably.

In Chinese medicine, *A. pilosa* is the species used, and its name, *xian he cao*, translates as "immortal crane herb," which gives an idea of the reverence in which it is held. It is used in surgery and trauma treatment to stop bleeding, and has been found to be effective against *Trichomonas* vaginal infections and tapeworms, as also for dysentery and chronic diarrhea.

Dr. Edward Bach chose agrimony as one of his 38 flower essences. It is for people who soldier on, who say everything is fine when it is not, hiding inner turmoil behind a cheerful facade and ignoring the darker side of life. The out-of-balance agrimony person will sometimes resort to alcohol, drugs or adrenaline-producing sports to avoid dealing with life issues.

Use agrimony for...

Contemporary American herbalist Matthew Wood has written more deeply about agrimony than anybody else. He uses it as a flower essence, herbal tincture and homeopathic preparation, and has researched it in great detail, expanding on the traditional picture of the plant. Wood calls agrimony "the bad hair day remedy" – imagine the cartoon picture of a cat that

Agrimony, from Woodville's *Medical Botany* (1790–3)

Agrimony tea
- eyewash, conjunctivitis
- gargle for mouth and gum or throat problems
- in footbath for athlete's foot
- in bath for sprains & strained muscles

Agrimony tincture
- appendicitis
- urinary incontinence
- potty training
- cystitis
- weak digestion
- diarrhea or constipation
- tension
- irritable bladder
- asthma
- childhood diarrhea
- burns

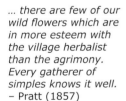

... there are few of our wild flowers which are in more esteem with the village herbalist than the agrimony. Every gatherer of simples knows it well. – Pratt (1857)

herb, as it rapidly stops bleeding and also relieves pain. It is thought that a high tannin and vitamin K content account for its remarkable coagulation properties. In the 1400s agrimony was picked in order to make "arquebusade water," to staunch bleeding inflicted by the arquebus or hand gun.

Agrimony works well for burns too – put tincture directly on the burn and take a few drops internally; repeat until the pain subsides.

Agrimony has an affinity for the liver and digestive tract, working effectively to co-ordinate their functions. John Parkinson – herbalist to King Charles I – wrote in 1640 that it "openeth the obstructions of the Liver, and cleanseth it; it helpeth the jaundise, and strengthneth the inward parts, and is very beneficiall to the bowels, and healeth their inward woundings and bruises or hurts."

All these are uses borne out today, and explained by the herb's bitter and astringent qualities.

Agrimony's other main affinity is for the urinary tract, being used to good effect to ease the pain of kidney stones, irritable bladder syndrome and chronic cystitis. It can be given safely to children for bedwetting and anxiety about potty training, and to the elderly for incontinence.

has had a fright or put its paw into an electric socket. He has found it works for people with mental and physical tension or work-related stress, with "pain that makes them hold their breath."

Agrimony is a go-to herb for treating intermittent fever and chills, or alternating constipation and diarrhea, working to help the body recover a working balance between extremes, by releasing the tension and constricted energy that cause such problems.

Pain is often associated with constriction, with one condition reinforcing the other. Agrimony can help release us from this self-perpetuating spiral, allowing body and mind to relax and restorative healing to begin as blood and energy flow return to normal. Agrimony is a wonderful wound

Harvesting agrimony

Harvest when the plant is in bloom in the summer, picking the flower spike and some leaves. For agrimony tea, dry them in the shade until crisp, and then strip the flowers and leaves off the stems, discarding the stems. Store in brown paper bags or glass jars, in a cool dry place.

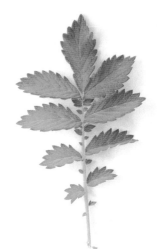

Agrimony tea

Use 1–2 teaspoonfuls of **dried agrimony** per cup of **boiling water**, infused for 10 to 15 minutes. The tea has a pleasant taste and odor, and was often used as a country beverage, especially when imported tea was expensive.

Dose: The tea can be drunk three times a day, or used when cool as an eyewash or gargle for gum irritations and sore throats.

Agrimony bath

Make a strong tea with a handful of **dried agrimony** infused in 1 pint of freshly **boiling water** for 20 minutes.

Poured hot into a foot bath, this soothes athlete's foot or sprained ankles; added to a hot bath it helps strained muscles after exercise, and general tension that has stiffened the muscles, back, and joints.

Agrimony tincture

To make agrimony tincture, pick the **flowers and leaves** on a bright sunny day. Pack them into a glass jar large enough to hold your harvest – clean jam jars work well – and pour in enough **brandy or vodka** to cover them. Put the lid on the jar and keep it in a dark cupboard for six weeks, shaking it every few days. Strain off the liquid, bottle, and label.

Amber or blue glass bottles will protect your tincture from UV light. If you use clear glass bottles, you will need to keep your tincture in a dark cupboard. It doesn't need to be refrigerated and should keep for several years, although it is best to make a fresh batch every summer if you can.

Dose: For tension or interstitial cystitis: 3–5 drops in a little water three times a day; as an astringent to tone tissues (as in diarrhea), half a teaspoonful in water three times daily.

The tincture can be used as a first-aid remedy for burns. First cool the burn thoroughly by holding it under water running from the cold tap for several minutes. You can just pour a little tincture onto the burn, but for best results, wet a cotton ball with the tincture and hold it in place until the burn stops hurting.

Bilberry

Vaccinium myrtillus **Blaeberry, Whortleberry**

Bilberries are one of the best herbs for the eyes and eyesight. They also strengthen the veins and capillaries, so are used for fragile and varicose veins.

The leaves are healing too, being effective for urinary tract infections and helping to regulate blood sugar levels.

**Ericaceae
Heather family**

Description: A short deciduous shrub with green twigs, pink flowers and bluish-black berries.

Habitat: Heathland, moors, and woods with acid soils.

Distribution: Circumboreal, across northern Europe, northern Asia, and in western North America.

Related species: North American blueberries are very similar to bilberries. There are several species, including highbush blueberry (*V. corymbosum*) and lowbush blueberry (*V. angustifolium*).

Parts used: Berries and leaves picked in summer.

Bilberry is an ancient source of food and medicine in Northern Europe, and picking bilberries takes the present-day forager as close to being a hunter-gatherer as one can get. Picking the berries is the perfect excuse to get out into wild nature. You have to crouch down to it on all fours to gather, especially on moorland where the plants are very low-growing.

Bilberry is not wild-harvested as a local cottage industry as much as formerly. Gathering bilberries in high summer was once a regular family and social occasion. The main food harvest, usually grain or potatoes, was about to begin, but the timing of early August was just right for a bilberry day.

Whether Fraughan Sunday in Ireland (from Gaelic for 'that which grows in the heather'), whort or hurt day in southern England, Laa Luanya in the Isle of Man, and equivalent August picking days in Wales, Scotland and the south-west, the pattern was similar. Whole communities would visit hill tops, woods,

lakes or holy wells, and the more assiduous would pick bilberries in rush or willow baskets. This was a rare day out, and it was a noisy, happy and often drunken occasion. It had predictable consequences, often with unmarried boys and girls, off the leash for once, taking the chance to slip away.

In Yorkshire, there was a more sober bilberry connection, with bilberry pies the traditional fare of funeral teas: berries mixed with sugar and lemon juice were baked in crusty pastry. Bilberry pies were known there as 'mucky-mouth pies' because they stained your hands and mouth blue.

Where commercial gathering was undertaken, as in Gwent, the process was sometimes eased by a toothed metal comb or rake, the *peigne*, named from a French tool, which could remove the berries from their stems. The fruit would be sold via dealers to jam-making factories, and sometimes for dyeing. In 1917 and 1918 the bilberry crop was requisitioned for wartime dyeing needs. In medieval times the bilberry was used as a purple dye and also tried as a writing ink and paint.

Bilberries have remained a favourite for their sweet, deep-toned and slightly astringent flavour. Commercial jam-makers appreciated them because they have no spines, fewer seeds than most other soft fruits and also more pectin.

This meant that less sugar was needed to set them, one pound of sugar setting two pounds of fruit (other fruit recipes usually specify about equal amounts of fruit and sugar). No wonder bilberry made a popular jam, one also rich in vitamins C and A, and healthier because of less sugar. The berries also went into wine and liqueurs.

Use bilberry for...
There's an interesting story about bilberry jam that neatly links its commercial and medicinal uses. Back in the early days of World War II, British pilots going on night missions chanced on the fact that eating bilberry jam sandwiches before flying seemed to improve their nightsight.

This all might seem "jolly prang" apocryphal, and indeed there is a wartime propaganda process in the background, but white-coat research has confirmed that taking bilberry stimulates production of retinal purple, known to be integral to night vision.

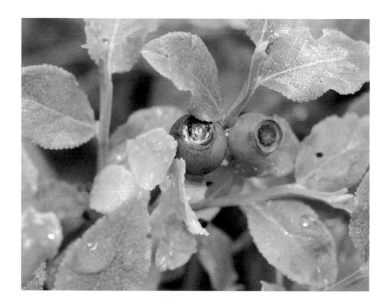

The berry's eyesight benefits are now recognized as also including treatment of glaucoma, cataract and general eye fatigue. Bilberry seems to work by its tonic effect on the small blood vessels of the eye, thereby improving the micro-circulation.

This is a relatively new feature of bilberry's repertoire. Mrs. Grieve, in her modern classic British herbal published in 1931, doesn't mention taking bilberry for eyesight. But, as you come to expect from reading Mrs. Grieve, she is thorough on historical uses.

So she mentions that the berries, being diuretic, antibacterial and disinfectant, as well as mildly astringent, are an old remedy for diarrhea, dysentery, gastroenteritis and the like. A bilberry syrup was traditionally made in Scotland for diarrhea. Eating a handful

Many a lad met his wife on Blaeberry Sunday.
– traditional Irish saying

This fruit and its relatives ... have been used traditionally for problems with visual acuity. And scientific research has validated this folk medicine approach.
– Duke (1997)

It is a pity they [bilberries] are used no more in physic than they are.
– Culpeper (1653)

… the first and most indispensable of all the tinctures in our family medicine chest.
– Abbé Kneipp (1821–97), on fresh bilberry tincture

Anthocyanins
These are a class of flavonoid compounds, found in high levels in bilberries. Anthocyanins are pigments that give red or blue color to blackberries, elderberries, hawthorn berries, cherries and many other fruits and vegetables.
These compounds are powerful antioxidants that are attracting a lot of attention in nutritional research. Their potential health benefits include easing the effects of aging, reducing inflammation and increasing insulin production. Anthocyanins also protect the blood vessels and have a range of anti-cancer effects.

of the dried berries works well too. The berry tea was used for treating bedwetting in children, and to dilate blood vessels of the body. The tea is valuable for varicose veins and hemorrhoids, strengthening vein and capillary walls. The berries mashed into a paste are applied to hemorrhoids.

Bilberry leaves are a valuable herbal medicine in their own right, with a different range of qualities, although often used in combination with the berries. The leaves are deciduous, and turn a beautiful red before they fall.

The particular and long-appreciated effect of the leaves is as an antiseptic tea for urogenital tract inflammation, especially of the bladder. This tea can also be drunk for ulcers, including of the mouth and tonsils.

Bilberry leaves are known to be hypoglaecemic, i.e., they reduce blood sugar levels, and are used successfully in treating late-onset diabetes. This is a slow-acting treatment, however, and taking the tea for long periods may lead to a build-up of tannins that is counter-productive. Some sources suggest using the leaf tea for only three weeks at a time; others say it is best with strawberry leaves.

Julie uses bilberry syrup for eyesight and vascular problems. She says: "A friend asked me to make up bilberry syrup for her elderly neighbor. This lady

had aching and discomfort in her legs from varicose veins but was about to go on a long walk, the pilgrimage to Santiago de Compostela in Spain. She completed it successfully, walking many miles, commenting that she could 'feel her veins tightening up' when she took the syrup."

Bilberry combines well with ginkgo tincture or glycerite for eye problems. Julie's father took this combination ever since he had surgery for a detached retina many years before. His eye surgeon was initially skeptical, but checked into the research and now regularly recommends both these herbs to his patients.

Julie has often used ginkgo and bilberry for macular degeneration or retinal tears. Two cases stand out, both people with small tears in the retina. These were not bad enough to warrant surgery, but were intensely worrying to the people concerned, who came to see her to learn if further damage could be prevented.

In both cases, the patients went back to their eye specialists after taking bilberry and ginkgo for several months, and the specialists said words to the effect of "but there's nothing there, we must have made a mistake when we looked at your eyes initially." Not everyone may be as fortunate, but bilberry certainly has an important role to play in promoting and restoring eye health.

Bilberry syrup

Place your **bilberries** in a saucepan with just enough **water** to cover them. Simmer gently for half an hour, then leave to cool before squeezing out as much of the liquid as possible using a jelly bag. For every pint of liquid, add 1 pound **demerara sugar**, and boil until the sugar has dissolved completely. Pour into sterile bottles, label, and store in a cool place.

Dose: 1 teaspoonful daily to maintain good eyesight and vascular health. For more acute problems, take 1 teaspoonful three times daily.

Bilberry glycerite

Fill a jar with **bilberries** and pour on **vegetable glycerine** to take up all the air spaces. Put the lid on and shake to get rid of any remaining bubbles, then top up again with glycerine. Keep the jar in a warm place, such as a sunny window ledge, by a range cooker or in an airing cupboard, for two or three weeks, then squeeze out the liquid using a jelly bag. Bottle, label, and store in a cool place.

Dose: 1 teaspoonful daily to maintain good eyesight and vascular health. For more acute problems, take 1 teaspoonful three times daily.

Berry brandy pot

Start out with **bilberries**, placing them in the bottom of a jar or crock and then pouring on enough **brandy (or whisky)** to cover. You can, of course fill the whole jar with bilberries, or you can leave room and repeat the process with **other berries** in layers as they come into season – raspberries, blackberries, elderberries, and lycium berries.

Leave until winter and enjoy as a rather alcoholic treat, which will be packed with antioxidants and do your eyes and your veins a world of good. The liquid can be poured off and added to your syrup or glycerite, or left and enjoyed with the berries as a dessert with cream or however you like them.

Bilberry leaf tea

Use a heaped teaspoonful of the **dried leaves** per cup or mug of **boiling water** and leave to infuse for 5 to 10 minutes.

Dose: Drink a cupful every few hours for an acute urinary infection, or one cup daily to help maintain blood sugar levels.

Julie often adds couchgrass (p. 54), horsetail (p. 96), pellitory-of-the-wall (p. 140) and cornsilk to her cystitis tea blends.

BILBERRY BERRY

Syrup or glycerite
• macular degeneration
• detached retina
• night vision
• cataracts
• capillary fragility

BILBERRY LEAF

Bilberry leaf tea
• urinary tract infections
• high blood sugar

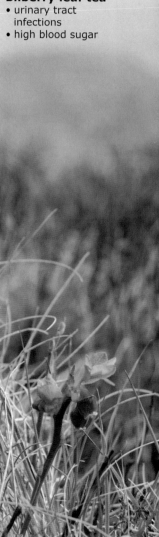

Bilberry flowers on the Long Mynd, Shropshire, England, April

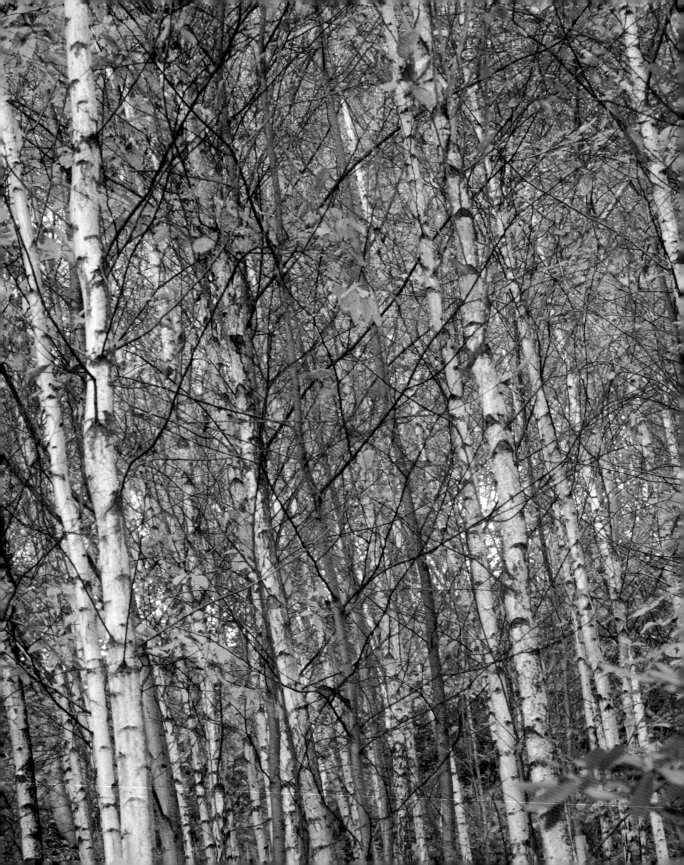

Birch *Betula pendula, B. pubescens*

Birch has a multitude of historical uses but is less familiar for its undoubted medicinal benefits. The sap makes a clear and refreshing drink that can be preserved as a wine, beer or spirit. The leaves produce a pleasant tea and an infused oil. In each form, birch is an excellent tonic and detoxifier, mainly working on the urinary system to remove waste products, as in kidney or bladder stone, gravel, gout and rheumatism. It reduces fluid retention and swellings, and clears up many skin problems.

Birch is one of the most useful of trees as well as one of the most graceful. From adhesives to wine, baskets to yokes and boats to vinegar, it has been a boon to people in the cold north for thousands of years. Its medicinal qualities have been historically valued and should be better known today.

Called the oldest tree in Britain, birch was a pioneer species when the ice caps retreated, moving in on the devastated land, growing quickly and then rotting to leave more fertile earth in which other species could take over. In its rapid life cycle birch pushes upwards too fast to develop a strong heart wood, but this makes it perfect for making buckets and canoes.

As a youngster (writes Matthew), "I was a suburban Hiawatha, and wanted to be a 'Red Indian.' I had read in my weekly comic, the *Eagle*, how my heroes had made birch bark canoes and wrote on birch bark paper. Birch was a common enough tree, but I never actually got down to making the boat or the paper. Soccer was more important."

But now these memories return, as Julie and I tap a birch in our garden. It is that time in spring after most of the frosts and before the birch buds and leaves emerge. The tree is now forcing its sap upwards in prodigious quantity, and you simply tap into the flow, thanking the tree after you have taken your share by closing off the wound.

Birch sap is rich in fructose whereas maple has sucrose. Sucrose is sweeter to the taste and the maple yields more per tree, so maple syrup is by far the bigger commercial industry. On the other hand, birch sap is cool, refreshing and clear. It tastes even better when reduced by simmering down into a golden-brown ambrosia. It's the sort of drink even the elves would envy!

**Betulaceae
Birch family**

Description: Deciduous trees with whitish papery bark that often hybridize.

Habitat: Woods, heaths, moors and gardens. Downy birch (*Betula pubescens*) prefers wetter places.

Distribution: Silver birch or European white birch (*Betula pendula*) and downy birch are native to northern temperate regions of Eurasia, and found as introduced species in North America. Sweet birch (*B. lenta*) is native to eastern North America.

Related species: Worldwide, several birch species have medicinal value. In Ayurveda, Himalayan silver birch (*B. utilis*) is used.

Parts used: Sap, tapped in early spring; leaves, gathered in spring and early summer. The bark is also used.

A stand of silver birch in the English Surrey hills, where the birch is so common it has earned the name "Surrey weed"

… birch water is the hope, the blessing and the panacea of rich and poor, master and peasant alike … almost unfailingly cures skin conditions … and countless chronic ills against which medical science is so prone to fail.
– Baron Percy (c. 1800)

Use birch for…
Birch sap, birch water or blood, had a folk reputation for breaking kidney or bladder stone and treating skin conditions and rheumatic diseases. It can be drunk in spring as a refreshing and cleansing tonic, clearing the sluggishness of winter from the system. The fermented sap also makes birch wine and country beers and spirits.

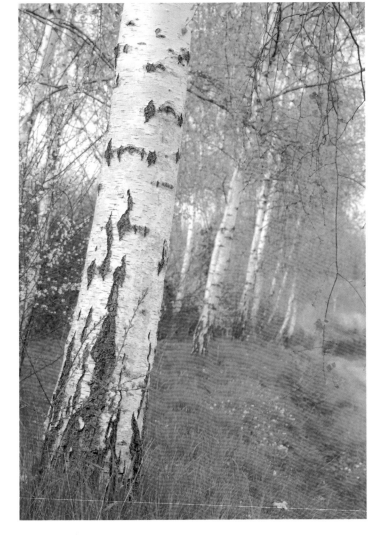

Besides being a source of tinder and paper, birch bark has been used for tanning leather, especially in Russia, and for preserving nets and ropes. Another product of this gracious tree is an oil tar from the bark. This is used commercially in birch creams and ointments for chronic skin conditions.

The fresh leaves or buds of birch offer a powerful but pleasant tea for general detoxing, urinary complaints, cystitis, rheumatic and arthritic troubles, and gout. Some herbalists add a pinch of sodium bicarbonate to improve the tea's ability to cut high uric acid levels. Any condition of fluid retention, such as cardiac or renal edema and dropsy, will be helped by the tea. Birch is rich in potassium, so that (like dandelion) it does not deplete the body of this mineral in the way that medical diuretics do.

Being such a good eliminator, birch tea is also effective as a compress applied directly to the skin for herpes, eczema, and the like.

You can easily make your own birch leaf oil by infusing the leaves in olive or sweet almond oil. This goes into commercial cellulite treatments, and can be used as a massage oil to relieve muscle aches and pains, fibromyalgia and rheumatism. Drink birch tea as well for maximum benefit.

Birch is regarded as safe medicinally and no side effects have been reported.

Birch leaf oil

Pick the **leaves** in late spring or early summer, while they are still fresh and light green. Put them in a jar large enough to hold them and pour in enough **extra virgin olive oil or sweet almond oil** to cover them. Put a piece of cloth over the jar as a lid, held on with a rubber band. This will allow any moisture released by the leaves to escape. Put the jar in a sunny place indoors and leave for a month but stir it fairly regularly, checking to see that the leaves are kept beneath the surface of the oil.

Strain off into a jug, using a nylon jelly bag or a large strainer (if you use muslin, it will soak up too much of the oil). Allow to settle – if there is any water in the oil from the leaves, it will sink to the bottom of the jug. Pour the oil into sterile storage bottles, leaving any watery residue behind in the jug, and label. Using amber, blue, or green glass will protect the oil from ultraviolet light, so if you use clear glass bottles remember to store your oil away from light.

This can be used as a massage oil for cellulite, fibromyalgia, rheumatism, and other muscle aches and pains. It can be also used on eczema and psoriasis – but remember that these also need to be treated internally, so ask your herbalist for advice.

Birch leaf tea

Pick the leaves in spring and early summer while they are still a fresh bright green. They can be used fresh in season or dried for later use. To dry, spread the leaves on a sheet of paper or on a drying screen, which can be made by stretching and stapling a piece of netting to a wooden frame. Dry them in the shade, until crisp when crumbled.

To make the tea, use 4 or 5 **leaves** per cup or mug of **boiling water,** and allow to infuse for 5 to 10 minutes.

Dose: Drink a cupful up to three or four times daily.

Birch sap

To collect the sap, drill a hole through the bark in the early spring, before the tree gets its leaves. Insert a tube into the hole – a straw with a flexible end works well – and put the other end in a bottle or collection bucket. After you have collected for about a week, make sure you plug the hole with a twig the right size so that the tree doesn't keep "bleeding."

The sap is a delightfully refreshing drunk as it comes from the tree, or it can be gently simmered down to taste to produce an amber ambrosia or further reduced to make a syrup.

Birch leaf oil
- cellulite
- detoxing massage
- aching muscles
- rheumatism
- eczema
- psoriasis

Birch leaf tea
- spring cleanse
- kidney stones
- urinary gravel
- cystitis
- gout
- arthritis
- rheumatism
- psoriasis
- eczema
- fluid retention
- fevers

Birch sap
- cleansing tonic

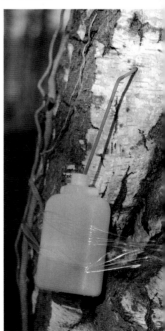

Our own crude birch tap: you can probably do better!

Blackberry, Bramble *Rubus fruticosus*

**Rosaceae
Rose family**

Description: A thorny, sprawling bush with white or pink flowers and black berries.

Habitat: Widespread in hedgerows, woods, and on waste ground.

Distribution: Widespread. Native to temperate Europe but naturalized in North America and Australasia.

Related species: Blackberry is actually an aggregate of many taxonomically difficult species. It is related to dewberry (*R. caesius*), which has fruits with fewer, large segments and a blue bloom, and raspberry (*R. idaeus*).

Parts used: Leaves, gathered in early summer, berries harvested when ripe.

Blackberry or bramble is one of the most familiar but also most aggressive of berry plants. The protective spines demand respect, but the berries and leaves offer medicinal rewards that repay the inevitable scratches of picking.

The poet Walt Whitman wrote this about blackberry in "Song of Myself" (1855):

I believe a leaf of grass is no less than the journey work of the stars/ ... and the running blackberry would adorn the parlors of heaven.

In more sober judgment, Jonathan Roberts's history of fruit and vegetables (2001) calls blackberry a "primitive thug." Sorry to say, Roberts is probably closer to the truth. Blackberry always has been an aggressive settler on waste or cleared land, using an array of effective spreading mechanisms.

It is promiscuous in hybridizing with similar thorny trailing plants of the rose family (over 2,000 blackberry "species" have been described in Europe); then, it has tasty berries to spread its seeds, which pass unharmed through birds and humans alike; its young shoots bend to the ground and start fresh roots; its thorns hook on to adjacent foliage and help spread the plant laterally; and its dense ground cover shuts off most competing plants.

The old ironic name of "lawyers" for blackberries was exported from England to the United States: in either case, once in their clutches you will never escape! (Perhaps the makers of the handheld wireless device of the same name hoped for the same sense of being captured by their product.)

Highlanders in Scotland had a high opinion of blackberry. Its Gaelic name was *an druise bennaichte*, meaning "blessed bramble." This referred to Jesus supposedly using a bramble switch when riding his donkey to Jerusalem to evict the moneylenders from the temple. Highlanders made wreaths of ivy, bramble, and rowan as protection against evil.

Blackberry has been spread from the temperate north around the world apart from the tropics. New Zealand has become overrun to

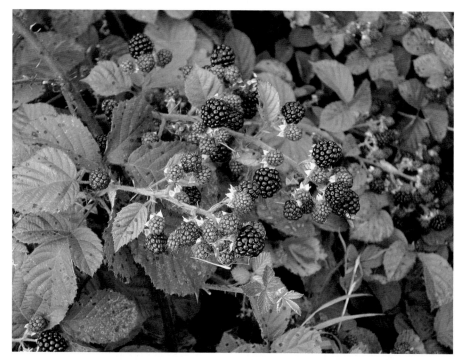

Blackberries are the most commonly used natural fruit in Great Britain. ... The fruit, so beloved of wine and jam makers, has rich medicinal properties, full of vitamin C and minerals, as are the leaves.
– Furnell (1985)

such an extent that there is a saying: there are only two brambles in New Zealand, one covering North Island and one South Island. In Australia it is a notifiable pest that must be destroyed wherever found; over 9 million hectares of land have been infested.

Blackberry hedges were used as defensive barriers around Native American settlements and in bygone Europe. Hedgerows containing blackberries make fields stock-proof, which is another reason why they are so widespread.

Sleeping Beauty, in the legend, was protected for a hundred years by a thicket of blackberry or perhaps wild rose – either would have been impenetrable after even two years by any but a true lover!

Going blackberrying or brambling is an ancient social activity worldwide, and family expeditions to gather the delicious fruit are well within living memory, though happening less in Britain these days. In the Ozark mountains, where communal picking persists, the blackberry harvest is called "black gold."

Perhaps because blackberry was and still is so successful in the wild it was only in the nineteenth century that it was grown as a commercial crop, in the United States. It was also in the States that Judge Logan developed a cross raspberry/blackberry, named the loganberry in his honour. The friendlier raspberry meanwhile had been domesticated in Britain by the sixteenth century.

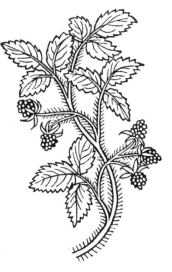

A medieval illustration of blackberry

We recommend you revive or continue the wild-picking habit because blackberries are so good for you and can be found almost everywhere. The ripe black fruit, as everyone knows, makes wonderful jams, jellies, preserves, pies, and cordials. The wine even stars in its own novel (*Blackberry Wine*, by Joanne Harris). But folklore dictates that you should not gather the berries after Michaelmas, because that is when the Devil spits or urinates on them. Or, we'd now say, the frost has got to them.

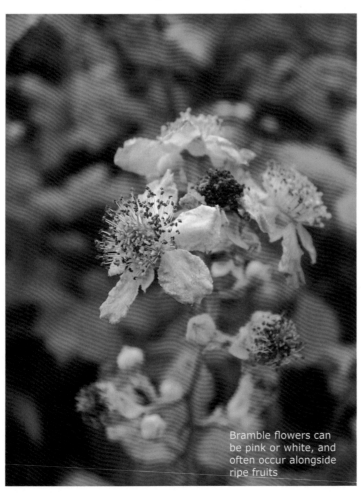
Bramble flowers can be pink or white, and often occur alongside ripe fruits

Use blackberry for...

In spring, blackberry shoots and the young leaves are a traditional European tonic, packed with vitamins and minerals, and used fresh as a tea. They can also be combined with raspberry leaves, young hawthorn leaves and birch shoots or leaves.

The leaves and unripe fruit are good medicine too, for their astringency. The leaves were chewed to allay headaches. Crushed blackberry leaves are exactly what you need as a styptic to treat small cuts incurred when picking the fruit; they also work for boils and swellings.

The main use of the leaf tea is as a folk remedy for diarrhea; the unripe red or green fruit can be used for the same purpose.

In the US Civil War of 1861–65 the ferocious hand-to-hand fighting in the woods was sometimes interrupted for "blackberry truces." Both sides would take time out to pick blackberry leaves for a tea to treat diarrhea and dysentery, which were rife in both armies.

The leaf tea is like a green tea, pleasant but with a tannin feel. It is also a welcome relief for problems of the mouth, such as ulcers and gum disease. It was once thought to strengthen teeth, and is an old remedy for soothing sore throats and treating colds and anemia. When cool, the tea makes a good skin lotion.

Bramble leaf tea

Bramble leaves should be picked in spring and summer while they are fresh and green. They can be used fresh for tea in season, or can be dried for the winter. Dry them in a shady place or indoors, until the leaves are brittle and crumble easily. Store in brown paper bags or in jars in a cool, dark place.

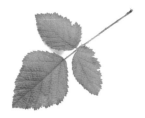

To make the tea, put a few **fresh leaves** or a rounded teaspoonful of crumbled **dry leaves** in a teapot. Pour on a mugful of **boiling water**, and allow to infuse for about 5 minutes, then strain and drink.

Dose: Can be drunk freely. Make double-strength to treat diarrhea, drinking a cupful every hour as needed.

Bramble leaf tea
- general health
- diarrhea
- mouth ulcers
- gingivitis
- sore throats
- colds
- flu and fevers

Blackberry spread

This is a traditional recipe, often called "blackberry butter," which is delicious with scones or on toast.

Put in a pan: **1 pound blackberries
1 pound tart apples, chopped up but not peeled or cored
grated zest and juice of a lemon**

Simmer gently for about 15 minutes, until soft and mushy. Rub the pulp through a sieve to remove the skins and pips. Weigh the pulp, and for every 4oz of pulp add 3oz of **sugar**.

Heat gently until the sugar has dissolved, then simmer and stir until the mixture is thick and smooth – this usually takes about 20 minutes. Pour into sterilized jars, seal, and label.

Blackberry oxymel

Pick blackberries when they are ripe, checking that the heel (the place where they come off the stem) is white or pale green – if this has gone purple or dark, it's not a good one to use.

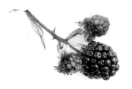

Put the **blackberries** in a china or glass bowl and pour on enough **white wine vinegar** just to cover them. Put a plate or a cloth over the bowl and leave it for a day or two, then crush the fruit with a potato masher. Strain the juice through a sieve or jelly bag into a measuring jug, then pour into a saucepan. Add half the volume of **honey,** then heat to melt the honey. Bring to the boil and boil for 5 minutes, bottle, and label. This syrup can also be frozen in an ice cube tray, and then stored in bags in the freezer.

To use: Mix one tablespoonful with a cup of hot water as a bedtime drink, or drink frequently to help relieve a cold.

Blackberry oxymel
- general health
- colds
- sore throats

Burdock *Arctium* spp.

Asteraceae (Compositae) Daisy family

Description: A biennial plant with large, soft, light green leaves and thistle-like red-purple flowers that form burrs with hooked spines. Can reach a sculptural 6 feet tall in its second year.

Habitat: Hedgerows, wood edges and waste ground.

Distribution: Native to Europe and Asia, but found in temperate regions around the world; taken to North America by European settlers.

Species used: Greater or common burdock (*Arctium lappa*) is the best-known species, but lesser burdock (*A. minus*) is more wide-spread in Britain. It is similar in appearance and used interchange-ably for medicinal purposes.

Parts used: Leaves picked in summer, roots dug in spring or fall, and seeds gath-ered in fall.

Traditionally combined with dandelion both as a soft drink and a medicine, burdock is a powerful cleanser and blood purifier. It is one of the foremost detoxing herbs, and is particularly effective for skin problems. The root is a food as well as a medicine, and is popular in Japanese cooking.

Burdock is a sturdy biennial, with a rosette of large leaves forming in the first year, as the tap root deepens. In the second year the stems shoot up, producing the thistle-like flowers or burrs that gave it the old name of beggar's buttons.

The roots are best used in the first fall or second spring, and are more tonic in the spring. Descending nearly a yard, the mature root takes energetic digging up, but younger roots are just as good.

Burdock can be grown in the garden (one has adopted us, and we are happy to host it), and if you use raised beds or drainage pipes the root is much less effort to harvest. The other advantage is that you will know where to dig for spring roots, as the leaves die back to very little in the winter and the plants can be difficult to find.

Burdock root was a food for our hunter-gatherer ancestors, and is a cooked vegetable in Japan, *gobo*; the dish is now popular in Hawaii and New Zealand. The delicious mild flavour is similar to artichoke or scorzonera.

Burdock has been called the velcro plant. This all comes from walking the dog: Swiss inventor George de Mestral noticed that after he and his dog had brushed by a large burdock, the plant's "hooks" had tagged onto "loops" in his wool trousers and in the dog's fur.

Using the technique of "biomimicry," De Mestral made two nylon pads, one of hooks and one of loops; the more you pushed them, the more they fused, but they pulled apart easily, just like the plant's fruits do in nature.

As space institute NASA later used his Velcro™-derived products for astronaut suits, burdock (by proxy) became the first space weed. It's the latest version of a story played out over the centuries, with immigrants' clothes and their livestock fur transferring the benefits and burdens of burdock across the seas to new lands.

In terms of the famous soft drink, a few specialist makers still use real roots in their dandelion and burdock mix but the mass market version has artificial flavorings.

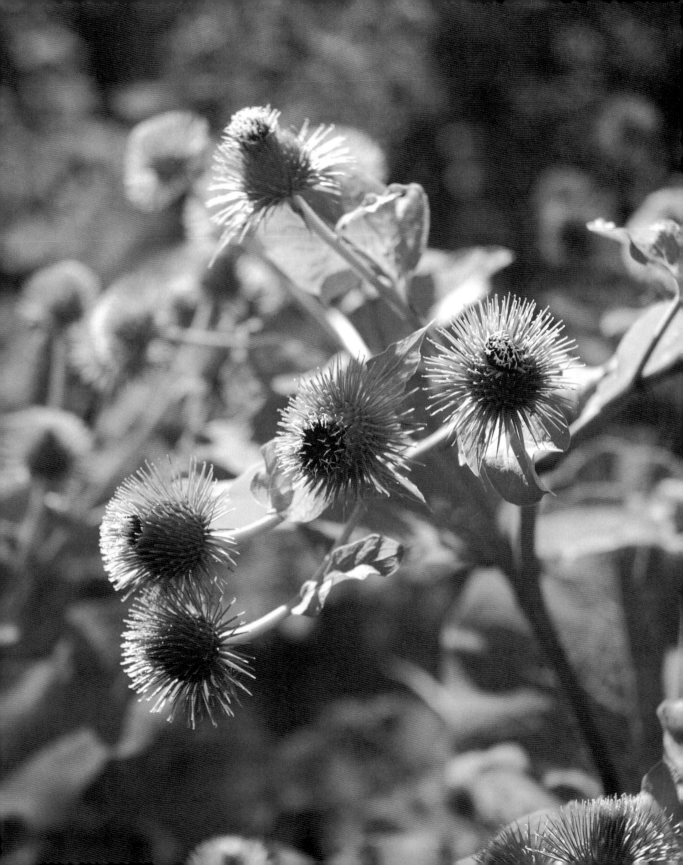

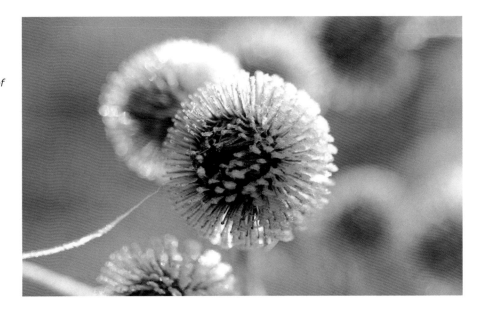

Burdock is a "deep food" and alterative that moves the body to a state of well-nourished health, promotes the healing of wounds, and removes the indicators of system imbalance such as low energy, ulcers, skin conditions, and dandruff.
– Green (2000)

Use burdock for...

Burdock is a significant detoxing herb in both Western and Chinese medicinal traditions. Known as a blood purifier, its special attribute is to stimulate the release of waste products from the cells. This is a powerful process at cellular level, and the metabolic wastes then need to be removed from the body.

Here dandelion comes in as a complement to burdock, with its diuretic and flushing qualities to the outside world via the kidneys and liver. Hence the classic mix of the two roots. Burdock also combines well with red clover or dock.

Herbal blood purifiers have the associated virtue of cleansing the skin. Burdock has a remarkable effect on skin conditions arising from imbalance, as in dry or scaly skin, and eruptions, as in acne,

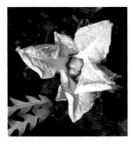

Burdock leaves emerging in early spring of the second year.

boils, eczema, and psoriasis. For all these it can be applied externally as a poultice or taken internally as a decoction or tincture (in small quantities as it's strong).

Burdock helps restore and maintain fluid balance in the body, both of water and of fats.

Burdock has been associated with medical conditions that seemed incurable, if not evil, at the time. Mixed with wine in the Middle Ages, it was given for leprosy; later it was used to treat syphilis (Henry VIII improved, but was not cured by it), epilepsy, and hysteria; in modern times research suggests possible benefits in treating HIV and cancer. Hildegard of Bingen was already using burdock root on her cancer patients in the 1100s. In each case burdock strongly supported the immune system.

Burdock root is used to break down excess uric acid in the joints that leads to gout. It also relieves arthritis and swollen prostate. Ask your herbalist's advice on the best combination of herbs for your own condition and constitution.

Another burdock benefit lies in its bitterness, which helps stimulate the digestive fluids and promote appetite and digestion. This underlies the tang of the famous drink and makes burdock palatable in anorexia.

Burdock leaf poultice
A simple poultice can be made from a whole burdock leaf. Steam it to soften the leaf, and apply as hot as can be borne to the affected place. Leave it there until it cools down and then heat again, or put a hot water bottle over it to keep it warm, and leave on for half an hour. The poultice will draw blood to the area, and as it is also antiseptic it will fight infection and accelerate healing.

The leaves can also be crushed with a rolling pin and applied as a poultice for minor burns; leave them in place until the pain subsides.

Burdock and dandelion root decoction
Simmer about an ounce each of fresh chopped **burdock and dandelion root** in 3 cups of **water** for 20 minutes. Strain and divide into three or four doses to drink during the day, hot or cold. To sweeten the decoction, add a tablespoonful of dried licorice root before boiling.

Burdock and dandelion toffee
Dig several roots of **burdock and dandelion**, preferably in spring. In each case strip the root bark off, and clean and chop up the inner part. Weigh out 3–4 ounces of each. Load into a saucepan and cover with **a pint of water**. Bring to the boil, simmer for 20 minutes, allow to cool.

Simmer again until the roots are tasteless (i.e., have surrendered their content to the liquid). This reduces the mixture by about half. Strain and add **1 tablespoon butter and 12 tablespoons of sugar**. Boil for 5 minutes then simmer for 20 minutes more. It will become toffee-like.

Test the toffee by pouring a drip of it onto a cold plate, as you would in testing jam: when it crinkles into soft threads, it is ready. Pour it into a buttered shallow tin. Before it sets totally, mark out squares and save the toffee slab in greaseproof paper; alternatively, stretch it out by hand into taffee: this is pale and pliable, ideal for balls, plaits etc.

Burdock leaf poultice
- bruises
- boils
- acne
- rheumatism
- arthritis
- gout

Burdock & dandelion root decoction
- acne
- eczema
- boils
- psoriasis
- detoxing

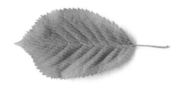

Cherry *Prunus avium, P. serotina*

Wild sweet cherries, also known as gaskins, geans, mazzards, and merrys, are not only delicious to eat but also good for your gout or arthritis. The fruit stalks and inner bark have medicinal virtues too, for treating dry coughs, sore throats, and bronchitis. It is a bonus that children seem to love the tea or syrup, leaving their parents to drink up the home-made cherry brandy.

Rosaceae
Rose family

Description: Tall trees with smooth, shiny and red–brown bark, peeling horizontally; bearing soft white flowers in spring; in summer mazzards have small red or yellow cherries, while black cherries have dark purple fruits.

Habitat: Edges of woods and fields, backyards.

Distribution: Wild sweet cherries are native to Europe and naturalized in North American; North American wild cherry or black cherry is naturalized in Europe.

Related species: The sour or dwarf cherry (*Prunus cerasus*) yields sour Morello cherries. It is native to Europe but naturalized in North America. Like sweet cherry, it is often cultivated. Chokeberry (*P. virginiana*) can be used like black cherry, but the fruit needs to be cooked and sweetened to be palatable.

Parts used: Fruit and fruit stalks gathered in summer, bark harvested in fall.

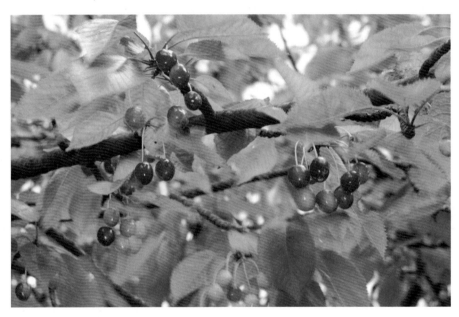

We all know and enjoy the cherry blossom and cherry fruit seasons, but using the bark of the wild sweet cherry (*Prunus avium*) medicinally may be a new idea to some readers. The official *British Herbal Pharmacopoeia* lists the powdered bark of the American cherry (*P. serotina*) as an antitussive, i.e., anti-cough, remedy, but we have found the wild equivalent to be excellent in its own right and recommend it to you.

Long used as a country recipe, a decoction or syrup of the inner bark of wild cherry, alone or with elderberry (as in our recipe), plums or sloes, remains a tasty and safe drink for sore throats and bronchitis that children find palatable. Its special affinity is for dry and irritating coughs. The stalks of the fruit also have a traditional use as a decoction for coughs, with similar effects to the bark. The fruit can be added for flavor.

The fruit has a reputation as a gout treatment, and a study of 633 gout sufferers (2012) indicated significant relief when using cherry fruit and extract. Cherries work well as a gentle laxative, but anyone who has gorged on fresh cherries will know that eating too many can cause diarrhea.

Cherries contain anthocyanins, which are potent antioxidants, as well as vitamins A, B, and C. They are cleansing and nourishing, and help to "build the blood" in cases of weakness and anemia. Cherries help with colds and recovery from illness, and taste so good you hardly need an excuse to eat them.

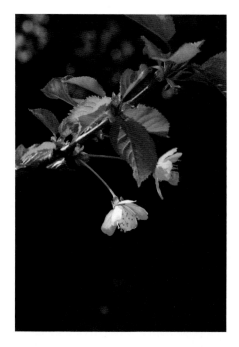

The cherry tree is the only fruit tree I know where people hold the bark in as high esteem as the fruit.
– Brill & Dean (1994)

A tree of virtuous blossom, virtuous timber, and rather less virtuous fruit, except for the purposes of cherry brandy.
– Grigson (1958)

Cherry brandy
Loosely fill a preserving jar with **cherries**. If they are sour, sprinkle with a little **muscovado sugar**, then top up the jar with **brandy**. Latch the lid down tightly and shake the jar well. Turn it upside down every few days to keep the sugar from settling at the bottom. After three months, strain and bottle. Enjoy at your leisure.

Cherry bark and elderberry cough syrup
Cut thin strips of **bark** from cherry branches in the fall when the leaves are dropping. One way to do this is to prune off a few small branches, then use a sharp knife to cut off all the bark. It is the greenish-white inner bark that is medicinal. Dry the bark in the shade.

Fill a small jar with the **dried bark** and top it up with **vodka**. Leave in a cool dark place for a month, shaking the jar occasionally, then strain. This is a cherry bark tincture.

To make the cough syrup, combine 1 part **cherry bark tincture** with 2 parts **elderberry glycerite** (recipe, p. 73). For example, for a 5 fl. oz. bottle of syrup you would use 1.7 fl. oz. cherry bark tincture and 3.4 fl. oz. elderberry glycerite.

Dose: 1 teaspoonful three or four times a day. Halve this for children.

Fresh cherry fruit
• anemia
• constipation
• gout
• arthritis

Cherry bark and elderberry syrup
• coughs
• sore throats
• bronchitis

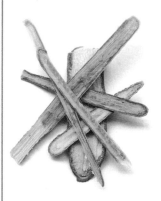

Chickweed *Stellaria media*

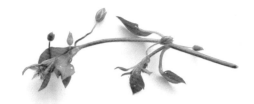

**Caryophyllaceae
Pink family**

Description: A floppy, sprawling annual plant with soft green leaves and tiny star-like white flowers.

Habitat: Gardens, hedgebanks and waste-ground.

Distribution: Native to Europe and Asia but now found as a weed worldwide.

Related species: There are over a hundred species in the genus.

Parts used: Above-ground parts, gathered whenever vibrant and green.

This is the best-known herbal remedy for itchy skin and hot skin inflammations of various types. Chickweed is a soothing, nutritious, and cooling herb, with a reputation for clearing stubborn, long-lasting bodily conditions.

It has special affinities for the eyes, lungs, and chest, and can be eaten as a food. As you'll see, it is far more than chickenfeed!

Chickweed has some less familar old names, like chick wittles, clucken wort, and chickeny weed, which confirm it is as a fowl favourite. This can be attested worldwide: for example, Julie's grandmother in Australia had chickens that loved their chickweed. Matthew's mother in England vouched for the relish with which her caged canaries used to nibble fresh chickweed flowers and seeds. Not surprisingly, it is also called bird seed.

But why should birds have all the fun? Chickweed is an excellent salad plant for humans, especially in late winter and early spring, when there's little else green and fresh available for foraging.

It tastes as though it is full of chlorophyll, has an earthy, slightly salty tang and is easily gathered. Its high vitamin A and C levels, saponins, and plentiful minerals, including iron, copper, magnesium, and calcium, make it one of the best spring tonics.

Chickweed has long been eaten fresh this way by country people, and it was once sold in the streets of London. Chickweed is tender and juicy, and has been called the tenderest of wild greens.

We often harvest it fresh for salad. Chickweed on its own is perhaps an acquired taste, but it is bland and goes well in a mixed salad. The tastiest way we have found to eat it is to make it into a pesto with pine nuts, which is surprisingly good (see recipe, p. 45).

Chickweed is available almost all year round, except in midsummer when it becomes fibrous and in midwinter when it disappears. It is one of the most genteel of weeds, easily pulled up and never rambunctious. Its presence signals fertile soil and it helps keep the soil moist. And once you find how good it is, you'll never seem to have enough of it!

One help in identifying chickweed among its *Stellaria* cousins is

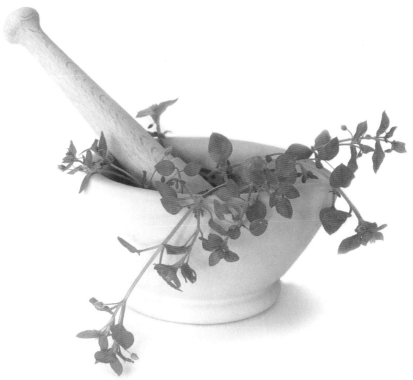

In late winter, it's a blessing for victims of F.W.S. (Forager's Withdrawal Syndrome) who crave a wild salad.
– Brill & Dean (1994)

Think of chickweed as being as soft as slippery elm, as soothing as marshmallow, and as protective and strengthening as comfrey root.
– Weed (1989)

its very commonness, virtually around the world. Chickweed is a very floppy plant and has smooth light green leaves, with one line of hairs up the side of the stem. In any event, other members of its clan have similar herbal attributes, such as lots of vitamins A and C and steroidal saponins, and can be used safely, if less effectively.

Use chickweed for...

Chickweed makes a good broth or tea for children and convalescents and can be taken in quantity. One American herbalist writes with gusto of taking "quarts of chickweed a day."

Herbally, the best-known external use for chickweed is to soothe itches, bites, stings, inflammations, burns, swellings, sunburn, bruises, splinters, and sore eyes. It makes a good and readily found first-aid or emergency remedy – pull up a handful and place directly onto the affected part.

If you have more time, crush some chickweed with a mortar and pestle, and bandage the paste against the wound or bite as a poultice. This is very cooling and soothing for sunburn.

Chickweed has the reputation of resolving skin problems where some form of heat is involved and where other herbs or creams have failed, especially when a cooling, drawing action is needed.

It is also known for clearing up long-standing or "indolent" damage, such as eczema, rheumatic joints, and varicose veins.

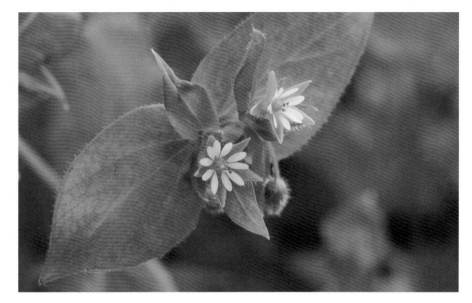

It is also safe for delicate organs that need cooling and soothing. One special affinity it has is for eye inflammations of most sorts, including itchiness from a contact lens. Dioscorides, the Greek scientist, described a chickweed recipe nearly two thousand years ago: he added crushed chickweed to corn meal to produce a paste that was poulticed onto the affected eye.

We mentioned before that chickweed contains saponins. Saponin means "soap-like." If you take a handful of the plant and rub it in your hands with a little water, you may not actually get a lather, but you'll feel the soapiness and it'll leave your hands lovely and soft, if smelling a little of chickweed.

Saponins work at a cellular level to increase absorption and permeability. What this means is that inflamed organ membranes, as in the liver, kidneys, and lungs, are helped by saponins to absorb healing nutrients, as well as allowing their wastes and blockages to be more easily removed. Add to this the cooling qualities of chickweed, and you have a wonderful, subtle herbal cleanser and restorer at work, far beyond the familiar and dismissive uses for "itchiness."

Chickweed works well internally on hot inflammatory problems like gastritis, colitis, congested chest, blocked kidneys and gallbladder, and piles. It has an affinity for the lungs, for sore throats, bronchitis, asthma, irritable dry cough, and other respiratory conditions. Also it has proven effective in anti- hepatitis B virus activity (2012).

Another quality you may come across is chickweed's reputed value as a slimming aid. Chickweed water or tea is an old wives' remedy for the overweight, and dried chickweed is added to some proprietary slimming formulas.

What do herbalists say? Some believe it does work, as the saponins help to dissolve body fat; others note it stimulates urination, so will assist in shedding body moisture, which would contribute to weight loss. As with many treatments, what works for one person may not be effective for everyone.

Chickweed has a valuable toning action for the body's internal organs. In American herbalist Susun Weed's words, it "sponges up the spills" and "tidies up the rips." She refers to its "deep mending skills," and to its ability to relieve, clear, protect, and nourish.

Chickweed can also be made into a flower essence, used to help release the past and focus in the present moment. To make a chickweed essence, follow the instructions for selfheal essence on p. 170.

Whether as a salad, tea or tincture, essence or vinegar, chickweed is effective, available, free, and safe.

Chickweed bath
- itchy skin
- shingles
- rheumatism
- rashes

Chickweed bath vinegar
- itchy skin
- shingles
- rheumatism
- rashes

Chickweed pesto
Pick a few handfuls of **chickweed**, removing any brown bits and roots. Break off the larger stems, as they have a very strong stretchy fiber at their core and are surprisingly stringy for such a floppy plant. Put the rest in a blender with a handful of **pine nuts**, a couple of cloves of **garlic** and enough **olive oil** to make it blendable. Blend until it is as smooth as you like it, then serve fresh on pasta with some **grated pecorino or parmesan cheese**. It can also be eaten with rice or other grains, or used as a sauce for vegetables.

Chickweed bath
For itchy skin, especially if this is over a large area of your body, try adding chickweed to a bath. Put a few handfuls of **fresh chickweed** in a sock, or tie in a square of muslin, and use a piece of string to hang this under the hot tap so that the water flows through it as you run your bath. Oatmeal can also be mixed with the chickweed for additional soothing. Once the bath is run, gently squeeze the sock or bag to release more of the contents. Alternatively, make a strong infusion of chickweed, strain, and add to the bath water.

Chickweed bath vinegar
Pick **chickweed** and put it in a blender, adding enough **cider vinegar** to blend. Strain and bottle. Your vinegar will start out a light lime green and change after a day or two to a lovely golden colour. Add a couple of tablespoons to bath water. This recipe combines chickweed's effectiveness at relieving itchy skin with vinegar's acidity, which helps restore the natural protective acid balance of the skin. It is particularly good if you live in a hard-water area.

Chickweed vinegar can also be used in salad dressings.

Cleavers *Galium aparine*

Rubiaceae
Bedstraw family

Description: A clambering annual covered in small hooks that help it "cleave" to anything it touches. Can be several yards high. Leaves are in whorls; small white flowers are followed by pairs of small ball-like fruit.

Habitat: Hedgerows, farmland, stream banks and gardens.

Distribution: Native to Eurasia and North America; widespread but introduced in the southern hemisphere.

Related species: The genus *Galium* also includes the bedstraws. Lady's bedstraw (*G. verum*) and hedge bedstraw (*G. mollugo*) can be used interchangeably with cleavers as medicinal herbs.

Parts used: Above-ground parts, gathered in handfuls from early spring until the plants flower in the summer.

Also known as goose grass, clivers, and sticky-willy, this common roadside plant clambers all over hedges and other plants in a green mass in high summer. It sends up bright green shoots from January onwards, being one of the first plants to sprout.

Cleavers is a wonderfully gentle lymphatic cleanser and a fantastic spring tonic, helping clean up our system after winter. It soothes irritated membranes of the urinary tract and promotes urine flow, and is useful for many mouth and throat problems.

Cleavers is the earliest of the traditional spring tonic herbs to sprout, appearing even before the end of the year in sheltered spots under hedges. By February it is making dense mats of intensely green whorled leaves. This is the time to harvest it to eat in salads, before it becomes tough and hairy. Pick the shoots and chop them finely. Nicholas Culpeper (1653) nicely summarises the traditional view:

It is a good remedy in the Spring, eaten (being first chopped small, and boiled well) in water-gruel, to cleanse the blood, and strengthen the liver, thereby to keep the body in health, and fitting it for that change of season that is coming.

By summer, cleavers romps all over the place, and its tiny white four-petalled flowers appear. At this stage, it will stick to anything, sometimes growing above head height. It can be used to make a quick makeshift collecting basket

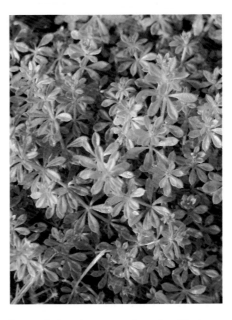

by twining it around on itself. As John Parkinson (1640) noted:

the herbe serveth well the Country people in stead of a strainer, to cleare their milke from strawes, haires, or any other thing that falleth into it.

To understand how cleavers works in the body, you need to know a little about the lymphatic system.

When our arteries carry oxygenated blood out to the far reaches of the body, the blood vessels branch smaller and smaller until only one red blood cell at a time can pass through.

These tiny blood vessels are the capillaries. Here, the red blood cells give up their oxygen and nutrients to the clear liquid around them, which then crosses the capillary walls into the cells.

The cells take the oxygen and nutrients, and in return give up their metabolic waste products to the fluid. This fluid doesn't go back into the blood vessels, but is collected by the lymphatic vessels, which are like a white bloodstream flowing back through the body toward the heart in parallel with the veins.

White blood cells in the lymphatic fluid start cleaning it up, and it passes through lymph nodes where the process continues. When it is all clean, the fluid rejoins the bloodstream at the point where the large vein enters the heart. Here it is pumped out to the lungs and the cycle begins again. If the lymph is clean and flowing well, the body will be healthy.

Use cleavers for...

Herbally, cleavers promotes the lymphatic flow and helps rid the lymphatic system of metabolic waste. In effect, it is like a pipe cleaner for our lymph vessels.

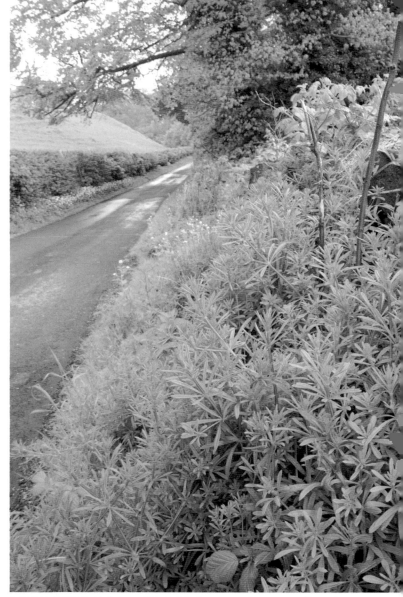

A spring tonic in the raw: cleavers in foreground, ramsons flowering across the road on left. In County Durham, northern England.

This quality makes it a useful remedy for swollen glands, tonsillitis, adenoid problems, and earache. Through its effect on the lymph, cleavers is reputed to help shrink tumors, both benign and cancerous (including breast cancer cell lines, 2016), and for removing nodular growths on the skin.

It is wonderful how strong and healthy you will become [on taking cleavers juice mixed with spring water]
– The Physicians of Myddfai (13th century)

Austrian herbalist Maria Treben (1980) favored cleavers tea as a drink and gargle to treat cancers of the tongue and throat. It is also used for other problems of the tongue, throat, and neck, and used by herbalists for goitre, other thyroid issues, and swollen glands.

Because it promotes the flow of urine, and cools and soothes, cleavers is used to reduce heat and irritation of the urinary tract. It relieves the scalding pain of urination associated with cystitis, and is a remedy for chronic recurrent bouts of urethritis, for kidney inflammation, irritable bladder, and prostatitis.

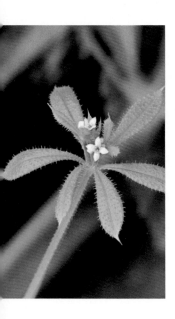

It is also effective in clearing grit, gravel or calcium deposits in the urinary tract. As a bonus, because cleavers is so good at cleaning the body internally, it also helps clear and nourish the skin.

Cleavers combines well with other familiar "weeds" – curly dock, nettle, dandelion and burdock – as in our "garden weed tincture" recipe. This tincture is an effective cleansing tonic for the whole body.

Cleavers loses some of its effectiveness when dried, and works best fresh. Picking your own in the spring and using it daily while in season is a great way to give yourself a gentle annual spring-cleanse. Try chopping a little young cleavers to mix in with salads or add to soups. The juice can be blended with fruit smoothies.

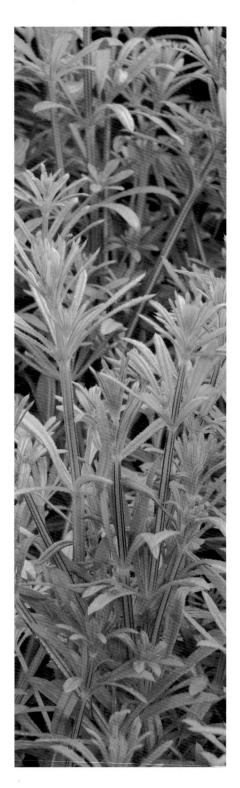

Cleavers poultice

The fresh, bruised plant is an excellent poultice for nettle rash, sores, blisters, burns, or any hot inflammation of the skin. Just pick a handful of cleavers, crush it with a mortar and pestle, and apply to the skin.

Cleavers cold infusion

Making a cold infusion is our favourite way to take cleavers. Simply fill a large glass with **freshly picked cleavers**, top up with **water** and let sit for a few hours before drinking. A glass a day is good in spring and early summer to keep your lymph clear. You can keep topping the glass up with fresh water for a couple of days before you need to replace the cleavers with fresh plant material.

Cleavers succus

A succus is simply a sort of syrup made by mixing fresh plant juice with honey or vegetable glycerine to preserve it for winter use. Measure your fresh **cleavers juice**, and add an equal amount of **vegetable glycerine** or **runny honey**. Mix well, then bottle and label. It tastes just like the smell of fresh-mown grass.

Dose: Take 1 to 2 teaspoonfuls two or three times a day.

Cleavers ointment

Stir the **fresh juice** into **anhydrous lanolin** until it is soft and a pale green color. Use a fork for this. It's hard work at first, but gets easier as the lanolin starts to absorb the juice. This is a particularly good application for dry, cracked, or chapped skin.

Garden weed tincture

Here's a great way to turn a morning's weeding into something really useful – a whole-body tonic to improve your health generally.
Weed out and wash:
Cleavers – best collected before they set seed
Dandelion plants – root, leaves, and all
Nettle tops (before they flower) and **nettle root**
Curled dock roots
Burdock roots
Chop the herbs and put them in a large, wide-mouthed jar, packing them in fairly tightly. Pour on enough **vodka** to cover them, and leave for a month, shaking occasionally. Strain off. If you have a fruit press, use it to get the maximum liquid out of the roots; otherwise just use muscle power to squeeze it out using a jelly bag. Bottle and label.

Dose: 1 teaspoonful twice a day.

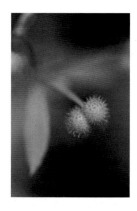

Cleavers in salads
• spring tonic

Cleavers poultice
• sunburn
• burns
• psoriasis
• open sores
• blisters
• nettle rash

Cleavers cold infusion
• swollen glands
• painful breasts
• fluid retention
• tonsillitis
• breast cysts
• bladder irritation
• burning urine

Cleavers succus
• swollen glands
• fluid retention
• tonsillitis
• breast cysts
• bladder irritation
• burning urine

Cleavers ointment
• dry chapped skin
• chapped lips
• burns

Garden weed tincture
• skin problems
• weak digestion
• anemia
• low energy

**Boraginaceae
Borage family**

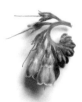

Comfrey *Symphytum officinale*

Description: A lush, hairy, fast-growing plant with yellowish-cream or dull purple flowers, and a winged stem.

Habitat: Moist, marshy places.

Distribution: It is native through Europe to Siberia, and introduced to North America and other temperate regions.

Related species: There are a number of species, often found as garden escapes. They can all be used externally, but only *Symphytum officinale* should be taken internally. Russian comfrey (*S. x uplandicum*) prefers drier ground, and is a hybrid between common comfrey (*S. officinale*) and rough or prickly comfrey (*S. asperum*). Tuberous comfrey (*S. tuberosum*) has pale yellowish-cream flowers. White comfrey (*S. orientale*) has pure white flowers, while creeping comfrey (*S. grandiflorum*) has reddish flowers, which fade to yellowish-cream. Because comfreys hybridize, it can be difficult to tell them apart.

Parts used: Leaves, root.

Comfrey's old name of knitbone refers to its strong healing action for broken bones. It will also knit flesh together, speeding the healing of wounds. Applied as a poultice or ointment, it can be used to treat bruises, dislocations, and sprains. Despite much controversy, comfrey is safe if correct guidelines are followed.

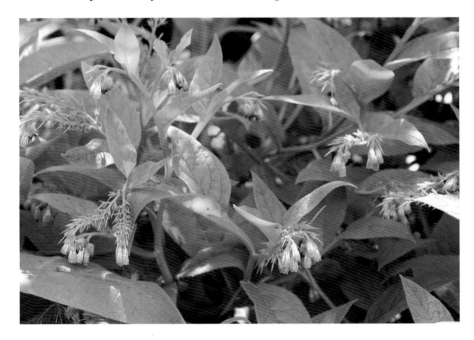

Comfrey has a long history of use for its healing and anti-inflammatory effects on bone fractures, arthritis, inflamed joints, cuts, wounds, and other injuries.

This herb had such a reputation for repairing tissue that it became popular for less virtuous brides to bathe in comfrey before their wedding day to restore their virginity!

Comfrey's scientific and common names both refer to its healing qualities. *Symphytum* is from the Greek *symphyo*, or make grow together, and *phyton*, or plant; "comfrey" is said to be from the Roman word *conferre*, to join together.

In addition to medicinal benefits, comfrey is often grown as a fodder plant for animals, as a fertilizer, and to add to compost. The most commonly grown comfrey for these purposes is Bocking 14, a sterile clone of Russian comfrey (*S. x uplandicum*).

Use comfrey for ...

In the past, comfrey was widely used for healing ulceration in the digestive tract, since it is mucilaginous and soothing as well as healing. It was also used for bronchitis and other chest complaints, to soothe the irritation and promote expectoration of mucus.

Today, other herbs tend to be preferred for these conditions, owing to the possible dangers of the pyrrolizidine alkaloids contained in comfrey – see box on p. 52. Comfrey nonetheless remains valuable as one of the best herbs for healing broken bones, snapped tendons, sprains, strains, and bruises.

Once a bone has been set by a qualified person, apply a fresh comfrey poultice. If the fracture is in plaster, take the comfrey up to the edges of the plaster. In addition, use homeopathic comfrey (Symphytum 6x) internally as directed by a homeopath, or – as long as you are not pregnant or breastfeeding – you can drink a couple of cups of comfrey leaf tea a day until the bone heals. Use a leaf or half a large leaf per cup of tea, infusing for 5 minutes.

Comfrey can also be applied to varicose veins, as a poultice. For wounds and ulcers that are open, place mashed comfrey on the skin around the affected part. Comfrey can help heal old wounds such as surgical scars, being applied as a fresh poultice or using the infused

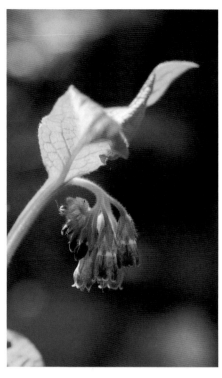

Comfery roots scrapd & boyle in milk is good to eat at night going to bed for a strayn or crik in the back; and boyld in ale to the thickness of a poultice [is] good to aply to a strayn.
– handwritten recipe from Norfolk, eighteenth century

It does not seem to matter much which part of the body is broken, either internally or externally; comfrey will heal it quickly.
– Dr. Shook (quoted by Dr. Christopher, 1976)

oil or ointment. It is also effective on bruises and other injuries to the muscles, ligaments, and tendons.

Comfrey's powerful healing effects are partly explained by its allantoin content. This chemical stimulates cell proliferation, which speeds up the healing process, and is also an anti-inflammatory that supports the immune system.

Comfrey is so good at "knitting" that it must not be used on broken bones until they have been set, or it will start bonding them together in the wrong position. Likewise, do not apply it on deep wounds, which can close at the top before the deep part has healed underneath. St. John's wort is better for deep puncture wounds.

Cautions: Do not use comfrey root internally, and do not take comfrey leaf for longer than six weeks at a time. Do not use internally if pregnant or breastfeeding, or give to young children.

Mistaken identities: Foxglove (*Digitalis purpurea*) leaves can easily be confused with comfrey before the plants flower.

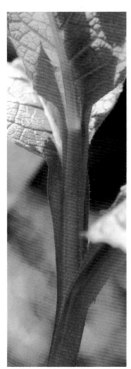

Common comfrey's leaves run down the stem to the joint below, giving the stem a winged appearance

Several recent randomized clinical trials substantiate the efficacy of topical comfrey preparations in the treatment of pain, inflammation and swelling of muscles and joints in the case of degenerative arthritis, acute myalgia in the back, sprains, contusions and strains after sports injuries and accidents, also in children aged 3 and over.
– Staiger (2012)

Common comfrey is the commonest comfrey in wetter habitats, but the flower colour is very variable, ranging from creamy white through pink to dull purple. The leaves run down onto the stem, with the upper leaves extending right down to the next set of leaves, giving the stem a winged appearance (see photo).

Russian comfrey is the most common comfrey in drier places. Its flowers are bright blue or purple, and the upper stem leaves don't run down the stem, or do so only slightly. **Rough comfrey**, its other parent plant, has bluish flowers and the upper stem leaves have short stalks and never run down the stem.

Comfrey and the pyrrolizidine alkaloid controversy

Comfrey has come into disrepute in recent years because it contains pyrrolizidine alkaloids. This is a large group of chemicals, some of which are toxic to the liver and can cause hepatic veno-occlusive disease. Poisoning has been reported in people eating other plants with high levels of these alkaloids, and there are a few reported cases of liver damage that appear to be based on the use of comfrey root.

Some herbalists argue that comfrey has been used traditionally and safely for hundreds of years without any problems, but the other side of the argument is that damage could occur gradually over time and not be attributed to the herb.

Another factor is the fact that Russian comfrey has been promoted for its benefits as a fertilizer and in making compost, especially for organic gardeners. It is wonderful for this purpose, but the problem from a medicinal point of view is that this is now the comfrey that most people have growing in their gardens.

Its levels of pyrrolizidine alkaloids are much higher than those of common comfrey, the "official" species of herbalism. Russian comfrey and rough comfrey, both introduced but now naturalized in North America, contain echimidine, the most toxic of the alkaloids, and are best limited to external use.

Russian comfrey is a hybrid between common comfrey and rough comfrey. It appears likely that comfrey was safe to use in the past when only common comfrey grew everywhere. Today the species hybridize readily and can be difficult to tell apart, but see above for guidelines.

We suggest erring on the side of caution by not using comfrey root internally (it contains higher levels of alkaloids than the leaves). A recent German clinical study supports topical external use.

Common comfrey leaf can be taken internally for short periods, not exceeding six weeks at a time. This is long enough to heal a broken bone. Do not take internally during pregnancy, while breastfeeding or if you have liver disease.

Bisset and Wichtl (2001) say that a high level of consumption of the leaves "as a salad is five or six leaves a day," would be within toxic range. Using a couple of leaves a day to make tea should be all right for short-term use, and external use on unbroken skin is considered safe.

Fresh comfrey poultice

Dig up **comfrey roots** and scrub them well. Cut them into shorter lengths and put them in a blender with an equal amount of **fresh comfrey leaf**. Add just enough water to make it blendable, and blend until you have a gooey mess. Spread this onto a piece of gauze and apply to the body part affected, covering with a piece of muslin or cling-film. The gauze makes the poultice easier to remove. Replace poultice daily until healed.

The leaves can also be used on their own as a poultice, but the hairs on them can irritate the skin. To avoid this, blend the leaves with a little water or pound them in a mortar and pestle, and then sandwich the leaf mush between two pieces of muslin before applying to the skin. The muslin will protect the skin from the irritating effects of the leaf hairs, and allow the juices to seep through.

Infused comfrey oil

Pick **comfrey leaves** and let them dry in the shade; then crumble them up and put into a jar big enough to hold them. Pour in **extra virgin olive oil**, and stir well. Top up the jar with a little more oil, put the lid on and place in a sunny part of the garden or on a windowsill for two weeks. Strain off the oil and bottle it, or use it to make an ointment (below).

Comfrey ointment

Put 10 fl. oz. of **infused comfrey oil** (above) in a small saucepan with **1 oz. beeswax**. The beeswax melts faster if you grate it or slice it up. Warm up on low heat until the beeswax melts. Allow to cool slightly, then pour into jars and leave to set before putting the lids on and labeling.

Comfrey poultice
- broken bones
- sprains
- sports injuries
- bruises
- surgical scars

Infused comfrey oil & ointment
- arthritis
- rheumatism
- bursitis
- tendonitis
- phlebitis
- mastitis
- glandular swellings
- pulled muscles
- injured joints
- back injuries
- tendons
- ligaments

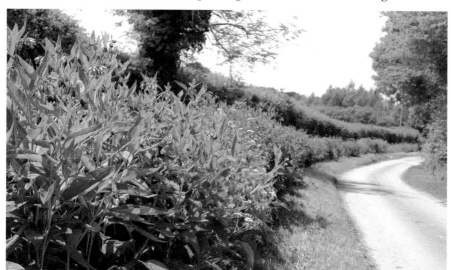

Russian comfrey (*S.* x *uplandicum*) in a country lane in Norfolk, England, July

Couch grass *Elymus repens*, syn. *Elytrigia repens*, *Agropyron repens*

This invasive grass is both gardener's foe and herbalist's friend. The couch grass rhizomes that gardeners hate possess soothing, diuretic and antibiotic qualities that have long been valued for making a tea to treat urinary problems, including cystitis, kidney stones, and prostate enlargement.

Poaceae
Grass family

Description: A grass, up to 3 feet tall, with a thin flowering spike, dark green pointed leaves and untidy creeping rhizomes.

Habitat: Lawns and gardens, roadsides and fields.

Distribution: Widespread worldwide, in a large range of habitats. Common across North America. Declared an invasive weed in many US states.

Related species: Bermuda grass (*Cynodon dactylon*), common in warmer areas, is also sometimes known as couch grass, and is used medicinally.

Parts used: Rhizome.

Similar species: The flower spikes of perennial rye-grass (*Lolium perenne*) look very similar to couch, but the leaves are shinier and there are no creeping rhizomes.

Garden weeds often attract colorful names that leave little doubt about gardeners' opinions. Couch grass is no exception, its other common names including twitch, quick grass, quack grass, scutch grass, dog's grass, witch grass and foul grass. It quickly spreads in most soils by vigorous white rhizomes (*repens* means creeping) just below the surface and forms a strong, dense root network that crowds out other plants.

Yet its herbal use goes back to classical times, and the love/hate relationship must also be as old. Culpeper, in 1653, puts it like this: "although a gardener be of another opinion, yet a physician holds half an acre of them [dog's grass or couch grass] to be worth five acres of Carrots twice told over."

The name "couch," according to the herbals, derives from an Anglo-Saxon word, *civice*, for vivacious and long-lasting. Perhaps the herbalists won naming rights here, and it's best to celebrate the vigor of the plant and hope this might transfer to us when we use it.

A successful colonist in garden and field, as are all of our familiar weeds, couch grass has an almost unstoppable capacity to spread. The pale runners or rhizomes give off side branches at intervals of only a few inches, and at each node the plant sends up a new shoot and drops a new web of fine roots. The leading runner is described by one writer as a lance that forces its way through any obstacle, including within your prized blooms. And if you leave the tiniest particle of the plant as you pull it or dig it up, it will invariably grow back.

Couch grass can be confused with perennial rye grass (*Lolium perenne*), but this has a wavier flower stalk and alternating darkish green spikelets set close to the stalk. Couch grass has distinct, very flat pale green spikes set at an acute angle to the stem.

At least couch grass is valued in dryland Australia, being planted there to create durable golf courses, grass courts and cricket squares. The binding quality of its rooting system has also been embraced in securing sand dunes, alongside specialist sand grasses.

And while gardeners in Britain may curse and burn their twitch, in mainland Europe it has often been used as a food for cows and horses, and sold as a tisane or tea for human use.

Mike Jones, a coffee plantation manager in Kenya for 26 years, used to spend a month a year getting his workforce to dig out the local couch grass by the deepest roots and burn it, or else it would climb to the top of the coffee bushes. When Julie sent him some couch grass, he said: "It comes as a bit of a surprise to learn we could have made ourselves a 'cup of tea' out of it."

What has so often been discarded should be more generally valued because it can ease a lot of suffering, and even prevent the need for surgery in some cases. A patient of Julie's, a keen gardener, said when prescribed couch grass, "but I've burned wheelbarrow loads of it!" He resolved to make better use of it in the future.

Use couch grass for...
The same rhizomes that cause all the gardener's woes are dug up by herbalists, then cleaned, dried and cut into lengths of a few inches. Brewed as a tea, the resulting infusion is mild and pleasant to drink.

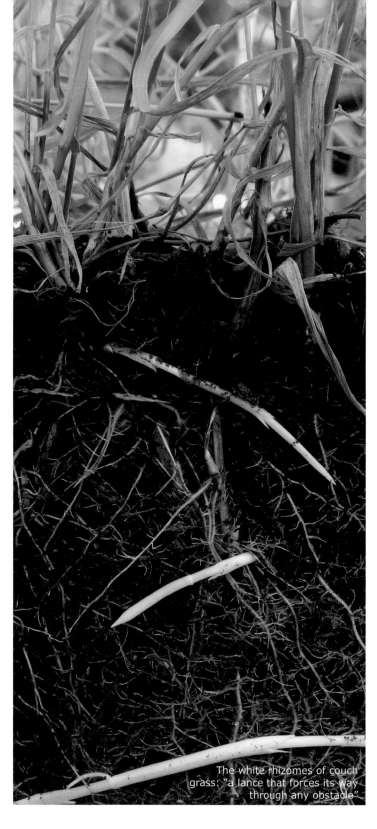

The white rhizomes of couch grass: "a lance that forces its way through any obstacle"

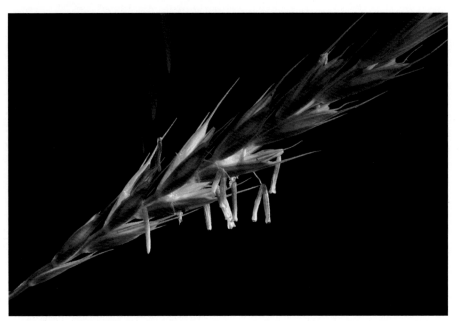

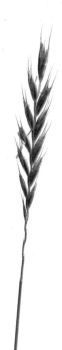

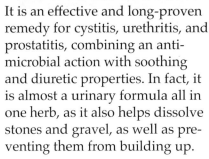

It is an effective and long-proven remedy for cystitis, urethritis, and prostatitis, combining an antimicrobial action with soothing and diuretic properties. In fact, it is almost a urinary formula all in one herb, as it also helps dissolve stones and gravel, as well as preventing them from building up.

John Parkinson, writing in 1640, said that couch grass (or Quich grasse, as he called it) not only dissolved stones in the bladder, but opened "obstructions of the liver and gall," indicating that it might help dissolve gallstones as well.

But it has wider modern uses too. Commission E, the expert panel that judges the safety of herbal medicines for the German government, has approved couch grass in the treatment of bronchitis and laryngitis as well as for bladder infections and kidney stones. It is also used together with other herbs for gout and rheumatism.

There are various other instances of couchgrass being employed in European medicine for liver and gallbladder problems, including jaundice.

Dogs and cats will seek it out as a natural purgative (hence "dog's grass"). Horse owners add couch grass rhizomes to feed to improve their horses' coats.

Couch grass is untidy in habit, with dead brown leaves typically growing in a clump alongside the flowering spikes, as the image opposite shows, but in supporting its claim on your attention, we invite you to take a look at the geometric beauty of the flowers in close-up (above).

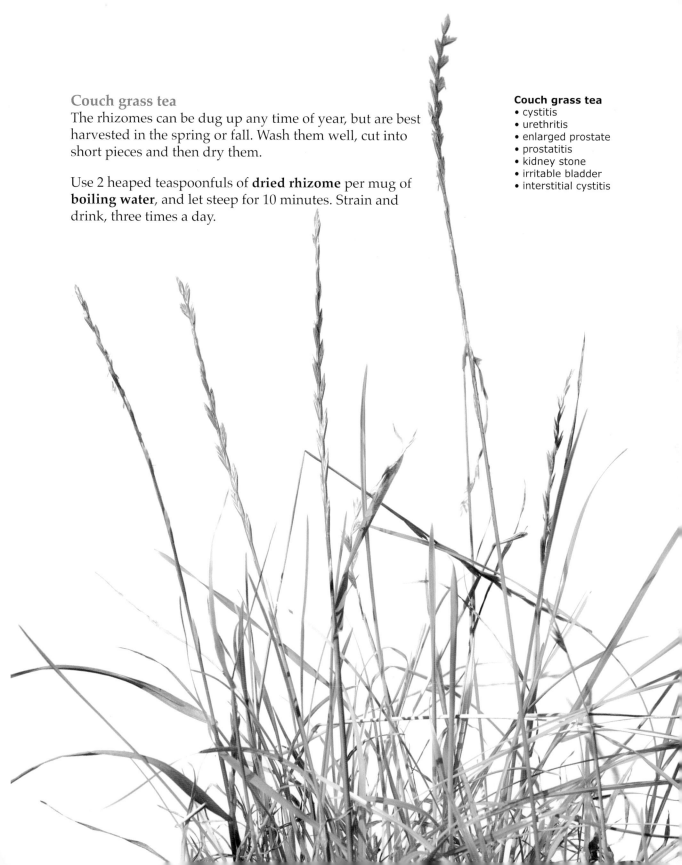

Couch grass tea

The rhizomes can be dug up any time of year, but are best harvested in the spring or fall. Wash them well, cut into short pieces and then dry them.

Use 2 heaped teaspoonfuls of **dried rhizome** per mug of **boiling water**, and let steep for 10 minutes. Strain and drink, three times a day.

Couch grass tea
- cystitis
- urethritis
- enlarged prostate
- prostatitis
- kidney stone
- irritable bladder
- interstitial cystitis

Curled dock, Yellow dock *Rumex crispus*

**Polygonaceae
Dock family**

Description: A perennial dock growing to a yard tall. Leaves are long and parallel-sided with wavy margins; its tap roots have a brown outer covering and are yellow within.

Habitat: Grassland, disturbed ground, farmyards, roadsides, river banks, coastal shingle and mud.

Distribution: Native to Europe and Africa, curled dock is one of the most widely distributed plants in North America and the world.

Related species: The other widely distributed species is common or broad-leaved dock (*R. obtusifolius*), with which yellow dock will hybridize. Broad-leaved dock can be used inter-changeably with curled dock – the thing to look for is a yellow root in either species, which indicates the presence of the medicinal compounds.

Parts used: Root, dug up in fall; leaves.

The two common docks are among the five official "injurious weeds" in Britan, but curled dock has long-recognized redeeming qualities as a detoxifying liver and bowel herb, a laxative and a blood cleanser. The root is effective for many chronic toxic skin conditions, including acne and boils, eczema and sunburn, not forgetting the most famous use of dock leaves for relieving the burning caused by nettle stings.

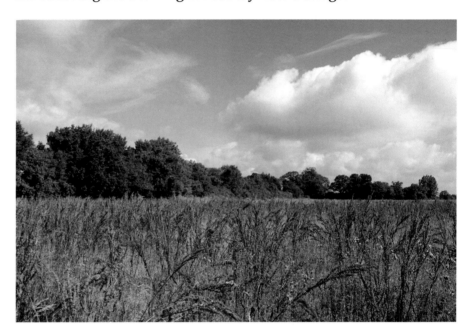

We have included dock in this book even though it is the root that is most used, as it is such a common weed across the world. Found in almost every field, garden and lawn, it is likely you have some growing on your own plot that you can dig up for medicine.

Dock's tap roots are long, slender and deep, going two feet down; any stray piece left in the soil can sprout into a new plant. Each dock can produce 30,000 or more seeds a year, and these can lay dormant for up to fifty years. It is no wonder it is hard to eliminate.

In addition, curled dock and common or broad-leaved dock hybridize freely. It is an almost unstoppable weed, yet one with redeeming medicinal benefits.

Dock's botanical success is official: both common British species are classed as injurious weeds in the Weeds Act 1959 (along with common ragwort, spear thistle and creeping or field thistle). The Act stipulates that farmers should take steps to prevent the spread of these five weeds: a scene like the one opposite of a fallow field filled with curled dock in fall ought to be harder to find than it still is.

Use curled dock for...

The one thing everybody knows about dock is that you rub its leaves on the skin when stung by nettle. This practice goes back centuries, being mentioned in the Anglo-Saxon leech-books and in Chaucer's *Troilus and Criseyde*, suggesting docks have always been freely available. Formerly, a chant was sung when applying the dock: in Ireland, it was "docken, docken, cure nettle"; in Cornwall, "dock leaf, dock leaf, you go in; sting nettle, sting nettle, you come out."

It is a cooling and astringent treatment, especially the sizeable leaves of broad-leaved dock, although we prefer treating nettle rash by plantain leaves. Digging up a few dock roots, pulping them and applying as a poultice, and renewing this every few hours, is another old nettle standby, as is a root tea. In South Africa, Tswana women warm up dock leaves and apply them to swollen breasts during lactation; they also use the root pulp to treat piles.

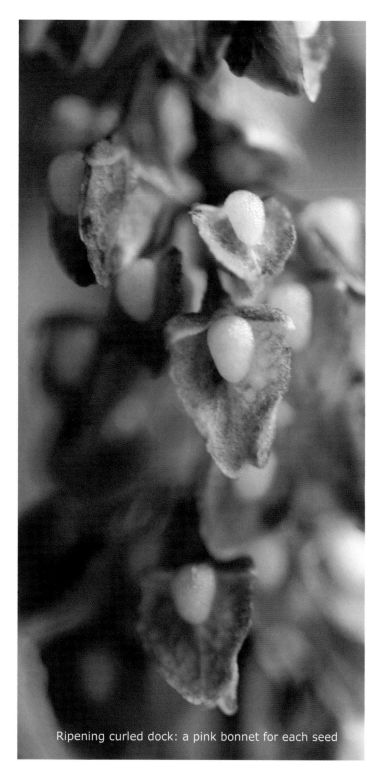

Ripening curled dock: a pink bonnet for each seed

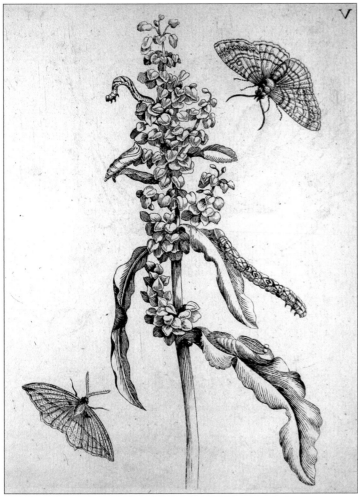

Curled dock, by Maria Merian (1717)

Probably the most general practice in all of folk medicine, occurring throughout the British Isles, is rubbing a dock leaf on the skin to ease a sting.
– Allen & Hatfield (2004)

Conclusively, [Rumex root extract] could be considered as potent carbohydrase inhibitor, anti-cancerous and anti-oxidant.
– Shiwani et al. (2012)

The reputation of dock as a "blood cleanser" is also ancient, being known in Chinese medicine, Indian Ayurveda and in classical Greece, whence comes dock's old family name "lapathum" or blood purifier. It was found that dock transmutes iron in the soil into organic iron in the plant (a real case of alchemy!); old herbalists added iron filings to soil near dock to "enrich" it. This property makes dock effective for iron-deficiency anemia and for period problems, especially in younger women.

Dock also has a laxative effect in which it stimulates gut motions; indeed it was once used as a purgative. It is a good natural remedy for constipation, reflux and acid stomach, and has been called a "superlative remedy" for enteritis, colitis, diarrhea and dysentery.

Dock's twin qualities to cleanse and to lower heat make it an ideal liver detox treatment, including for jaundice and "liver stagnation," when the flow of bile is congested, and for disorders of the spleen and lymph. A healthy liver means a healthy skin, and dock works on both; use small quantities over a long period.

One Anglo-Saxon recipe for reducing a groin swelling was to pulp dock leaves in grease, wrap in a cabbage leaf that had been warmed in hot ashes, and apply as a plaster. Culpeper (1653) suggested boiling roots in vinegar for bathing itches, scabs and "breaking out of the skin." Modern external uses have added chronic acne, boils, bites, cuts, sunburn, easing rheumatic aches and soothing inflamed gums (using a powder of dried roots).

Dock root gives a gluten-free flour, once a famine food. The young leaves of curled dock cook as a tasty spring vegetable with a light lemony taste, and are good in nettle soup. Avoid too much raw dock, though, as it contains oxalic acid, which is toxic in quantity.

Harvesting dock

Dig up the roots in late summer or fall. Large older plants are more likely to have a strong yellow colour to their roots. Scrub them well, and cut off the tops.

Curled dock tincture

Fill a jar with chopped-up **dock roots**. Pour **vodka** in until the roots are covered and put the lid on tightly. Keep in a cool dark place for a month, ideally shaking the jar every day or two.

Strain off, using a press or squeezing through a jelly bag. Bottle the liquid, remembering to label it. This tincture will keep for about five years in a cool dark place.

Dose: Half a teaspoonful once or twice daily as a cleansing tonic.

Take when the bowels are sluggish, for anemia and poor absorption of nutrients (if the edge of your tongue shows scalloping from your teeth), for skin problems and any time you feel a bit slow and tired.

Curled dock tincture
- poor absorption
- anemia
- skin problems
- sluggish bowels
- liver congestion
- constipation

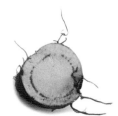

Curled dock root in cross-section, showing the yellow color

An East Anglian cure for jaundice
(collected by Elizabeth Hicks, late eighteenth century)

Take 1 oz of red Doc. Seed dry, boil it in 3 pints of water till 1 pint is nearly wasted then strain it of and add 3 gill glasses of white Wine.
Dose take a gill glass 3 times a day when the stomach is the emptiest, this will be 4 days in taken, then stop 2 days and repeat the Medicine which will with the Blessing of God compleat the Cure be the Jaundice ever so bad.

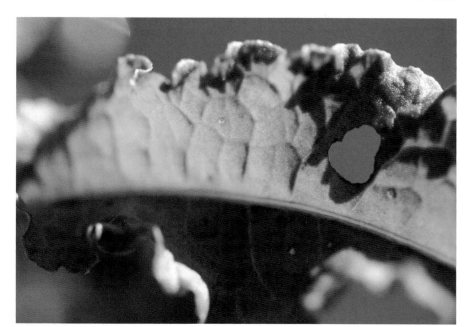

The wavy leaf edge (and typical snail hole) of curled dock

Dandelion *Taraxacum officinale*

Dandelion is a wonderful food as well as a beneficial medicine. It supports overall health by gently working to improve the functioning of the liver, gallbladder, and urinary and digestive systems. It is excellent for cleansing the skin.

Next time you spend an hour removing dandelions from your garden or lawn, turn them into medicine instead of throwing them out, and rejoice in the fact that they will always grow back!

Asteraceae (Compositae) Daisy family

Description: A familiar weed of lawns, with bright yellow flowers, seed "clocks," a bitter white latex in the stem and a long tap root.

Habitat: Lawns, fields and roadsides.

Distribution: Worldwide in temperate zones.

Related species: *Taraxacum officinale* is actually a group of several hundred plants. These are divided into nine sections and are very difficult to distinguish. Most common forms of dandelion belong to the *Ruderalia* section. They are all safe medicinal plants. In Chinese medicine, *T. mongolicum* is used to clear heat and toxicity.

Parts used: Leaves, roots, flowers, and sap.

Dandelions: where to begin? They do so much! They were once much used in Britain as a spring tonic, and still are in Europe. In the US fresh dandelion leaves for salads was a $2m a year industry in 2009.

Dandelions have followed European settlers around the world, though it is probably native in China and most of Asia. Most people know them as lawn weeds, but we're prepared to upset the gardeners to say: consider the benefits of a lawn of brightly blooming dandelions. Can grass give you salad, tasty fritters, wine, a coffee substitute, tea, useful medicine and more besides?

This plant is almost indestructible: it is a perennial and, unusually, it is self-fertilizing; its deep tap roots make it hard to dig out, and any pieces left will regenerate. Its seeds soar miles on little parachutes, whether or not helped by children playing the "clock" game. It flowers almost all year long.

Any amount of mowing, herbicide, and flamethrowing fail to eradicate this sunny plant from the garden. Really, you'll be happier if you view dandelions as a culinary and medicinal gift, a superb "cut and come again" crop, rather than as an annoying weed!

An old companion of man, it has accumulated many names. Blowball and telltime refer to the seeds, priest's crown to the stem after the seeds have flown, and swine's snout to the unopened flower. And "dandelion" itself? The "teeth of the lion" (*dent de lion*) explanation, from the appearance of the saw-edged leaves or perhaps the tiny florets, is found in many languages. But there is also a case made for an older link to the sun.

In many cultures the lion has been the animal symbol of the sun since antiquity, as in the astrological sign Leo. Dandelions are yellow discs, like the sun, and open and close along with it. So, perhaps

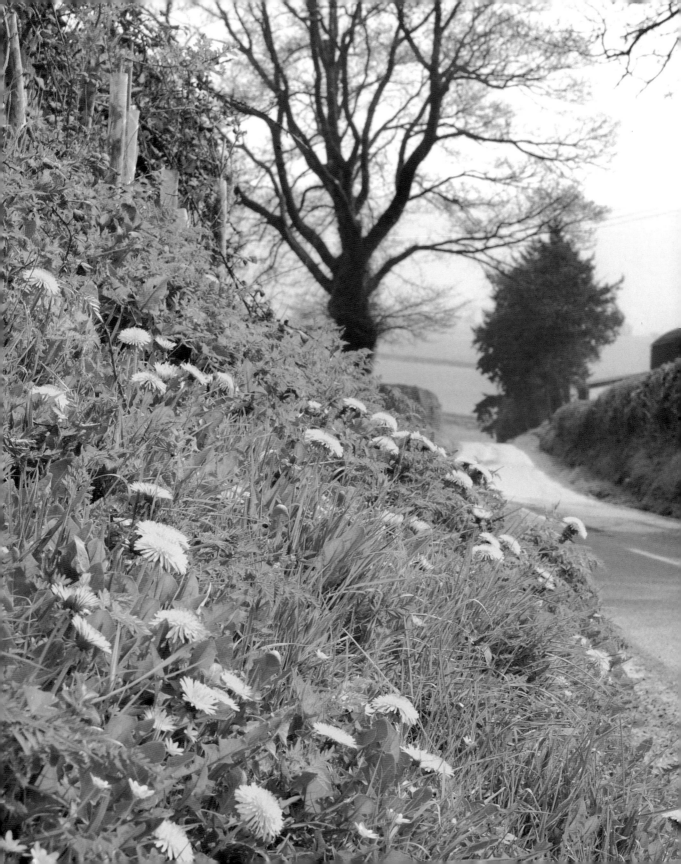

the old name might mean "rays of the sun" rather than "teeth of the lion"? In any case the Chinese, who have long used the dandelion, have even better names for it: two are "yellow-flowered earth-nail" and "golden hairpin weed."

Use dandelion for...
It is high in minerals, especially potassium, and vitamins A, B, C, and D. The young leaves boiled up into a tea or eaten fresh in salads are detoxifiers, clearing blood and lymph by increasing elimination through the kidneys and bowels. This in turn benefits overall health.

If dandelion says "think spring," it also suggests "think liver." It has

a reputation as a safe liver herb, especially where there are toxins and heat in the blood. The plant's chemicals cause the gallbladder to contract, releasing bile, stimulating the liver to produce more.

Liver-related conditions aided by dandelion include jaundice and hepatitis, gallstones and urinary tract infection, painful menopause, PMT, and menstruation; improvements are achievable in the pancreas, spleen, skin and eyesight.

A herbal monograph on dandelion lists two pages of remedies, from abscess and acne to varicose veins and venereal warts; to this author it is a "self-contained pharmacy."

It is the bitterness in dandelion leaves that makes them so good for your digestion. The bitter taste stimulates secretion of digestive fluids, including stomach acid, bile, and pancreatic juices. Dandelion promotes the appetite, and is recommended for those who have been ill or have lost enthusiasm for food in advanced age.

Roasted dandelion root is a well-known and caffeine-free coffee substitute. We grind the roasted root with a few pods of cardamon just before brewing; it's also tasty with cinnamon and fennel seed. The root can also be eaten as a boiled vegetable.

The flowers don't look very edible, but they are surprisingly good eaten straight off the plant, mild

An ancient connection with man: dandelions at Avebury stone circle, England, April

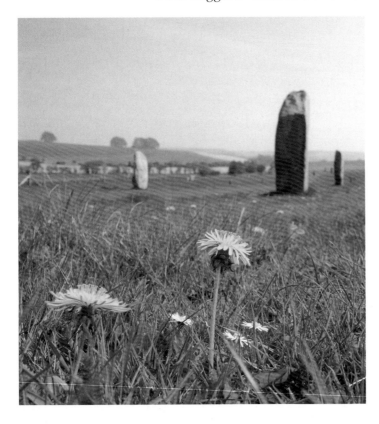

and slightly sweet. Eating a few dandelion flowers often relieves a headache too. They are delicious washed, dipped wet into flour and fried in butter until golden brown. This needs to be a lunch dish, as the flowers only open when the sun is shining, and they are too bitter when picked in the evening.

One of Julie's first paid jobs as a girl in Jackson Hole, Wyoming, was collecting paper bags full of dandelion heads for a neighbor to make dandelion wine. This wine is a beautiful golden colour, like distilled sunshine. The flowers also yield a refreshing dandelion "beer" and a face wash.

The sap or latex of the stems was once used in patent medicines, and was said to remove freckles and age spots, corns and warts, to help hair grow, and treat bee stings and blisters.

Dandelion is known as "piss-en-lit" in French, "pissabed" in English, and is justly renowned for its diuretic properties, that is, increasing the flow of urine. What is less familiar is how well it strengthens the urinary system. It is effective in treating bed-wetting in children and incontinence in older people. All parts of the plant have this effect, but especially the leaves.

With most diuretic drugs potassium is lost from the body and has to be supplemented, but dandelion is naturally high in potassium. It can safely be used long term

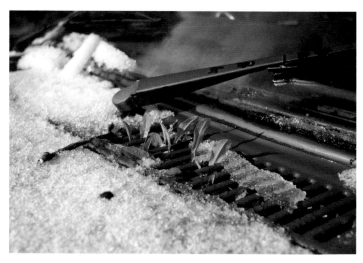

without causing imbalance. The leaves boiled with vegetable peelings make a potassium-rich broth.

Dandelion's diuretic effect makes it a good herb for treating swollen ankles, for fluid retention and high blood pressure. It can also be used to alleviate shortness of breath in the elderly.

As a medicine the whole plant is invaluable for liver and gallbladder problems, and for skin complaints including eczema and acne. Its action helps reduce high blood pressure, high cholesterol and the pain of arteriosclerosis and joints, digestive problems, chronic illness, viral infections, and heart and lung irregularities.

Dandelion can form part of a natural cancer treatment, and taken regularly as a food and medicine may help prevent some cancers, especially melanomas (2010), and other chronic illnesses by keeping the body clean, toned and healthy.

Dandelions will grow almost anywhere, from cracks in pavements to car hoods. They are wonderfully adaptable survivors.

Dandelions may well be the world's most famous weed. Up until the 1800s, [American] people would actually pull the grass out of their yards to make room for dandelions and other useful "weeds" such as chickweed, malva, and chamomile.
– Mars (1999)

DANDELION SAP
• warts
• calluses
• corns
• rough skin

Dandelion tincture

The root or the leaves can be tinctured separately for specific uses, but for general use we prefer to use the whole plant. Dig up **dandelion plants**, wash the dirt off and remove any dead leaves. The plants can be left whole or chopped up. Place in a jar large enough to hold them, and pour enough **vodka** in to cover the plants completely.

Put the jar in a cool place out of sunlight. If you chop up your plants, the tincture can be ready in as little as two weeks, otherwise leave it for a month before straining, squeezing the residue in a jelly bag or piece of muslin to get all the liquid out. Pour it into clean amber or blue glass bottles, label, and store until needed.

Dosage
• For general health maintenance, take half a teaspoonful twice daily.
• For acute skin eruptions, take 10 drops in water frequently throughout the day until the skin clears.
• For digestive problems, recuperation from chronic illness, sluggish liver, arthritis, gout, eczema, and psoriasis, take half to 1 teaspoonful three times daily in water.
• For over-indulgence in food or drink, take 10 drops in water every hour until you are feeling better.

Dandelion salad
• sluggish liver
• constipation
• urinary problems
• fluid retention

Dandelion tincture
• skin problems
• sluggish liver
• constipation
• urinary problems
• fluid retention
• arthritis
• gout
• hangovers
• chronic illness

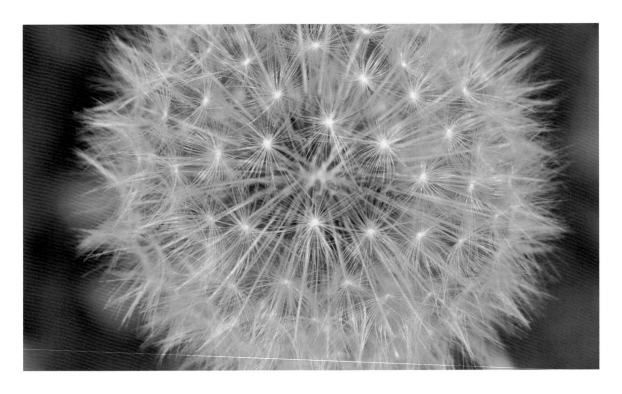

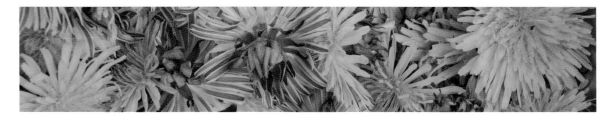

Dandelion flower beer

Pick 100 **dandelion flowers**. Boil 4 pints of **water** with three and a half ounces of **light brown sugar** until the sugar has dissolved. Allow to cool until tepid, then pour over the dandelion flowers in a large container. Add **a lemon**, finely sliced.

Cover the container with a clean cloth and set aside in a cool place for three or four days, stirring occasionally. Strain and pour into tightly corked bottles. The beer will be ready to drink in just a few days.

Dandelion flower infused oil

Pick enough **dandelion flowers** to fill a clean, dry jam jar. Pour in **extra virgin olive oil** slowly, allowing it to seep down around the flowers until the jar is full and there are no air pockets left.

Cover the jar with a piece of cloth held in place with a rubber band, and put the jar in a warm sunny place. It can be left outdoors during the day if the weather is clear, and brought in at night, or left on a sunny window ledge. The cloth cover lets any moisture escape. You may need to prod the flowers down to keep them immersed in the oil, as they can go moldy if left in the air.

After a week or two, or when the flowers are limp and have lost their colour, strain off the oil. If you put the flowers in a cloth or jelly bag to squeeze out the oil you may get some juice as well, so you'll need to let the oil stand for a while in a jug. This will allow any water to sink to the bottom. The oil can then be carefully poured off into bottles, leaving the watery bits at the bottom of the jug.

Dandelion flower oil is an excellent rub for muscle tension and cold, stiff joints. It is good for dry skin, and can be rubbed into the delicate skin around the eyes. Don't forget this oil can be eaten too, adding a taste of sunshine to salads and other foods.

For external use, add essential oils to your home-made flower oil, using up to 20 drops per 3 fl oz of oil. The essential oils act as a natural preservative, and bring their own healing qualities to the mixture. Lavender, ylang ylang, and rosemary all combine well with dandelion.

DANDELION FLOWERS
Flower infused oil
- muscle tension
- muscle aches
- stiff neck
- arthritis

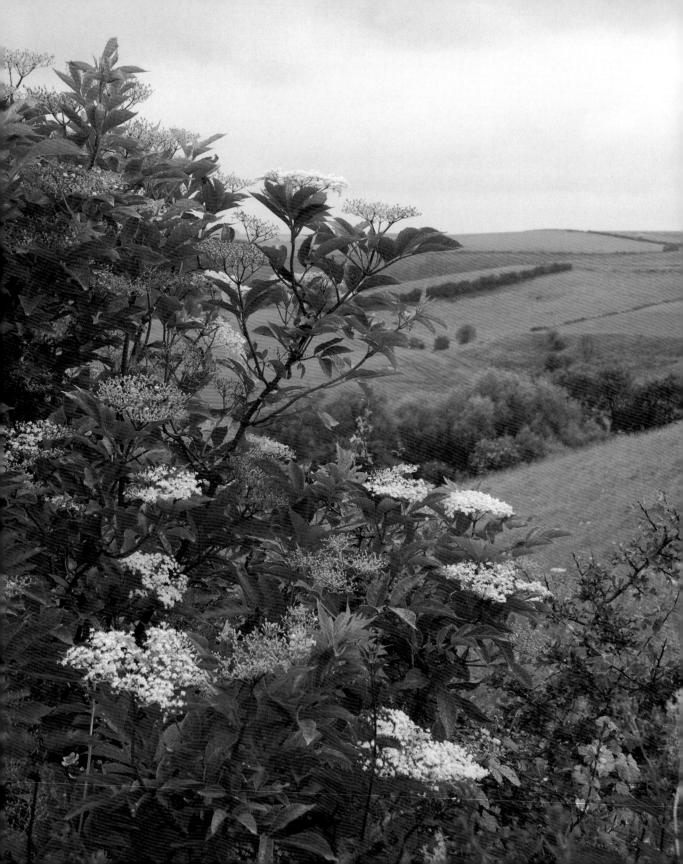

Elder *Sambucus nigra*

If ever the soul of a plant has been fought for, it is elder. An important herb through the ages, it has been described as a whole medicine-chest in one plant. Less used now than formerly, its flowers remain a wonderful fever remedy and delicious in drinks or desserts. The berries work against flu and colds, and help relieve coughs. The leaves, as an ointment, are good for bruises.

Few plants are as steeped in folklore, legend, and superstition as the elder. Its hollow stem was said to have been used by Prometheus to bring fire to man from the gods, and the Saxon *aeld* ("fire") may have given elder its name. The same empty stem was a ready-made flute, and the genus name *sambucus* was chosen by Linnaeus for a flute made of elder.

Elder was faerie and pagan. If you were in the company of the tree on Midsummer night you would see the Faery King ride by. Another version of our name "elder" was from Hylde Moer, the elder or earth mother – when an elder planted itself in your garden it meant the mother had chosen to protect your house from lightning and your cattle from harm. You must never cut down an elder or burn it, because the mother was present, without asking her leave.

So entrenched was the cult of the elder mother that the Church vilified elder with its most powerful negative associations: Christ was said to have been crucified on an elder tree and Judas to have hanged himself on one.

And if that seemed to stretch credulity, judging by the tree's weak branches, there was something else: God had cursed elder by making its once large black berries small and its straight branches twisted. Such sanctioned hostility was borne out in a verse on elder quoted by Robert Chambers in his *Popular Rhymes of Scotland* (1847):

Bour-tree, bour-tree, cookit rung,
Never straight, and never strong,
Ever bush and never tree
Since our Lord was nailed t'ye.

Its rank smell has always been held against elder. The leaves were once sold as a fly repellent, and it was bad luck to have the flowers indoors. An English rhyme went:

Hawthorn blooms and elderflowers
Fill the house with evil powers.

The plant was redolent of sex and death, the greatest taboos, yet a

Adoxaceae / Moschatel family (formerly in the Caprifoliaceae)

Description: A shrub or small tree, with fragrant clusters of creamy white flowers in summer, followed by black berries in fall.

Habitat: Hedgerows, riverbanks, woods, and waste ground.

Distribution: Native to Europe, introduced to North America.

Related species: American black elder is now considered a subspecies (*Sambucus nigra* spp. *canadensis*), as is blue elder (*S. nigra* spp. *caerulea*). They can be used interchangeably with black elder, but the raw fruit may be more likely to cause stomach upset in some people. The North American red-berried elder (*S. racemosa*) has been used medicinally but again eating the raw berries is not recommended.

Parts used: Flowers, berries; leaves externally.

(opposite) Elder coming into flower, Lincolnshire Wolds, England, June

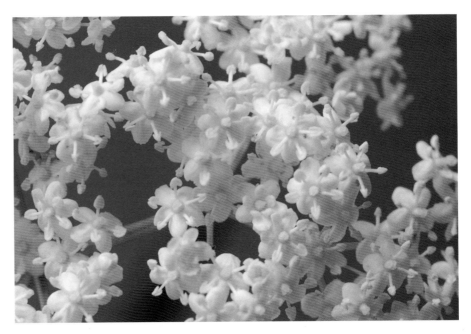

scientific Puritan like John Evelyn could see beyond this to its medicinal virtues: "though the leaves are somewhat rank of smell and so not commendable in sallet, they are of the most sovereign virtue." An extract of the berries, he went on, would "assist longaevity and was a kind of catholicon against all infirmities whatsoever … every part of the tree being useful."

The battle for control of elder has always swung like this. It was a tree of life, yet a devil's tree; it was needed, hence a good herb in the monastery garden; it was feared, so it was a witch's plant.

Yet survive it has, in town and country alike, on any patch of waste ground. Of all the wild plants in this book elderflower is the one harvested for commercial use, for cordials and other drinks.

Elderflower drinks are also widely made at home, and drug stores often run out of citric acid during the elderflower season!

Strangely, the berries are often ignored as food these days, but they make a lovely wine and are delicious cooked with apples (and were once widely used to adulterate wine and true ports).

Use elder for...
Elder blossom is one of the best herbs for encouraging sweating to break a fever, when drunk as a hot tea, as Julie recalls:

"I was visiting my parents once in Namibia when my mother came down with a slight fever. I had seen an elder blooming in a nearby park, so dosed her with a tea of the fresh flowers before tucking her in bed. The elder worked so well that she became drenched in sweat and thought she had malaria. But a blood test was clear."

The flower tea "clears the channels" in the body, promoting elimination via the skin and urinary tract, and supporting the circulation. Elderflowers cut congestion and inflammations of the upper respiratory tract, breaking up catarrh. They can reduce symptoms of hayfever, used with nettle tops.

Elderflower products are also used internally and externally to help clean the skin. A distilled water of the flowers made a eyewash in the 1600s, and helped remove freckles and spots, and was used to cool sunburn; it will still work today.

Elderberries are well known for reducing the length and severity of colds and flu, and can be used to help prevent infection. They are an excellent winter standby.

Elder leaf ointment
Warm half a pint **extra virgin olive oil** in a small pan and add a couple of handfuls of chopped **elder leaves**. Simmer gently until the leaves are crisp, then strain. Return the oil to the pan. Melt 1 oz **beeswax** in the oil, then pour into ointment jars. Leave to cool and set before putting the lids on and labelling. Use for bruises, sprains, and chilblains.

Harvesting elderflowers
Pick elderflowers on a dry sunny day, choosing those that smell lemony and fresh. In damp weather or in shady places the flowers can have an unpleasant smell. Pick the whole head of flowers. If you are drying them for tea, spread the heads on brown paper to dry, and then use a fork to strip the blossoms off the stems.

Elderflower tea
This can be made with fresh flowers, but as their season is relatively short, the dried flowers are usually used.

Use 1 heaped teaspoonful of **dried flowers** per cupful of **boiling water.** Cover and allow to infuse for 3 to 5 minutes. Strain and drink hot and frequently for the early stages of a cold or fever, to promote sweating. For this, it combines well with equal parts of yarrow and mint. For hayfever, use in combination with nettle leaves.

Drink cold for its diuretic effect and for menopausal hot flushes, or use as a face wash.

ELDER LEAF Ointment
- bruises
- sprains
- chilblains

ELDERFLOWER Hot tea
- fevers
- colds and flu
- promotes sweating
- use in bath
- hay fever

Cold tea
- night sweats
- promotes urination
- hot flushes
- fluid retention
- use as a face wash

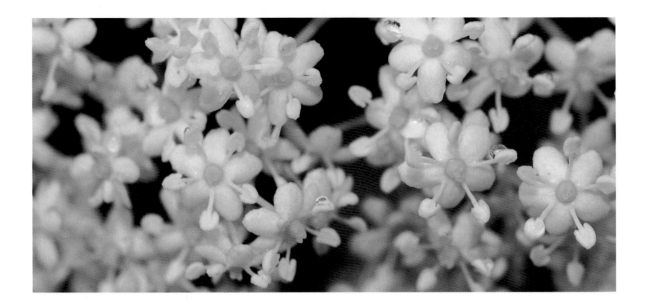

ELDERFLOWER
Glycerite
• sore throats
• stuffy noses
• hot flushes
• face lotion

Cordial
• hot flashes
• colds
• sore throats

For a cold
Elder flowers dry boyled in milk & drink it at night. It weill sweat & do much good.
– Book of culinary recipes 1739–79

Elderflower glycerite

Pack heads of **elder blossom** into a large jar, then fill with **vegetable glycerine**, stirring to release any air bubbles. Put the lid on and place the jar in a warm place, on a sunny window ledge or by a range cooker, and leave for two weeks. Strain using a jelly bag or a press. Bottle the liquid, label and store in a cool dark place. You can use this glycerite as is, or add elderberries in the fall (see next page).

Dose: 1 teaspoonful as needed for sore throats. For a clear complexion and smooth skin, mix half and half with rosewater and use freely as a face lotion.

Elderflower cordial

Pick 30 heads of **elderflower** on a dry sunny day, choosing those that smell lemony and fresh.

Boil **2 lbs sugar** in **4 pints of water** for about 5 minutes in a large saucepan. Pour into a large ceramic bowl and add **2 oz citric acid**, a **chopped lemon** and a **chopped orange**.

Add the **elderflower heads** and stir well. Cover with a clean cloth and leave for 4 days, stirring every day. Strain through a jelly bag and bottle. For long-term storage, the cordial can be frozen.

To drink, dilute to taste with cool sparkling water. It can also be made with hot water to encourage sweating in colds and fevers.

Harvesting elderberries

Pick bunches of elderberries when they are ripe and black but still firm and shiny. The easiest way to strip them from their stems is to use a fork.

Elderberry glycerite

Fill a large jar with **elderberries**, and pour in **vegetable glycerine** or elderflower glycerite to fill the gaps until the jar is full. Place in a warm spot, on a sunny window ledge or by a range cooker, and leave for two weeks. Strain and squeeze the juice out of the berries, using a jelly bag or a press. Bottle the liquid, label and store in a cool dark place.

This can be used on its own for coughs and sore throats or mixed with cherry bark syrup (see p41).

Elderberry syrup

Put **ripe elderberries** into a large saucepan with half their volume of **water**. Simmer and stir for twenty minutes. Allow to cool, then squeeze out the juice using a jelly bag or fruit press.

Measure the juice, and for every pint of juice add half a pound **muscovado sugar**, a **stick of cinnamon**, a few **cloves** and a few **slices of lemon**. Simmer for 20 minutes, strain and pour while hot into sterilized bottles.

Dose: Take 1 teaspoonful neat every few hours for colds and flu, or use it as a cordial and add boiling water to taste for a hot drink.

**ELDERBERRY
Glycerite**
• coughs
• colds
• flu

Syrup
• coughs
• colds
• flu

... To press and make their eldern berry wine/ That bottled up becomes a rousing charm/ To kindle winters icy bosom warm/ That wi its merry partner nut brown beer/ Makes up the peasants christmass keeping cheer.
– John Clare, 'October', *The Shepherd's Calendar* (1827)

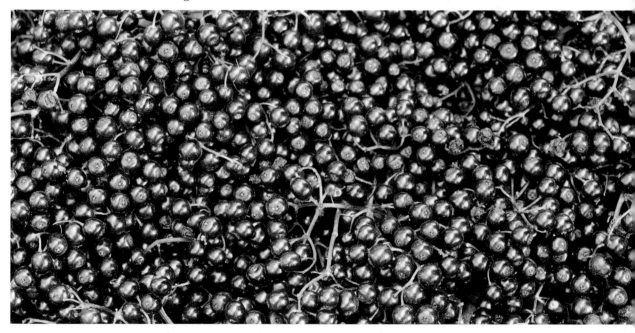

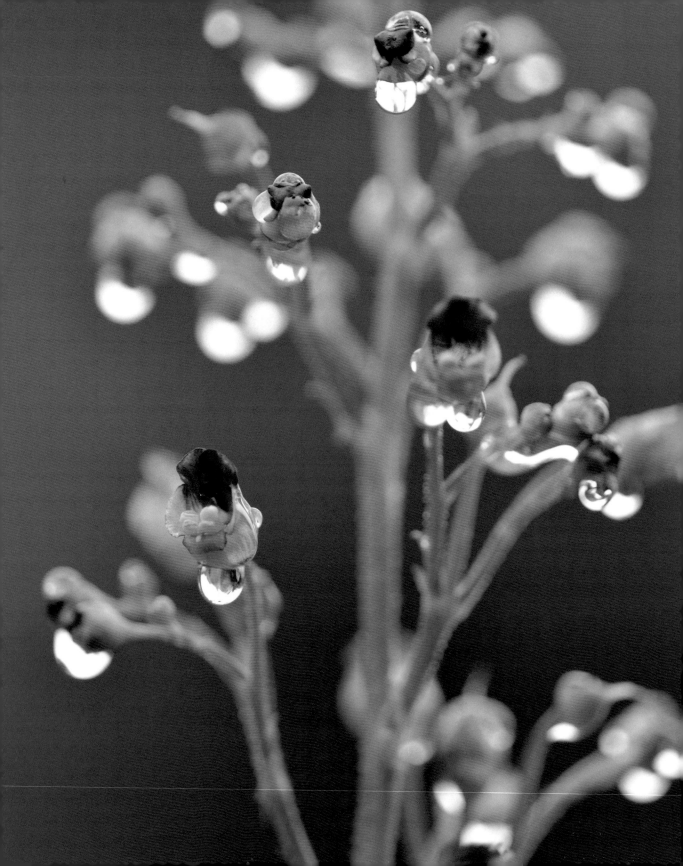

Figwort *Scrophularia nodosa*

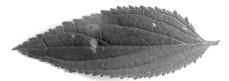

Figwort, also known as common or knotted figwort, has an impressive bearing, as do its other Scrophularia relatives the mulleins and foxglove. Figwort looks wonderful in the rain, its red-brown flower hoods dripping moisture. It also had hidden "signatures" for the herbalist to discern, once competed with the "king's touch" to treat scrofula, and has anti-cancer potential.

There is no doubt about figwort's place in the world. Its names have always spoken to its truth. An old Roman name was *cervicaria*, meaning "of the neck." Later translations of "throatwort" suggest the same location for the plant's therapeutic effect.

The family name Scrophularia, applied from medieval times, was for herbs used to treat scrofula, the painful and purulent tubercular swellings of lymph glands of the neck. The rural name kernellwort suggests the same meaning.

Figwort's Latin species name *nodosa* means swelling or swollen, and can refer to neck nodes or also to "figs" or hemorrhoids, swellings around the anus. The roots of figwort have small tubers, and the old name for hemorrhoids or piles, from the visual resemblance, is figs.

Figwort thus has a double identification of its root tubers and their healing action on scrofula and piles. The knobbly flower buds are also sometimes taken to suggest nodes. This was the doctrine of signatures in action.

We have coincidental examples in figwort's history of how ancient observation preceded medieval signatures theory. Around two millennia ago, the Greek physician Dioscorides and unnamed Chinese physicians were independently discovering the same scrofula-treating qualities of Scrophularia species, *S. nodosa* in the West and *S. ningpoensis* in the East.

The best-known English-language textbook on the Chinese *materia medica* says that the root of Ningpo figwort "Softens hardness and dissipates nodules: for neck lumps due to phlegm-fire as well as severe throat pain and swelling" – a trans-continental confirmation of experimental plant medicine.

A time-honoured remedy for scrofula, or the king's evil, was the royal touch. From King Edward the Confessor (d. 1066) until Queen Anne (d. 1714) English monarchs would graciously confer the royal touch on the afflicted.

**Scrophulariaceae
Figwort family**

Description: Tallish (to 4 ft), rather striking perennial, with angular branches and square stems; its broad-based leaves have serrated edges and taper to a point; flowers are small, knobbly, with lower green sepals and an overhanging red-brown upper lip.

Habitat: Damp woodland, by rivers and ditches or drier patches.

Distribution: Widespread across North America, Eurasia, China.

Related species: Over 200 species worldwide. *S. marilandica* is an equivalent North American species used medicinally, as is *S. ningpoensis* in China.

Parts used: Whole plant, including roots, harvested in summer.

The doctrine of signatures: Figwort or figment?

Does the appearance of figwort indicate its therapeutic potential? Are the "figs" or tubers of figwort a sign that it can treat piles or scrofula, or is this coincidence rather than meaningful or even divine purpose?

Actually, for figwort, the method worked, and the plant has proven to treat the symptoms it "signed."

So can we still dismiss signatures theory as pre-scientific wishful thinking? It's no worse a simplification than, say, that of modern phytochemical research, which legitimizes use of standardized extracts of single elements of plants that can be commoditized and marketed. Signatures were at base a learning mnemonic, an "organizing construct" for a differently literate age.

All the same the method was subjective. Crucially, how did you know which element of the plant was being signed to you? American herbalist Michael Moore (d. 2009) points out that the figwort signature could equally have been for mouth problems (shape of flowers), heart disease (shape of some leaves), cuts (leaf serrations), ligaments (square stem) or clotting blood (red flowers).

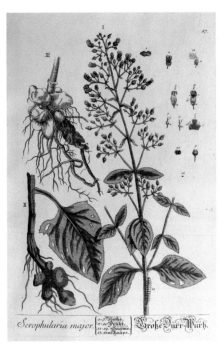

Figwort by Elizabeth Blackwell (1737), here in a revised German edition, 1750s

In 1597, royal chaplain William Tooker described Elizabeth I's royal healing touch: "her very beautiful hands, radiant as whitewashed snow, courageously free from all squeamishness, touching their [sufferers'] abscesses not with fingertips, but pressing hard and repeatedly with wholesome results."

Herbalist John Pechey was equally impressed in 1707: "This, [figwort] and some other Herbs, do good in the King's Evil; but nothing has been found so effectual, as Touching … the Goodness of God, who has dealt so plentifully with this Nation, in giving the Kings of it … an extraordinary Power in the Miraculous Cures thereof."

Use figwort for…

While the plant's smell is unappealing – an old name is "stinking Christopher" – the tubers can be eaten. In 1627, when the port of La Rochelle in France was besieged, its Huguenot inhabitants (the town's population dropped from 27,000 to 9,000 in the 14-month siege) lived on figwort tubers, leading to figwort's honorary name *l'herbe du siège*.

Coming back to medicinal matters, it's unlikely we would encounter a case of scrofula these days, as antibiotics generally do an excellent job. But would we use figwort roots for treating piles? Yes, although our garden has more prolific lesser celandine or pilewort (*Ranunculus ficaria* or *Ficaria verna*: note the *ficaria*, "figs" again), which we use as an infused oil or ointment, made in springtime when it flowers.

For lymphatic cleansing another wild-gathered herb is cleavers (p46). Cleavers makes a pleasant cold infusion (the plant picked and left overnight in cold water), but a less appealing tincture or syrup than the warmer-tasting figwort.

Figwort can be drunk as an infusion of the leaves or the liquid applied topically to skin problems, like eczema and psoriasis, when there is itching, discharge, and heating. External and internal treatment can be combined, with a splash of figwort infusion added to a bath.

As an ointment figwort can be applied to external ulcers, and as a poultice the leaves soothe burns and swellings. A decoction of the root eases throat problems, swollen glands (as in the historic uses) and painful menstruation.

A figwort syrup is sometimes called a "deobstruent," or remover of obstructions, in gently clearing the glandular system or sluggish liver. American herbalist Peter Holmes calls figwort "a prime agent for the body's glandular system as a whole, […] can be used for any glandular disorder."

Writing in 1979, the British herbalist Malcolm Stuart stated that "Figwort is an interesting medicinal plant which deserves closer modern examination." He instanced figwort's cardio-active glycosides, and its potential for heart therapy is being explored.

Most research effort has gone into the anti-cancer properties of Scrophula species: *S. striata* has been shown (2010) to inhibit 1321 cell line proliferation; *S. atropatana* (2017) has cytotoxic and apoptotic effects on some breast cancer cells as does *S. oxysepala* (2015) on MCF-7 breast cancer cells.

S. deserti (2003) has shown anti-diabetic and anti-inflammatory activity, while the wound-healing tradition of *S. nodosa* (2002) has been confirmed. As one modern commentator puts it, figwort is "an alterative with some 'bite.'"

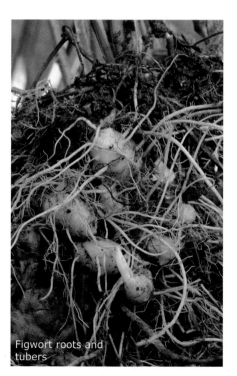

Figwort roots and tubers

Harvesting figwort
Figwort tops can be harvested when flowering, or anytime during the summer when the leaves look fresh. To harvest the tubers, gently lift the plant with a garden fork to expose the roots. Break off a few tubers, leave some for the figwort, then replant.

Figwort tuber tincture
Wash the tubers and slice them. Leaves and tops can be added. Put them in a glass jar and pour enough vodka over to cover them. Put away in a dark place for about a month, shaking bottle occasionally, then strain, bottle and label.

Dose: 1 teaspoon 3 times a day.

Figwort tincture
• swollen glands
• weeping eczema
• psoriasis
• piles
• painful breasts
• boils
• abscesses

Cautions: Figwort is contraindicated if you have rapid heartbeat (tachycardia)

Guelder rose, Crampbark

Viburnum opulus

Guelder rose is able to relieve muscle tension, both in skeletal muscles and in the smooth muscle of the intestines, lungs and uterus. It is used on its own for cramps and muscle spasms, including uterine cramps, back pain, fibromyalgia, and irritable bowel syndrome, and in formulae for high blood pressure, arthritis, and nervous tension.

Adoxaceae / Moschatel family (formerly in the Caprifoliaceae)

Description: A large shrub or small tree with palmate leaves, white blossoms and vivid red berries.

Habitat: Hedgerows, woodlands, damp places and scrubland.

Distribution: Native to Eurasia and North America.

Related species: There are around 150 species in the genus worldwide. Black haw (*V. prunifolium*) from the eastern USA has similar herbal uses.

Parts used: Bark, harvested while the tree is in leaf.

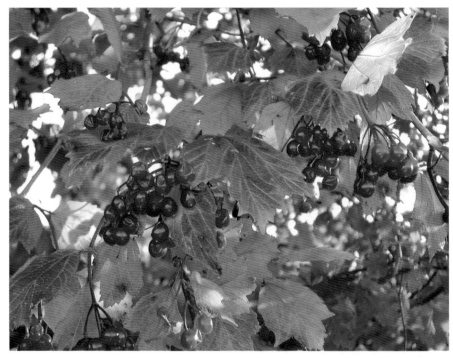

This beautiful native tree should be more widely planted in gardens for its all-year generosity. It has showy creamy-white flowerheads in early summer, while in late summer and fall the berries ripen to a stunning scarlet, their translucence lending them a gorgeous glow, and the foliage colours intensify as the weather cools. The berries are edible, and make a delicious jelly. And if you need more reasons to grow Guelder rose, there are all the medicinal uses of the bark!

Luckily, it is also a common tree in damp woodlands and hedgerows. It has been used medicinally for centuries (Chaucer mentions it), and the name could derive from the town of Guelders, on the former German–Dutch border. Another possibility comes from its superficial similarity to elder, in the same family, reflected in the old common names water elder and white elder. Gerard calls it rose elder or Gelders rose. Crampbark is a more recent name, well capturing its principal use today.

Guelder rose really helps in rheumatic conditions where the pain is from tension rather than inflammation, easing the pain and improving blood flow to the affected area. It is a great remedy to take at the first onset of both migraines and tension headaches, and by relaxing the blood vessels it helps with high blood pressure, Raynaud's syndrome, restless legs, cramps and menstrual pain.

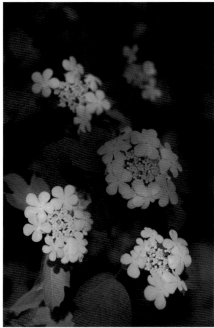

Guelder rose: the small yellowish flowers in the centre are fertile while the large white flowers surrounding them are sterile.

… possibly one of the best herbs known for preventing miscarriage due to stress and anxiety, and is specifically used for relaxing the uterine muscles … among my favorite remedies for menstrual cramps.
– Gladstar (1993)

… will speedily quiet the uneasiness and relieve the pains of uterine and abdominal cramps and is a remedy for nervous disorders and spasms of all kinds.
– Dr. Christopher (1996)

Harvesting Guelder rose

Guelder rose bark can be harvested any time of year, but is usually harvested in the spring or early summer. Use a small knife to remove the bark in short strips, taking care not to take too much from any branch and not to ring the limb, or it will die. The bark can be used fresh, or dried for later use.

Decocted Guelder rose tincture

Put the pieces of **bark** you have harvested in a small saucepan, and add enough **water** to just allow them to float. Bring to the boil, then turn down the heat and simmer gently for 10 minutes. Leave to cool, then strain off the liquid. Measure it, add an equal amount of **vodka** and pour into a jar with the bark pieces you've just boiled. If you are making the tincture in autumn, you can add a few ripe berries to the jar too. Keep the jar in a cool dark place for a month, shaking it every day if you can remember. Strain off the liquid, bottle and label.

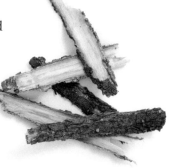

Dose: Half to 1 teaspoonful in water, two to three times a day. For acute conditions, you can add 3 tsp to a glass of water and sip frequently. The tincture can also be used as a liniment rub for aching muscles.

Hawthorn
Crataegus monogyna, C. laevigata (syn. C. oxyacantha)

Rosaceae
Rose family

Description: Thorny shrubs or small trees with clusters of white or pink flowers in spring followed by deep red berries in the fall.

Habitat: Hedgerows, scrub, and woodland margins.

Distribution: Throughout Europe, introduced to North America and Australia. Hawthorn (*C. monogyna*) is the more common species in Britain. Midland hawthorn (*C. laevigata*) is known as smooth hawthorn in North America. They can be used interchangeably. The pink and red flowering hawthorns found in gardens and parkland are generally varieties of Midland hawthorn.

Related species: There are over 200 species worldwide, found in northern temperate regions. Several of these are planted as ornamentals in parks and gardens. Chinese haw (*C. pinnatifida*) is used in Chinese medicine to calm the spirit.

Parts used: Flowering tops, leaves, and ripe berries.

Hawthorn is a superb heart and circulatory tonic, protecting and strengthening the heart muscle and its blood supply. It improves blood circulation around the body, and can be used to treat a wide range of circulatory problems.

Hawthorn also affects the emotional side of what we think of as "heart," by calming and reducing anxiety, helping with bad dreams and insomnia, and smoothing menopausal mood swings.

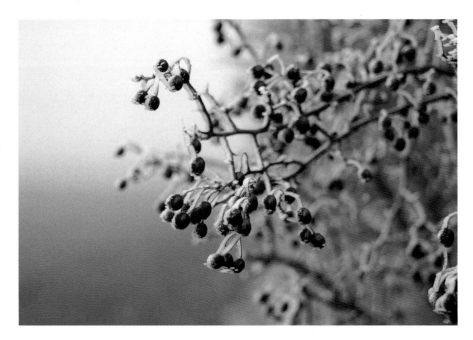

Hawthorn is *the* hedgerow plant of the British Isles. It is the most commonly found species in hedges and spinneys, both historically and in present planting; its very name means "hedge-thorn." It bounds fields and keeps stock in, it grows steadily, is readily plashed and managed, survives poor soils and high winds, and was long a sacred, protective presence.

Hawthorn is well known today as a herbal remedy for the heart and circulation, but this is a relatively new use. Old European herbals mainly talk of hawthorn for "the stone" and for drawing out thorns and splinters, and an occasional use for treating gout and insomnia. It's perhaps surprising that it wasn't thought of for the blood, because the berries are such a

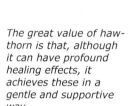

deep blood-like color, and color was often taken as an indication of healing possibilities. Anne Pratt's mid-Victorian survey of British flowering plants (1857) expressed a conventional, and what could be called a pre-modern, view of hawthorn's value:

The chief use of the Hawthorn is for those green impenetrable hedges which bound our meadows and lanes, which are so hardy that they are not even killed by the sea breeze, and which when whitened by their flowers are one of the greatest beauties of the rural landscape…

The modern tale of hawthorn (there are many ancient ones too) begins with a Dr. Green in County Clare, Ireland, in late Victorian times. The doctor had singular success in treating heart disease, but refused to divulge the secret of his medicine. When he died, in 1894, his daughter disclosed that he had been using a tincture of ripe hawthorn berries.

Dr. JC Jennings of Chicago wrote up the story for the *New York Medical Journal* in 1896, and the use of hawthorn tincture for a variety of heart problems quickly caught on on both sides of the Atlantic.

Here is a case history recorded by another Dr. Jennings, this time MC, and published in *A Treatise on Crataegus* in 1917. It is suggestive of the high esteem in which some doctors had soon come to hold hawthorn for heart treatments:

Mr.B., aged 73 years. I found him gasping for breath when I entered the room, with a pulse rate of 158 and very feeble; great oedema of lower limbs and abdomen. A more desperate case could hardly be found.

I gave him fifteen drops of Cratae-gus *in half a wineglass of water. In fifteen minutes the pulse beat was 126 and stronger, and breathing was not so labored. In twenty-five minutes pulse beat 110 and the force was still increasing, breathing much easier.*

He now got ten drops in same quantity of water, and in one hour from the time I entered the house he was, for the first time in ten days, able to lie horizontally on the bed. I made an examination of the heart and found mitral regurgitation from valvular deficiency, with great enlargement.

This clinical success would have been a surprise to earlier generations of doctors and herbalists, as well as to contemporaries. Hawthorn had always had a mixed reputation in popular lore, and for it to be a demonstrably useful heart herb was unexpected.

There is something exciting about wild plants with white spring flowers and dark berries in the autumn. Both elder and hawthorn were fertility symbols of pre-Christian British peoples, and both plants were long ago absorbed by the incoming religion.

Hawthorn was appropriated as forming Christ's crown of thorns

The great value of hawthorn is that, although it can have profound healing effects, it achieves these in a gentle and supportive way.
– Conway (2001)

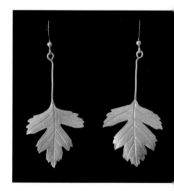

Hawthorn earrings made in fine silver by Julie Bruton-Seal

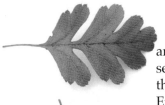

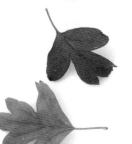

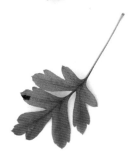

and as being the "burning bush" seen by Moses. The Glastonbury thorn was the best known of the English holy hawthorns.

In its old name of May, hawthorn was the very plant of May Day's plaited crowns and the maypole, much tamer echoes of earlier rites; yet this abundant, fertile spring plant was and still sometimes is unlucky to bring into the house.

Perhaps it was the smell of the flowers, which gives some people hayfever or was said to have lingered from the Great Plague of London; it was also reminiscent of the taboos, of death and putrefaction, but also of sex. On the other hand, an old proverb gave a softer view of hawthorn's erotic power:

The fair maid who, the first of May,/ Goes to the fields at break of day,/ And washes in dew from the hawthorn tree,/ Will ever after handsome be.

Use hawthorn for…
Long the plant of the heart in folklore, we know now that hawthorn works in several ways as a restorative of the physical heart. Its flavonoids and procyanidins have a wonderful capacity to dilate the coronary arteries and strengthen heart muscle without raising blood pressure or the beat.

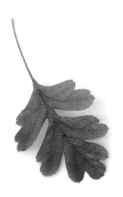

The berries, leaves, and flowers can treat angina, enlargement of the heart from overwork or excessive exercise, and heart damage from over-use of alcohol.

It is important to state that heart disease is a life-threatening illness, and should be treated under the advice of a primary healthcare practitioner – your doctors or a qualified professional herbalist. If you are taking beta-blockers, only use hawthorn under supervision.

Unlike digitalis and numerous commercial preparations, hawthorn is a prophylactic with few side effects. It can – and we'd say should – be made part of personal regime to forestall future problems with the heart and circulation.

Hawthorn helps stabilize blood pressure and to dissolve cholesterol and calcium deposits, making it good for arteriosclerosis, or hardening of the arteries, and plaquing.

When a fatty plaque comes loose from an artery wall it can rapidly lead to a blockage. If the artery involved is the coronary artery, which feeds the heart muscle, this blockage will mean a heart attack; if a plaque blocks an artery in the brain, it will cause a stroke. Arteries anywhere in the body can be affected, but problems often go unnoticed.

Hawthorn is an effective treatment for intermittent claudication, where the blood vessels of the legs aren't supplying enough oxygen to the muscles, resulting in pain on walking. Similar conditions, such as Buerger's disease and Raynaud's disease, also benefit from hawthorn's gentle effects.

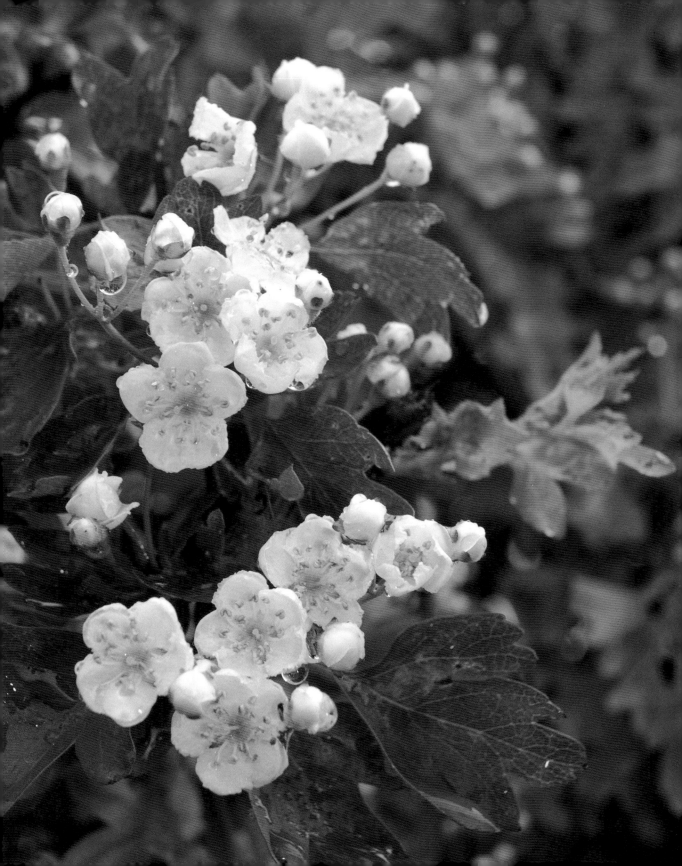

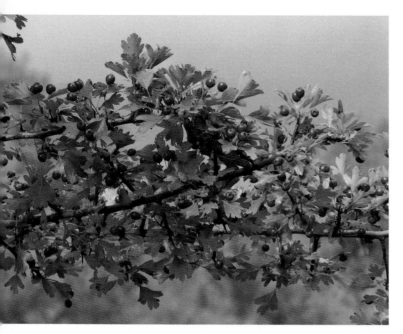

Hawthorn combines well with yarrow in cases of constriction of the blood vessels with a risk of thrombosis or clotting. As a general heart/circulatory tonic, use alongside ramsons or garlic, and ginger. If the circulation is sluggish, take it with horseradish; for memory, with ginkgo; and to improve the peripheral circulation of the limbs, with lime blossom.

Hawthorn research on human subjects has focused on mild forms of heart failure (e.g. (2010a)), with clinical improvement in left ventricular ejection, heart pressure rates, and well-being, plus good toleration, safety, and lack of herb–drug interactions. More advanced forms of cardiovascular disease are being examined (2010b) too, but ever-higher dosage of what is essentially a cardiotonic herb is not the magic bullet that heart research is seeking (2013). Herbal experience suggests hawthorn treatment earlier and prophylactically, as a daily tonic.

Hawthorn enhances the functioning of the heart and circulation during exercise, and taken in moderation can improve athletic performance. Moreover, taking hawthorn calms the spirit, and gives good results in menopausal mood swings, restlessness, and anxiety; it will help quieten overactive children who have ADHD.

Hawthorn berry leather

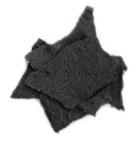

Pick ripe **hawthorn berries** and place in a saucepan with half their volume of **water**. Simmer gently for about 15 minutes and allow to cool. Blend the mixture briefly to loosen the pulp from the seeds or mash it with a potato masher, then rub the pulp through a coarse sieve.

Pour this strained pulp into baking trays so that it is a quarter of an inch thick, and put the trays in an oven at the lowest temperature setting to dry. If you have a food dehydrator, you can put the fruit leather trays in that, following the manufacturer's instructions. Leave until the pulp is dry and leathery, and can be peeled off the trays without being sticky. Cut up and store in airtight jars. Eat about a 1 inch square every day to help keep your heart and circulation healthy.

Hawthorn berry syrup

Put 1 lb **berries** in a large saucepan with 1 pint **water**, and slowly bring to a boil. Mash a little with a potato masher. Turn off the heat and leave to stand overnight. Bring to a boil again, then turn down the heat and simmer gently. The berries quickly lose their deep red colour and turn a dingy sort of yellow. Don't worry if the decoction smells somewhat fishy at this point – the syrup will not taste like it smells.

When the mixture has sweated down to half its volume, allow to cool and then squeeze out the juice. Weigh the juice and put back into the saucepan with an equal weight of **sugar**. Bring rapidly to the boil, then pour while still warm into sterilized bottles. The finished syrup often has a strawberry-like flavour. You can use honey instead of sugar for this syrup, but the honey version does not keep as well.

Dose: 1 teaspoonful daily as a heart tonic or use as a flavouring.

Hawthorn tincture

The best hawthorn tincture is made in two parts, using the flowers and leaves gathered in spring and then adding the berries in the fall when they are ripe (or vice versa). Either tincture can also be used on its own, with the berry tincture tasting the best.

In spring: Gather the **flowering tops** when the blossom is young and fresh. Remove any large twigs, and pack into a jar. Fill the jar with **vodka**, put the lid on and shake the jar to remove any air bubbles. Put the jar in a cupboard for about a month, until the blossom and leaves have lost their colour, then strain off the liquid and bottle it.

In fall: Put the **berries** in a blender with enough **hawthorn flower tincture** to cover, and blend to a mush. Pour the mixture into wide-mouthed jars – this is important because hawthorn berries have so much pectin that the whole mixture will set solid, and you'll find it impossible to get it out of a narrow-necked bottle. Leave the jars in a cool dark place for a month, then poke a knife into the jar to chop the contents enough to get them out. Squeeze the liquid out using a jelly bag – this is good exercise! If you have a juice press, use that as it will be a lot less work.

Bottle and label your tincture. This will keep for several years, although it's best to make a fresh lot every year if you can.

Dose: 1 teaspoon once a day as a general tonic; 1 teaspoon three times a day or as advised by your herbalist for circulatory problems.

BERRIES
Hawthorn fruit leather
- heart tonic
- circulatory tonic

Hawthorn berry syrup
- heart tonic
- hardening of the arteries
- abnormal blood pressure
- mild angina
- menopause
- palpitations
- anxiety, restlessness

FLOWERS, LEAVES & BERRIES
Hawthorn tincture
- heart tonic
- hardening of the arteries
- abnormal blood pressure
- palpitations
- irregular heart beat
- mild angina
- anxiety, restlessness
- intermittent claudication

Caution: Only take hawthorn alongside beta-blockers and other cardiovascular drugs if you are under the professional supervision of an herbal or medical practitioner.

Honeysuckle, Woodbine *Lonicera periclymenum*

Honeysuckle is esteemed for its superb scent and lovely flowers but should also be valued as a cooling herb. It has benefits for menopausal hot flashes, flu, fevers, heat stroke, urinary tract infections, and other hot conditions. The flowers have similar qualities to aspirin and are strongly antiseptic, being effective against a range of micro-organisms.

**Caprifoliaceae
Honeysuckle family**

Description: A twining deciduous shrub with fragrant white, yellow, and red flowers followed by red berries.

Habitat: Hedgerows, woodland and scrub.

Distribution: Native to Europe, where it is widespread. Introduced to North America.

Related species: There are around 180 honeysuckle species worldwide, several with medicinal qualities. Japanese honeysuckle (*L. japonica*) is a popular garden plant now naturalized in Australia and North America, with similar medicinal uses to woodbine.

Parts used: Flowers, harvested when in bloom during late spring, summer or fall.

Honeysuckle must be among the best-loved of wild and garden plants. It has the sweetest and most intoxicating of fragrances, and its attractive white, yellow, and red flowers keep on blooming through spring and summer. It forms lovely bowers that offer dappled shade around the front door of many a cottage; it is irresistible to the bees and hawk moths that pollinate it; and honeysuckle's scarlet berries in autumn are a food source for many birds.

Its intertwining habit has made it the very symbol of love in many cultures. Honeysuckle flowers were once thought too dangerous to keep indoors because the scent would give forbidden thoughts to young ladies. Shakespeare knew well its mythic power, using it as an image of lovers sleeping enfolded in each other's arms in *A Midsummer Night's Dream*.

Honeysuckle was probably more common in Shakespeare's day, as England was so heavily wooded. The very old common names woodbine or woodbind recall this origin, and the twining habit. Modern foresters are not quite so taken with the way honeysuckle twists around hazel stems, leaving permanent grooves that lower the commercial value. These twisted hazel stems, though, were once highly prized for making into twirly walking sticks that were said to help suitors win the woman of their dreams.

The Elizabethans would have been as taken by the plant's medicinal properties as its beauty or romantic associations. They would not have known that its leaves and flowers are rich in salicylic acid, a compound similar to aspirin. But they would have been well aware that an infusion of the flowers or leaves was good for headaches, fevers, bronchial complaints, and rheumatism, as it is today.

Modern herbalists favor the flowers over the leaves, but the bitter berries are seldom used, except in serious vomiting or diarrhea. Any of the yellow-flowered varieties of honeysuckle are effective in treating heat

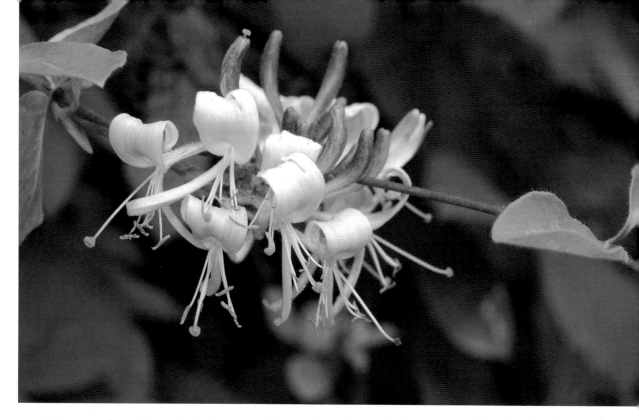

conditions, perhaps the principal benefit of the plant today. The effect is cooling for menopausal hot flashes, fevers, sunstroke, and urinary tract infections.

Honeysuckle is also used for spasm in the respiratory system in such conditions as asthma, croup, and bronchitis. It is antiseptic and effective against many micro-organisms, reinforcing its value for sore throats and respiratory problems. A traditional Chinese formula, *shuang huang lian*, mixes honeysuckle, forsythia, and skullcap for respiratory complaints. The late American herbalist James Duke rated honeysuckle second only to eucalyptus for sore throats.

We favor the flowers steeped in honey, though a tea of the dried flowers is also good, drunk often or poured into a hot bath.

The oyle wherein its flowers have been infused and sunned, is good against cramps, convulsions of the sinuses, and palsies and other benumming cold griefe.
– Parkinson (1640)

Honeysuckle flowers infused in honey or glycerine
Pick **honeysuckle flowers** and buds and put them in a jar, then fill it up with **runny honey** or **vegetable glycerine**. Put the jar on a sunny windowsill or in another warm place and leave it for two weeks. You may need to push the flowers down into the liquid every few days to keep them covered, or they will go brown. Strain, bottle, and label.
Dose: 1 teaspoonful as needed for sore throats, or 3 times a day.

Honeysuckle flowers in honey
• sore throats
• tonsillitis
• flu
• colds
• hot flashes
• bronchitis

Hops *Humulus lupulus*

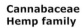

A bitter sedative herb best known for its role in brewing and as an aid to sleep, hops also stimulate digestion and affect hormones.

The medicinal use of hops preceded that in brewing, in both cases via the female flower cones, the strobiles. Used mainly in the form of a hops pillow or tincture, hops' estrogen-like compounds reduces libido in men while increasing it in women.

Cannabaceae
Hemp family

Description: A perennial climber, with separate male and female plants.

Habitat: Hedgerows, edges of woods.

Distribution: Native and widespread in North America and Europe.

Related species: There are several subspecies of hops, and two other species are found in Asia.

Parts used: Female fruiting cones (known as strobiles).

The manifold vertues of Hops do manifest argue the wholesome-nesse of beere above ale; for the hops make it a physicall drinke to keepe the body in health, than an ordinary drinke for the quenching of our thirst.
– Gerard (1597)

Hops is considered by herbalists to be one of the most calming and relaxing herbs known to mankind.
– Dewey (1996)

While often thought to be of exotic origin, hops are native to Europe as well as North America. They were named *lupulus* ("small wolf") by the Romans, who wrongly thought hops strangled host plants on which they grew, like wolves strangled their prey. In Italy, hops were a food: the buds and tendrils still make an interesting soup, omelette and asparagus-like boiled vegetable. Hops are rather bitter, however, and John Evelyn's opinion (1699) – 'rather *Medicinal*, than fit for *Sallets*' – holds good today.

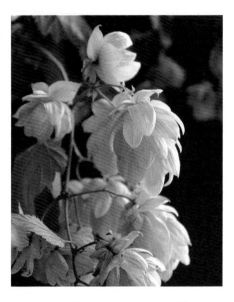

Hops were already cultivated for brewing in France and Germany by the eighth and ninth centuries. But ale held its place over beer in Britain until the seventeenth century; indeed, Henry VIII had banned the use of hops for a while. The Briton's ale was tradionally flavored by plants such as ground ivy (old names alehoof and tunhoof), bog myrtle, yarrow and sage, but hops had a critical edge: all these other herbs did not preserve the brew for as long.

As beer gained ground, and hops became a commercial cash-crop in the southeast and parts of the English Midlands, the plant's medicinal virtues became obscured. But then another king, George III, gave the reputation of hops a boost. His insomnia was relieved by the suggestion of his prime minister, Lord Addington, to try out a hops pillow. It succeeded, and the fashion for this effective sleep aid was royally set.

Hops are now used in some 60 commercial sedative formulas in Britain, and this is the "official" use. This herb gently sedates without narcotic side effects, and soothes the smooth muscle of the stomach and bowel. It is thus a specific for nervous stomachs, IBS, and Crohn's disease. It works to relax hyperactivity in children (using half doses of hops tincture). For sleeplessness, it combines well with wood betony, vervain, skullcap, red poppy, California poppy, and passionflower. Avoid if you suffer from nervous depression.

The one fact everyone knows about hops is causing "brewer's droop" in men; less familiar is the plant's role in increasing libido in women. Both reactions relate to hops' estrogen-like compounds. Female hop pickers used to suffer disruptions in menstruation from constant contact with the plant. But used in balance with a woman's constitution hops are a good treatment for hot flashes and in menopause. They also help control premature ejaculation in men.

As a bitter and a tonic, hops have an appetite-stimulating effect that can be beneficial in cases of anorexia. They calm and relieve the spasms of irritable bowel syndrome and increase urine flow (ask any beer drinker!).

Hops pillow

Pick **hops** strobiles (the flower cones) and dry them in a cool shady place. Make a small bag for the pillow out of **cloth**, leaving one end open – any size you like, but 8" x 10" works well. Fill the bag loosely with the dried hops (or add lavender if you wish) so that the finished pillow will be 1 inch thick, then stitch up the open end. Place this under your regular pillow to help with sleep.

The hops will gradually lose their volatile oils and therefore their effectiveness, so for best results replace the contents of your pillow every three months. Use hops that have been stored in the dark, in an airtight container. If your dried hops turn pinkish or reddish, their oils have been exhausted, and they should be discarded.

Hops tincture

Pack dried **hops** cones into a jar, and fill it with **vodka**. Put the jar in a dark place for two weeks, shaking it every few days. Strain off the liquid, bottle, and label.

Dose: 1 teaspoonful taken in the evening to help with sleep. For menopausal hot flashes, half a teaspoonful morning and evening. For lack of appetite or sluggish digestion, a few drops pre-meals.

Hops pillow
• insomnia

Hops tincture
• hot flashes
• insomnia
• lack of appetite
• sluggish digestion

Cautions: Hops should not be taken if you suffer from depression. Taking hops can affect the menstrual cycle.

Horse chestnut *Aesculus hippocastanum*

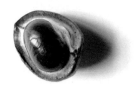

Description: A tall tree, up to 130 ft, with palmate leaves in spring and huge candelabras of white–pink flowers in summer, then conkers in fall.

Habitat: Gardens, parks and roadsides.

Distribution: Native to western Asia and southeast Europe, but widespread as a planted and natural-ized species in Western Europe and in eastern North America.

Related species: The red horse chestnut (*A. x carnea*) is used in a flower essence. North American buckeyes (*Aesculus* spp.) are related, but sweet chestnut (*Castanea sativa*) is not.

Parts used: Conkers, collected in fall; leaves in spring.

Familiar for its nuts, or conkers, horse chestnut is a beautiful introduced tree. It also has significant medicinal uses, notably for supporting weakened veins, as in varicose veins, hemorrhoids and capillary fragility. It is used for two Bach Flower Essences and in commerical quantities for allopathic and homeopathic remedies for irregularities of the veins. It also has some surprising other uses.

A shapely tree, with glossy brown sticky buds in winter, lime green hand-shaped leaves in spring, then soft and frothy Folies-Bergère-like pink and white flowers in summer, and hard spherical auburn nuts, conkers, in fall – no wonder the all-season beauty of horse chestnut was such a hit when the tree was introduced into England in the early 1600s.

At first a tree of kings and own-ers of great estates, it later came to belong to everybody as Britain's municipal tree of choice, planted ornamentally in every avenue and park, in every Chestnut Villas of every Victorian city.

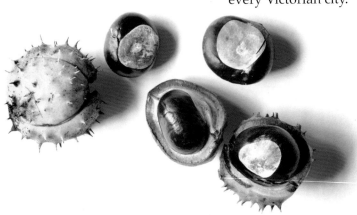

Recent estimates of the national horse chestnut 'park' give a figure of over 400,000 trees. It was and is admired for its looks – the wood of horse chestnut is soft and spongy, poor for carpentry or building.

The tree's scientific and popular names may derive from its use in Turkey, one of the countries of ori-gin of the first specimens to reach Western Europe. The Turks mixed flour from the conkers with oats to improve the breathing of broken-winded horses.

Other plant historians suggest that "horse" is meant as a derogative comparison to the native and tasty sweet chestnut (which is unre-lated botanically). Horse chestnut conkers do contain a complex bitter chemical, escin (aescin in UK spelling), as the plant's active prin-ciple, and this is said to be toxic to humans in very large quantities.

Surprisingly varied uses have been found for the tree. The bark was used as a quinine substitute

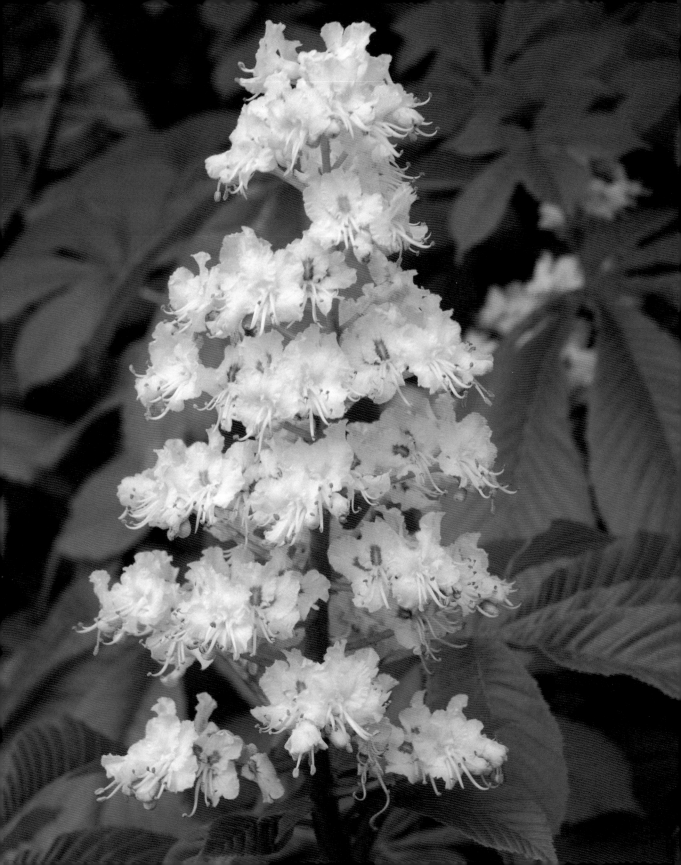

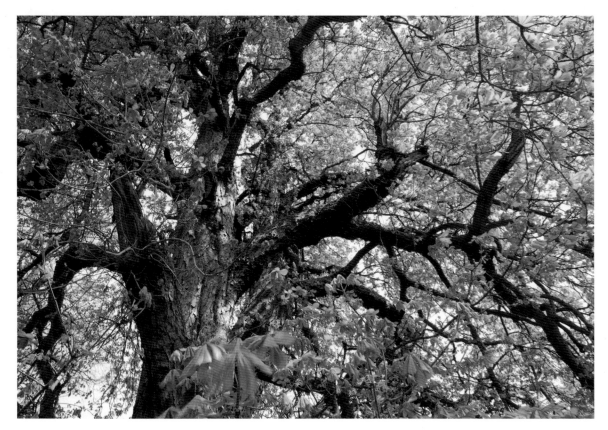

[Aescin, found in conkers] ... *reduces leakage and is used in the treatment of oedema (lower leg swelling) and has proved to be as effective as compression stockings. It strengthens and tones the blood vessels and is becoming very important in the treatment of varicose veins and chronic venous insufficiency (CVI) ... Haemorrhoids respond well too...*
– Howkins (2005)

for malaria and other fevers, while the flower buds made an ersatz flavoring for beer. Conkers produce a good soapy lather for shampoo and to clean clothes, stop mold, and repel clothes moths.

And, little known today, conkers were used for explosives during the First World War. With other sources of acetone unavailable, British children collected 3,000 tons of conkers secretly in summer 1917 (their schools received a certificate). The research chemist seconded to the government's chestnuts plan, Chaim Weizman, then in Manchester, would become first president of Israel in 1948.

Other new "explosive" chestnut issues include worries about a leaf miner moth damaging (but not killing) mature trees, and the charge that children are at risk while playing with conkers if they chew or eat them. Sadly, the game is now banned in some English schools, but it would need concerted force-feeding to reach toxic levels of escin, and the bitter taste is already off-putting to children.

Use horse chestnut for...

Horse chestnut is a leading herbal treatment for weakened veins, including varicose veins, hemorrhoids, acne rosacea and chronic venous insufficiency (CVI). It has an unusual capacity to strengthen small blood vessel walls by reducing the size and number of the pores; it also works well on wrinkles by tightening the skin (an alternative to Botox, perhaps?), and for fluid retention or edema.

Horse chestnut is taken both internally as a tincture and externally as a cream, oil or lotion. Internal use should be in small doses and under the supervision of a herbalist, in case of stomach irritation.

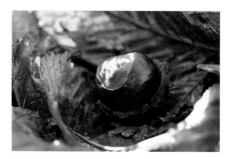

Aesculus has unique action on the vessels of the circulatory system. The herb appears to increase the elasticity and tone of the veins while decreasing vein permeability.
– Hoffmann (2003)

Commercially, it is grown for horse chestnut seed extract (HCSE) and a homeopathic remedy. It also makes two Bach Flower Essences, chestnut bud and white chestnut.

Conker tincture
Collect the **conkers** as soon as they fall to the ground in early fall. They will usually come out of their green spiky husks by themselves. While fresh, they are quite soft, but they soon harden and are much more troublesome to cut. Use a serrated knife and be careful in chopping them up, as they can skid out from under the knife blade.

Put the chopped conkers in a jar and pour in enough **vodka** to cover them. Leave in a dark cupboard for a month, shaking every few days. It is normal for the alcohol to extract a milky sediment from the seeds. Strain and bottle, or use to make the lotion below.

Internal use: 5 drops in water twice a day, or as recommended by your herbalist. **External use**: add a splash to your bathwater.

Horse chestnut leaf oil
Pick **leaves** in spring before the flowers open. Chop them up and put them in a jar large enough to hold them. Fill the jar with **extra virgin olive oil**. Stir to remove any air bubbles, and top up with more oil if necessary. Put on a sunny windowsill to infuse for a month, then strain off the oil into a jug. Allow this to settle for half an hour. Carefully pour the oil into jars, leaving any watery sediment behind at the bottom of the jug. Apply directly to the skin or use to make the lotion below.

Horse chestnut lotion
Chill equal amounts of **conker tincture**, **horse chestnut leaf oil** and **castor oil** in the fridge overnight, then blend until creamy. Bottle. Shake well before use, as it may separate on standing. Apply twice a day.

Conker tincture
- varicose veins
- thread veins
- fragile capillaries
- restorative bath

Horse chestnut leaf oil
- varicose veins
- thread veins
- fragile capillaries

Horse chestnut lotion
- varicose veins
- thread veins
- fragile capillaries

Cautions: May cause digestive irritation when taken internally. If you are pregnant or breastfeeding, or taking blood-thinning medication, only take under professional supervision.

Horseradish *Armoracia rusticana*

Brassicaceae (Cruciferae) Cabbage family

Description: A perennial, which forms large patches. The leaves are dock-like, but bright green with parallel veins and wavy edges, and often full of holes from snails. In summer there may be trusses of white flowers.

Habitat: Along road-sides, on waste ground and in kitchen gardens.

Distribution: Widely cultivated. Often a garden escape, it spreads by strong lateral roots, and is hard to remove once you have it.

Parts used: Roots.

Horseradish root is hot and pungent, and the same qualities that make it the chosen accompaniment to roast beef also power its medicinal uses. It stimulates digestion, is an active eliminator of the waste products of fevers and colds, clears the sinuses and is warming for rheumatism and muscle aches.

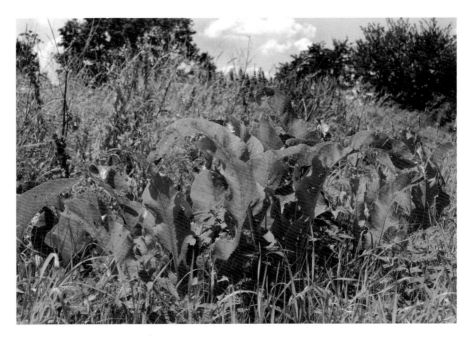

... it is also a good remedy in strong bodies, both for the Cough, the Tissicke and other diseases of the lunges ... the roote bruised and laid to the place grieved with the Sciatica-gout, joynt-ach, or the hard swellings of the spleene and liver, doth wonderfully helpe them all.
– Parkinson (1640)

Horseradish is this book's example of a hot, pungent and stimulating herb. Lacking native ginger or galangal, horseradish is a good British heating herb, although the mustards have similar virtues.

Horseradish is a bit of a show-off, a hot cabbage originating in southern Russia, with large, coarse, wavy-edged leaves that glisten in the rain. It has small and pretty white flowers, but its main claim to fame is its long and sturdy white tap root. And this hides its healing secrets.

The root is the part used medicinally, as it is to make Britain's customary sauce for roast beef. We readily break our own rules about using roots for several reasons: horseradish is abundant, if not invasive; a few roots are all you need for a year's supply as a standby medicine; and it regenerates quickly from the smallest fragment of root left behind.

It was a medicine long before it became a condiment, but works in a parallel way in both uses. The outer layer of root is beige and inoffensive, but as soon as you cut into the tissues beneath you are assailed by a hot and biting smell that makes your eyes water.

In small amounts the grated root, usually preserved in vinegar or a cream sauce, lifts the gastric enzymes into overdrive to break down the cell structure of cooked beef and prevent indigestion. Note that larger amounts can inflame the stomach lining in some people.

A mustard-like peroxidase is being created and released, stimulating digestive and other reactions. The mucous membranes in the mouth and throat react immediately, clearing blocked sinuses.

This vigorous response indicates the value of horseradish in promoting elimination in flus, fevers, coughs and catarrh. Be aware that it is an active process, with

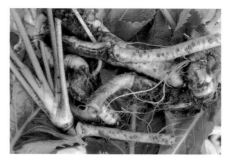

hot sweats. Indeed, a 2016 study recommends horseradish enzymes for targeted cancer treatments.

The cut root rubbed on stiff or aching joints and muscles will bring warmth to the skin. Rheumatic conditions can be eased using a poultice, but people with sensitive skin may react by blistering. The plant's antiseptic and antimicrobial qualities offer relief for boils.

Bear in mind the root's strength and volatility. "Horse" in the name means "coarse" or "rough," while an earlier English name, red cole, likened the fiery taste to red-hot coals. John Pechey summed up (1707): "horseradish provokes the appetite, but it hurts the head."

Horseradish syrup
- coughs
- colds
- fevers
- sinus congestion

Horseradish sauce
- sinus congestion
- sluggish digestion

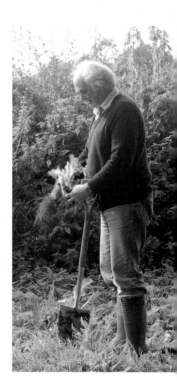

Horseradish cough syrup
Grate a **horseradish root** into a bowl (outdoors if the fumes are strong). Whatever amount you make, cover this with **sugar.** Stir well, and leave for a few hours until a syrup develops. Strain off the liquid. If it is too fluid, heat until it reduces to the consistency you like. Pour into a bottle. It is strong, so dosage is no more than 3 tablespoons a day.

Horseradish sauce
Chop **fresh horseradish root** and put in a blender with enough **cider vinegar** to blend. Store in the fridge. Use as a condiment, or chew a teaspoonful to clear blocked sinuses. The vinegar can be strained off after a week or two to use in the formula given on page 209.

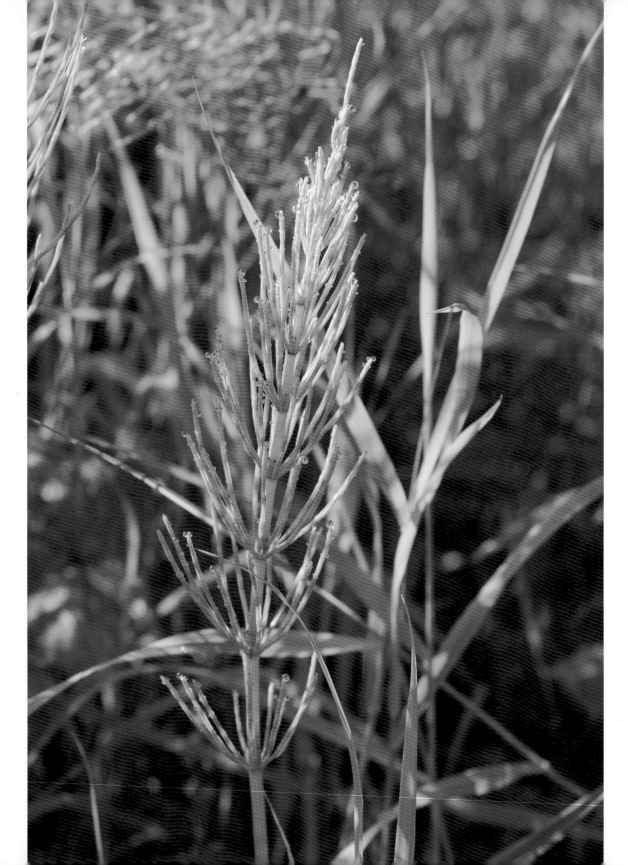

Horsetail *Equisetum arvense*

Horsetail is one of the oldest of plants and a long-used folk remedy for the urinary system, cystitis, incontinence, bedwetting, and prostate problems. It is the leading source of plant silica, and so helps where this mineral is deficient, as shown by symptoms like brittle nails, thin hair, and allergies. Externally, it is good for rheumatism, chilblains, and skin problems, and helps wounds, joints, and sprains to heal.

When we say horsetail is old we do really mean old: relatives of our one foot-tall common plant grew a hundred feet tall and were the forest trees of the Carboniferous age, roughly 270–370 million years ago. You can see fossilized traces of proto-horsetail in lumps of domestic coal today, and apart from size the prehistoric and modern look uncannily alike.

The name *equisetum* refers to "horse" and "bristle," giving rise to the common name. To the Romans it was "hair of the earth,"

Horsetail is now esteemed as the main source of silica in the plant world. In effect little more than a skeleton of silica, it contains 30% or more of this element, depending on the soil; the burnt ash has over 80% silica.

Such a rich natural source of silica was recognized long ago. Old names of horsetail include pewterwort, shave-grass and bottlebrush, which hint at its ability to scour but not damage pewter, and safely polish wood and glass. The plant was sold in London streets up to the eighteenth century for such purposes. It is said that powdered horsetail ash mixed with water is still the best silver cleaner.

Another unique quality of the plant is that it doesn't have leaves or flowers as such, and spreads by means of spores, like a fern. In spring, fertile stems grow up from deep underground rhizomes. These stems are bare with cone-like heads full of spores – "drumsticks poking out of the ground," says one author. Another writer thinks it "resembles moth-eaten asparagus." The softish stems die back and are replaced in summer by segmented, stiff and infertile stems with narrow leaves sprouting from nodes, something like pine needles on a bamboo.

While the spore stems can be eaten, and were favored by the Romans as a tonic salad, the silica-rich summer stems are better used for cleaning your pots and for their herbal qualities.

Equisetaceae
Horsetail family

Description: A leafless non-flowering perennial with hollow, jointed stems, growing up to a foot tall. It looks like a miniature Christmas tree, and has spreading green teeth on the stem sheath.

Habitat: Roadsides, gardens, and waste ground.

Distribution: Widespread in Europe, Asia, and North America. Introduced to the southern hemisphere.

Related species: Two other of the nine species found in the British Isles have a traditional medicinal use: wood horsetail (*E. sylvaticum*), similar to field horsetail but more delicate and drooping at the tip; and rough horsetail (*E. hyemale*), which has no branches. The other species are not used for medicine.

Parts used: Above-ground parts harvested in summer.

Use horsetail for...

A key virtue of horsetail is that its silica is water-soluble, meaning that it can be readily transported around the body in solution form. Taken as a tea or syrup, it reaches your nails and joints, hair and skin; externally it makes a good poultice and hair rinse, or can be added to the bath or body lotion.

Horsetail may help if you have weak or brittle nails, thin hair with split ends, chronic cystitis or bladder irritation, multiple allergies, or weak joints and connective tissue.

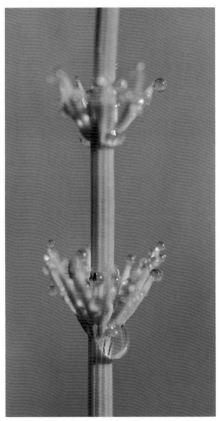

A young field horsetail (*E. arvense*) collects the early morning dew. Note the green joints, an identifying characteristic.

Horsetail can, in certain cases, work wonders in rebuilding joints and other connective tissues.

One case of horsetail's value was told by a massage therapist who thought she might have to give up her work on account of pain and weakness of the wrist joint. Taking horsetail corrected this, and indeed also led to her fingernails growing much faster. She had to cut them more often to remain a smooth operator!

There is a tradition of horsetail being used to strengthen bones and teeth, and it is often found in formulae for osteoporosis and bone fractures. It helps in the healing process following surgery, including after episiotomy (2015).

Horsetail seems to work by strengthening the channels in the body, including the arteries and veins, and assists the free passage of fluids. One of its common names, bottle brush, could refer to its shape but could as easily relate to this clearing of channels.

Horsetail is mildly diuretic, meaning it can clear the kidneys without exhausting them. It is useful in teas for cystitis, incontinence, and other bladder issues, and can help with the problems associated with prostate enlargement. It is also known as a wound herb, releasing pus and damaged cells from infected wounds. Another way it works on wounds is to slow down the bleeding.

Harvesting horsetail

Pick horsetail in early summer, cutting the plant several inches above the ground so that it can grow back. For teas, dry it quickly, so that the plants don't turn brown. Crushing the plants lightly with a rolling pin helps the moisture escape. When dry, cut up into short pieces.

Cystitis tea blend

Combine roughly equal parts by volume of dried **horsetail** and **couch-grass**, and whichever you have on hand of the following: **bilberry leaves, yarrow** or **pellitory of the wall**.

Use a rounded teaspoonful of the mixture per mug of boiling water in a teapot, and leave to brew for 10 minutes.

Dose: Drink a cupful every two hours for acute cystitis, and continue with three cups a day for a while until you are completely over the cystitis.

Horsetail tea

Add **a rounded teaspoonful of dried horsetail** and **half a teaspoonful of sugar** to **2 cups of water** in a small saucepan. Bring to the boil, turn down the heat and simmer gently, uncovered, until the liquid has reduced by about half.

Dose: Drink a cup occasionally to keep your skin, nails, and hair strong and healthy.

Make triple strength and add a cupful to hot baths and foot baths to help heal sprains and other injuries. It is remarkably effective.

Horsetail syrup

This recipe keeps well, is convenient to take, and tastes good.

A couple of handfuls of fresh horsetail (about 2 oz)
1 pint water
Three and a half oz sugar

Place the ingredients together in a pan, boil, then reduce heat and simmer for half an hour until the horsetail turns dark green and becomes soft. Strain off the liquid and return it to the pan with an additional 5 oz sugar. Boil for 5 minutes, allow to cool, then bottle. Makes about 13 fl oz syrup.

Dose: Take one teaspoonful a day for two or three weeks, then take a break for a week before resuming if needed.

Horsetail tea
- cystitis
- incontinence
- bedwetting
- weak nails
- skin problems
- brittle hair
- benign prostate hyperplasia

Horsetail bath
- rheumatic pains
- skin problems
- chilblains
- sprains

Horsetail syrup
- incontinence
- bedwetting
- weak nails
- thin or brittle hair
- chronic cystitis
- benign prostate hyperplasia

... it doth perfectly cure wounds, yea, although the sinues be cut asunder.
– Galen (1st century AD)

An excellent remedy, internally and externally, for the whole kidney and bladder system.
– Treben (1980)

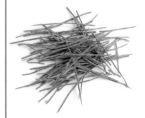

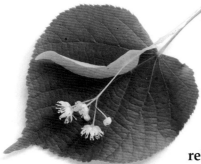

Lime, Linden *Tilia* spp.

The perfect remedy for stress, tension and over-work, lime blossom helps us relax and sleep well. It soothes irritation, boosts the immune system, and protects the heart by reducing cholesterol levels and relaxing the arteries.

Linden tea is widely enjoyed in France where it is drunk as a daily beverage for its pleasant honey-like taste and its health benefits. It is also wonderful for children.

Malvaceae
Mallow family
(formerly in the Tiliaeceae)

Description: Tall, elegant trees that bear deciduous, heart-shaped leaves and fragrant flowers in summer.

Habitat: Woods, hedgerows, parks, and gardens.

Distribution: Small-leaved lime, European lime, and large-leaved lime are native to Europe, but grown in parks and gardens elsewhere. American basswood is native to North America.

Species: Common lime (*Tilia* x *europaea*) is the hybrid of small-leaved lime (*T. cordata*) and large-leaved lime (*T. platyphyllos*). These are the species traditionally used in Europe. American basswood (*T. americana*) can be used in similar ways.

Parts used: Flowers, picked when the first flowers in each bunch have opened in summer.

There is nothing quite like walking under lime trees when they are in full flower in early summer, drowsily fragrant and loudly humming with the buzz of masses of honeybees. Bees adore lime blossom, and make a flavorsome honey from it that retains the calming effects of the flowers.

Linden's heady scent does have an uplifting effect on consciousness, and in folklore it was said that if you fell asleep under a lime tree you could wake up in fairyland. More practically, if you park your car under one in high summer, it will be covered with sticky droppings of honeydew from greenfly that live on the leaves.

The name lime can be confusing, as many of us think of lime fruit, a relative of the lemon. All that links the two is the color, which is similar in the leaves of linden trees and the citrus fruit. There is also no connection with limestone.

The blossom season is short and can easily be missed, especially if the weather is bad.

Use lime or linden for...
Medicinally, lime blossom is best known as a calming, relaxing remedy. It can be used to treat high blood pressure, and arterio-sclerosis, particularly where stress and anxiety are major factors. It is a circulatory relaxant, working to destress the arterial walls.

Relieving tension as it does, linden encourages a restful relaxing sleep, helping you wake refreshed and clear-headed. It was recommended as a sedative in Britain during World War II.

The tea, drunk hot, promotes sweating. This can be used to "break a fever," with sweating being the body's natural way of preventing a fever from burning too hot, while also helping eliminate toxins through the skin and

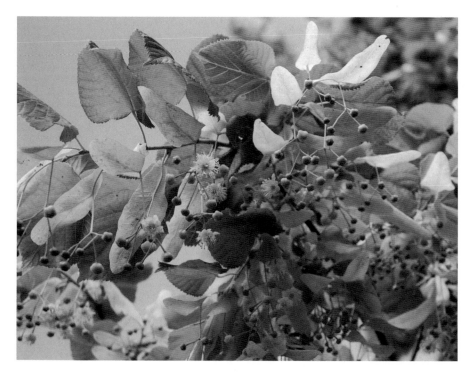

clearing them through the urine. If the linden infusion is drunk cool, it is cooling to the body and useful for treating the hot flashes associated with menopause. Cold linden tea makes a delightful light summer drink on a hot day.

Linden is also warming and relaxing to the digestive sytem. It can help whenever tension goes to the digestive tract, either through eating on the run or through general anxiety. Related tension conditions, like cramps, colic, and period pains, can also be alleviated.

Being a gentle remedy with a pleasant taste, linden is particularly good for treating children. It quietly calms an overactive or fractious child, soothing and relax-ing them. It is effective when they have nervous digestion or trouble sleeping, and can also be used for coughs and colds and flu, alone or with elderflower.

Externally, the tea can be rubbed into the skin to give relief in inflamed conditions such as boils, rashes, bites, scalds, and burns, or used for sore eyes. It is also soothing in a bath and or for massage.

Homeopathically, linden has much the same uses as the herb, being specific for children's toothache and women's pelvic inflammation. The inner bark of linden is known as bast (bass in the United States, giving basswood, another name for the tree). Bast can be made into a tea that is soothing for diarrhea.

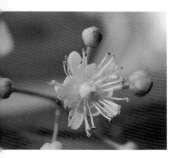

Hot linden tea
- nervous tension
- anxiety
- stress
- high blood pressure
- colds
- fevers and flu
- insomnia
- tension headache
- migraine

Cold linden tea
- hot flashes

Linden tincture
- nervous tension
- anxiety
- stress
- high blood pressure
- insomnia

Linden tea

Use the new flowers and unopened buds, with their stalk and leaf sheath. Pick on a dry sunny day, and avoid any blossoms with a blackish mildew growing on them. The lime blossom season is very short, with the blossoms only at their best for about a week, so if the weather is wet during this time you are better off tincturing the blossom than drying it.

Dry the flowers out of the sun until they are crispy. Once dry, you can remove the larger stalks and store the blossom in paper bags or jars in a cool dark place. If exposed to light, lime blossom will soon deteriorate. If it turns a pinkish color, it should be discarded.

Use a heaped teaspoonful of **dried blossom** per cup of **boiling water** in a teapot, and infuse for about 5 minutes. This is a good evening drink as it will relax without being too sedative. Drink a cupful one to three times a day for anxiety or restlessness. For colds or fevers, drink small amounts of the hot tea throughout the day to soothe, clear catarrh, and promote perspiration. Drink cold for hot flashes.

Linden tincture

Fill a jar with the **freshly picked blossom**, and top it up with **vodka**. Leave it in a cupboard for two weeks, shaking every few days. Strain, bottle, and label.

Dose: Half a teaspoonful 2 or 3 times a day.

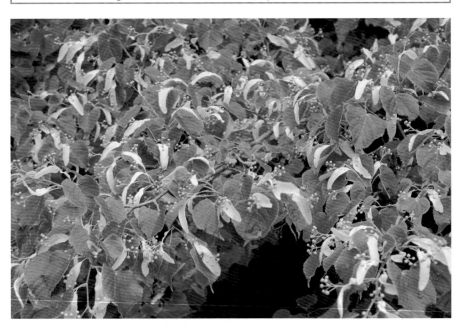

Small-leaved lime, Bardney Woods, Lincolnshire, England, June

Lycium *Lycium barbarum, L. chinense*

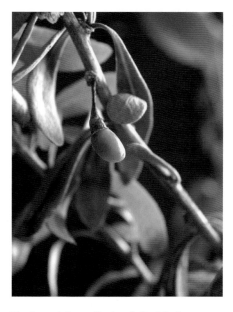

Marketed as goji berry, lycium has a reputation as an exotic health food or "superfruit." It is actually a naturalized plant in North America and Britain, known as the Duke of Argyll's tea plant, Chinese wolfberry, box thorn, or matrimony vine.

The berries make a rejuvenating tonic with a wide range of claimed benefits including improving eyesight and helping to reduce the side effects of chemotherapy in cancer patients.

Lycium originates in China and has been part of Chinese medicine for millennia. Its undoubted health benefits have become something of a fad in the West in the last two decades or so.

In Chinese cuisine worldwide young leaves and seedlings of lycium are used for soup, and the bark of the root medicinally for malaria and high blood pressure. However, it is the tasty orange–red berries, known as *gou qi zi* (or goji), that are prized.

In Chinese terms, the berries nourish and tonify the liver and kidney meridians, and address blood and *yin* deficiency. In practice this means the berries are useful for conditions as varied as dryness, sore back and legs, weak muscles and ligaments, impotence, dizziness, and vision problems.

What may be surprising is that this plant has actually been a naturalized plant in Britain since the 1730s. The story goes that the third

Duke of Argyll, Archibald Campbell (1682–1761), an avid plant collector, was sent a true tea plant, *Camellia sinensis*, and a lycium, but the labels were switched in the ship's hold. The name Duke of Argyll's tea plant (or tea tree) for lycium stuck and was kept even once the mistake was recognized. Other names lycium has attracted include Chinese wolfberry, box thorn, and matrimony vine.

Solanaceae
Nightshade family

Description: An arching, floppy shrub with small, stiff leaves and purple flowers, followed by scarlet berries in the fall.

Habitat: Hedgerows, gardens, and near the seashore.

Distribution: Native to Asia and possibly to eastern Europe. Found in most European countries and widely distributed in North America.

Related species: *Lycium chinense* (Chinese tea plant, Chinese desert thorn) and *L. barbarum* (Duke of Argyll's tea plant, matrimony vine) are very similar and may be used interchangeably. There are around 80 other species in the genus, found in the Americas, Eurasia, and Africa.

Parts used: Berries gathered in fall,.

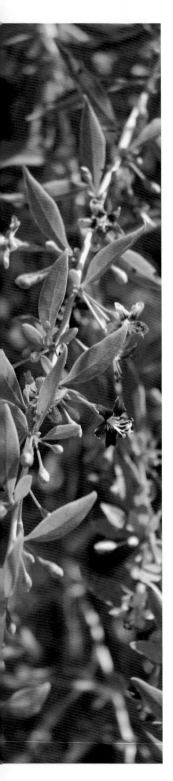

Use lycium for...

Lycium is both a food and a medicine, and the berries can be eaten daily, dried if fresh isn't available, with claimed improvement in strength, eyesight, and male sexual performance. They are safe even in quantity, with no reported safety issues, except when somebody has problems with nightshade family plants, such as potato or tomato.

The fresh berry is tasty and somewhat astringent, resembling a small persimmon, and when dried is like a sweet red raisin. We eat dried berries on cereal or hot with rice; in China lycium tea, coffee, wine, and beer are all made.

There has been considerable recent hype about the "superfood" benefits of lycium taken as a juice, but we make no comment here on the claims for commercial goji products. Full-scale research is lacking, and we base our comments on our own experience and that of herbalists whose opinion we respect.

One benefit of lycium that is generally accepted is to promote a healthy gut flora, while lowering "bad" LDL and VLDL cholesterol levels in the bloodstream. The berries serve to stabilize the capillaries, veins, and arteries throughout the body. They work on thread and varicose veins, and fragile capillaries that bleed under the skin. They also help to reduce narrowing of the arteries (atherosclerosis), thereby benefitting cold hands and feet.

This effect of lycium berries on capillaries is one reason they are good for the eyes; they also contain high levels of lutein and other carotenoids needed by the retina and for healthy eye functioning.

Regular use of lycium berries can help improve night vision, reduces excessive watering of the eyes and delays the onset of cataracts and glaucoma. The berries also stimulate lubrication of dry, red, or painful eyes, and prevent macular degeneration.

There are, further, indications that the berries enhance the beneficial effects of chemotherapy and radiation while also protecting cancer patients against the reduced white blood cell count that will often accompany these treatments. The berries support the liver against the side effects of medication and help relieve cachexia (malnutrition and other metabolic disturbances linked with cancer and AIDS). This liver protection also extends to exposure to toxic chemicals.

In addition, the berries, with plentiful antioxidants and high levels of vitamin C, reduce inflammation, enhance the immune function, and slow down tumour growth.

These are substantial and substantiated benefits for any herb, especially one that is now widely naturalized. Lycium has also attracted official attention. It was specifically named in 2003 by a

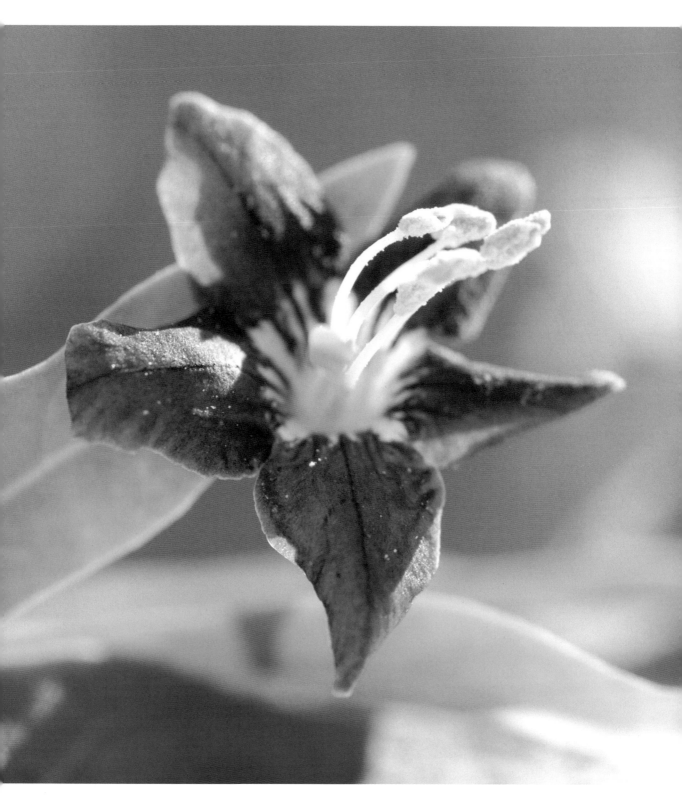

[Lycium fruit and leaf] *makes one feel happy and vigorous.*
– Lu Ji, *Shi Shu*, an ancient Chinese text

[do not eat lycium] *when travelling thousands of miles from home*
– Chinese saying, referring to sexual potency of lycium

Lycium in Lincolnshire: a sprawling hedge in the English village of Nettleton, June

government department looking at protecting traditional hedgerows. Then, in mid-2007, goji products were officially approved for sale as a food in the UK after demonstrating they had a proven history of use, mainly in the UK Chinese population, for many years.

In China it has long been claimed that lycium improves sexual performance, mainly in older men. Research has found that regular doses of the berries can raise testosterone levels when these are deficient. Many older men have this problem, so to this extent lycium may reduce impotence and can be seen as aphrodisiac.

Allied to the last use, lycium is renowned as anti-ageing, one Chinese name being "drive-away-old-age-berries." This is good news,

but marketing claims that one man, Li Qing Yen, lived for 252 years (1678–1930) because he took daily lycium are surely excessive.

Our descriptions of lycium's many and varied "virtues," in the old herbal phrase, should not cloud the fact that it is an effective general energy-restoring tonic treatment, which can be safely taken on a long-term basis.

For example, a serving of 3.5 oz of dried berries has been estimated to supply 100% of daily needs of iron and riboflavin (vitamin B2), and nearly all the selenium and calcium. It is reasonably strong in vitamin C but exceptionally rich in polysaccharides and zeaxanthin.

Goji is not a cheap commercial product, but it need not be expensive to use if you harvest

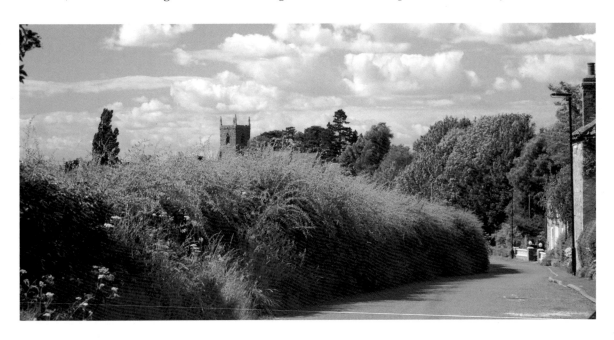

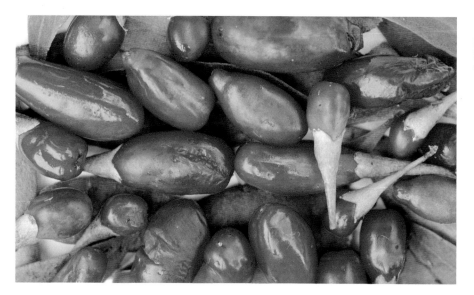

Both the berries and leaves of lycium can be eaten

from a local field side or plant your own lycium hedge. It is easy to grow from seed, but note that snails adore it and will devour seedlings. Once established, it is vigorous (it is used as a sand dune-fixer), and needs strong springtime pruning. This effort could repay you with a mass of beautiful purple flowers and brilliant scarlet berries later.

Lycium is interesting, with both ancient and very modern health applications. Goji berries and juice are a fashion of the day, with China exporting US $108m of these products in 2015. But even if this commercial fad declines, lycium is worthy of a place in your garden or to find in the outdoors, with much to commend it as food and medicine..

Harvesting lycium berries

The berries are picked in the fall when they are ripe. These scarlet, glossy fruits are enjoyed by a variety of wildlife, so you will have some competition. The best ones are often found where bramble and nettle help protect them, but they have no thorns themselves. They can be eaten fresh and have an unusual flavour, similar to persimmon with perhaps a hint of red bell pepper.

Lycium berry tincture

Put your fresh **lycium berries** in a blender with enough **vodka** to cover them, and blend briefly. Pour into a jar and leave in a cool dark place for a couple of days, then strain off the liquid. Bottle and label.

Dose: 1 teaspoonful 2 to 3 times a day.

Lycium berry tincture
- eyesight
- fragile capillaries
- varicose veins
- thread veins
- high cholesterol
- aphrodisiac
- fertility

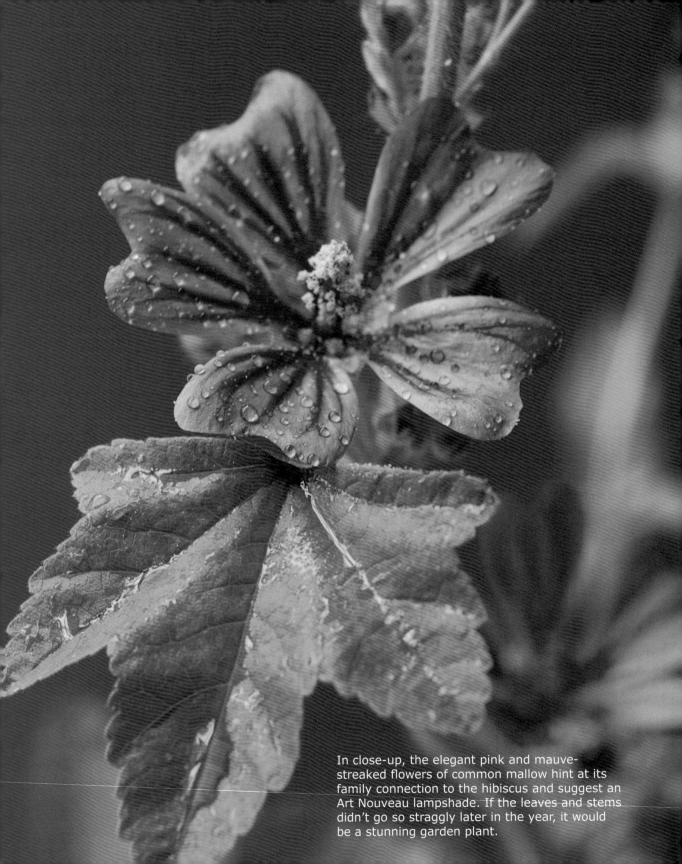

In close-up, the elegant pink and mauve-streaked flowers of common mallow hint at its family connection to the hibiscus and suggest an Art Nouveau lampshade. If the leaves and stems didn't go so straggly later in the year, it would be a stunning garden plant.

Mallow *Malva sylvestris*

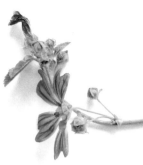

The common or tall mallow has suffered by comparison with its more famous cousin, the marsh mallow, the only member of the family to be an "official" herb. But marsh mallow is rare as a wild plant and moreover is dug up for its root, so for the many soothing, anti-inflammatory qualities of mallow, internal and external, the common form offers a highly effective alternative.

Malvaceae
Mallow family

Description: A sprawling perennial growing to 3 ft tall, with pinkish-purple flowers and ivy-shaped leaves.

Habitat: Roadsides, bare ground.

Distribution: Native to Europe and northern Africa, but widespread an an introduced species in North America, where it is known as tall mallow.

Related species: Marsh mallow (*Althaea officinalis*) is now quite rare in its native habitats but is easily grown as a garden plant.

Parts used: Leaves and flowers collected in summer.

The latest official list of British herbs, the *British Herbal Pharmacopoeia* 1996, describes only one mallow, the marsh mallow (*Althaea officinalis*), which has become rare in the wild in the British Isles. For commercial use it is now imported from eastern Europe. The confection "marshmallow" was once cooked from the roots of this plant but has long since ceased to be made of anything herbal.

Its abundantly found cousin, the common, high, blue or tall mallow (*Malva sylvestris*), has many of the same benefits, so, in the spirit of responsible wild herbal medicine, we recommend its use.

The common mallow does have its advocates, among them Maria Treben in twentieth-century Austria and the journalist and traveller William Cobbett in early nineteenth-century England. Cobbett offers a remarkable encomium of wild mallows, having learned of their value from a French military captive, a follower of Napoleon, in Long Island, New York.

The English farrier, A. Lawson, writing after Cobbett, quotes his own experience of using boiled mallow leaves to treat the badly swollen arm of a nearby farmer and to close a deep wound in a pig that had been gored by a cow's horn. Lawson quotes Cobbett with approval:

This weed is perhaps amongst the most valuable of plants that ever grew. Its leaves stewed, and applied wet, will cure, and almost instantly cure, any cut or bruise or wound of any sort…. And its operation is in all cases so quick that it can hardly be believed.

For her part, Treben writes of making up a mallow gargle to treat a man with cancer of the larynx. She used the residue of the mallow mixture, mixed with barley flour, as an overnight poultice for the man's throat. Within two weeks, he was well enough to consider a return to his profession of teaching. The man's medical specialist said of Treben, "this woman deserves a gold medal!"

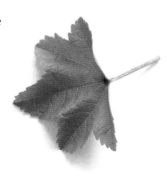

At an earlier date, Nicholas Culpeper had written movingly of saving his son from "inside plague" by using a mallow liquor [see panel on right]. In the sixteenth century and later, mallow had a reputation as *omnimorbia*, literally a cure-all. This could have been because mallow is laxative, and this was thought to rid the body of all disease.

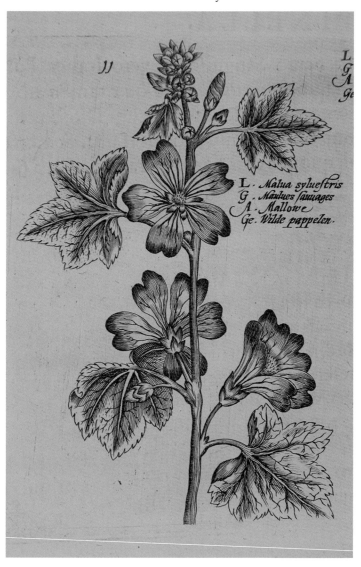

L. *Malua syluestris*
G. *Maulues sauuages*
A. *Mallowe*
Ge. *Wilde pappelen*.

Use mallow for...

While modern-day mallow users would scarcely claim it as a cure-all, they would also say it doesn't merit official oblivion. Mallow does have solid virtues, and most of these arise from its high mucilage content: common mallow flowers have around 10% mucilage and the leaves 7%. Indeed, all thousand or so members of the *Malva* family worldwide possess this gelatinous substance, including okra and hibiscus.

Mucilage, a word that is cognate with mucus, is extremely soothing to any inflamed part of the body, both outside and within. This includes dry coughs, colds, gastrointestinal upsets, stomach ulcers, and urinary tract infections. As one herbalist notes, when you cannot even swallow water, you can take a mallow tea. Further, it is very safe, in any quantity.

Maria Treben advocates mallow foot and hand baths for treating swellings following bone fractures.

One thing to watch out for in wild-gathering mallow is that its low-growing crinkly leaves tend to accumulate heavy metals from vehicle exhausts and also attract a mallow rust and various insect eggs. So it is a good idea to do your picking well away from busy roads and examine carefully any leaves and flowers you collect.

Mallow from *Hortus Floridus* (1614–16), by Crispijn van de Passe

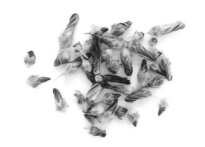

Mallow is sometimes eaten as a soup, though it is rather "gloupy," and the unripe seed heads make a slightly astringent addition to salads. These seed capsules have long been known as "cheeses," but because of the circular shape rather than the taste. The flowers were chewed to relieve toothache.

Always with mallow, though, you come back to its unrivalled soothing benefits. But do remember that large doses can be laxative as well as purgative! Cicero (106–43 BC) angrily reports being accidentally purged by eating a stew of mallow mixed with beet – and he laments that he had already forgone the oysters in an effort to be good.

You may remember, that not long since there was a raging disease called the bloody-flux; the college of physicians not knowing what to make of it, called it the plague of the guts, for their wits were at Ne plus ultra about it.

My son was taken with the same disease, and the excoriation of his bowels was exceeding great; myself being in the country, was sent for up; the only thing I gave him, was Mallows bruised and boiled both in milk and drink; in two days (the blessing of God being upon it) it cured him.

And I here, to shew my thankfulness to God, in communicating it to his creatures, leave it to posterity.
– Culpeper (1653)

Harvesting mallow

Pick the leaves before the plant flowers or whenever they are a bright healthy green. They are best used fresh, although they can be dried.

Pick the flowers and flower buds in summer. They can be used fresh or dried by spreading them out on a sheet of paper in a cool airy place. Mallow flowers turn from pinkish purple to blue as they dry. They can be used on their own as a soothing tea, and make a pretty addition to other herbal tea blends.

Mallow poultice

Chop or chew a fresh mallow leaf and apply to swellings, wounds and cuts. The poultice can be held in place using a sticking plaster or bandage for as long as it is needed. It reduces inflammation as it soothes and heals, so is good for insect bites, boils, and abscesses.

Mallow tea

Use a rounded teaspoonful of the **dried or fresh flowers** or a couple of **fresh leaves** per mugful of boiling water. Allow to infuse for about 5 minutes, then strain.

Dose: Drink a mugful 3 times a day as needed to soothe the digestion, or coughs and sore throats.

Mallow salad

Mallow leaves and petals make a mild and pleasant addition to a leafy green salad, and make it warmer and more soothing to the digestion.

Mallow poultice
- swellings
- insect bites
- boils & abscesses
- cuts
- bruises

Mallow tea
- indigestion
- irritable bowel
- dry, sore throat
- dry cough
- mild constipation

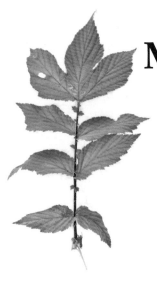

Meadowsweet *Filipendula ulmaria*

The story of meadowsweet, queen of the meadow, links mead, Cuchulainn, Queen Elizabeth I, and the invention of aspirin.

This is the number one herb for treating stomach acid problems, while also benefitting the joints and urinary system. Meadowsweet is effective for fevers and flu, diarrhea, headaches and pain relief generally. It well earns its name "herbal aspirin."

**Rosaceae
Rose family**

Description: A perennial of up to 4 or 5 feet tall, with serrated leaves, silvery beneath, and fragrant masses of creamy-white flowers in high summer.

Habitat: Marshes, streams, ditches, and moist woodland.

Distribution: Widespread in its native Europe, introduced to northeastern North America.

Related species: There are ten species in the genus worldwide.

Parts used: Flowering tops; less often, leaves and roots.

A European wild plant, fortunately more common now there is less crop spraying on field edges and hedgerows, meadowsweet has some delightful country names, including queen or lady of the meadow, maid of the mead, bride-

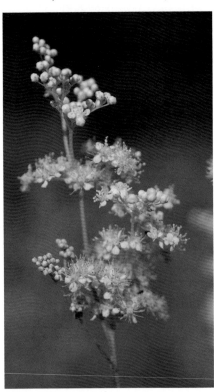

wort and sweet or new mown hay. But plant historians suggest the origin of the common name is more to do with mead the honey drink than meadows as such. Meadsweet is another old name, and William Turner's herbal (1568) has "medewurte," a term also used by Chaucer two centuries earlier.

The creamy billows of meadowsweet's flowers have indeed been used for centuries as a flavoring for mead, wine, beer, and syrups, and still make a good choice.

Everybody says the smell is full of summer echoes, but some do find it rather overpowering. Matthew is one of these, and says:

I owe a lifelong debt to meadowsweet as this was the very first long word I uttered. At about three years old, according to my mother, when I was saying almost nothing else, out pops this word I'd heard on family walks in the Trent marshes. These days I'm more likely to swear, though, as I get hayfever if I'm too close to the flowers.

In herbal medicine terms, the plant gives much more than it takes. A sacred herb of the Druids, meadowsweet was well known to Celtic communities as a malaria and fever treatment. The legendary hero Cuchulainn was given it to calm his fits of rage and fevers, as recalled in the plant's Gaelic name, "belt of Cuchulainn."

Use meadowsweet for...

The flowers and tops yield a beneficial herb tea or tincture that is particularly good for an upset stomach and diarrhea, and the whole plant was a traditional strewing herb of medieval and Tudor times. Charles I's herbalist, John Parkinson, wrote in 1640:

because both flowers and herbes are of so pleasing a sweete sent, many doe much delight therein, to have it layd in their Chambers, Parlars, &c. and Queene Elizabeth of famous memory, did more desire it then any other sweet herbe to strew her Chambers withall.

Willow has a longer record of use in pain relief, with Hippocrates, ' "the father of medicine," in the fifth century BC, using powdered willow bark and leaves to control headache and pain generally. But it was research on meadowsweet that led to chemical breakthroughs in the nineteenth century.

These included the identifying of salicylic acid, and culminated in the synthesis and manufacture of it as aspirin. The drug company

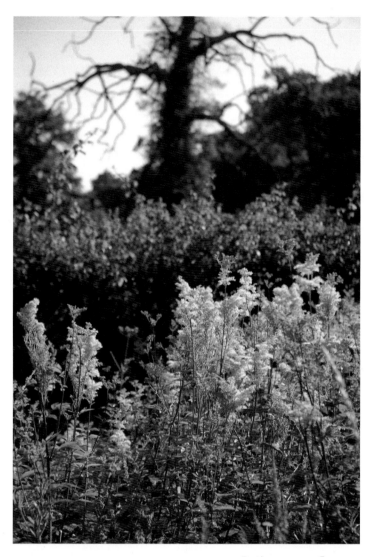

Bayer patented the name in 1899, basing it on the old Latin name for meadowsweet, *Spiraea*.

We now know that, like willow, meadowsweet contains natural salicylate salts. Aspirin itself is synthesized acetylsalicylic acid, which in concentration the stomach finds burning. This means pure aspirin can cause stomach pain and ulcers, but meadow-

Frothy, creamy flowers, erect reddish stalks, a ditch location: typical meadowsweet in high summer

Caution: If you are allergic to aspirin you may have a similar reaction to meadowsweet.

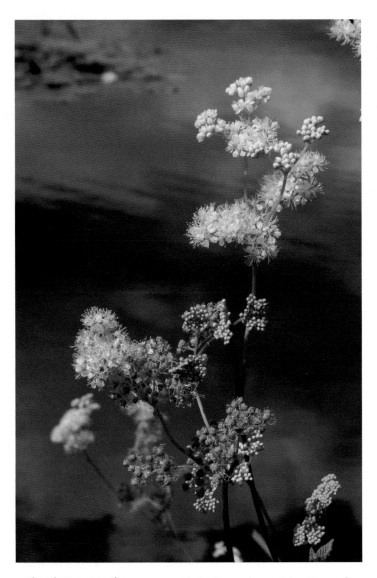

astringency. Instead of damaging the stomach, it soothes upset tummies and is a good remedy for children's diarrhea.

In terms of acid indigestion, reducing the acid levels in the stomach can assist in lowering such levels in the body overall. This might explain why meadowsweet is so effective in treating joint problems associated with acidity.

It has been used to good effect in dispelling uric and oxalic acid, thereby relieving some of the pain of articular rheumatism and gout. A stronger infusion is taken in such cases. Externally, cloths soaked in meadowsweet tea can also be applied to sore joints and bring extra relief; another soothing external use is for mouth ulcers and bleeding gums.

One other area of benefit is in the positive effect of the plant's salicylates for treating cystitis and urethritis, as well as breaking down kidney stones and gravel. The strong capacity of the plant to eliminate toxins and uric acid supports this action.

Meadowsweet always brings its analgesic and soothing properties to even the more vigorous aspects of its healing range, and as a relaxant it stops spasm and promotes restorative sleep. And even if you are feeling well, if you have the tea to hand, all you have to do is smell it, and you'll feel summer's heat and brightness return.

... the plant exerts the same effects and is prescribed for the same complaints [as aspirin], *but with the bonus of being a natural remedy.*
– Palaiseul (1973)

... an excellent "herbal aspirin."
– Cech (2000)

sweet's balanced combination of organic compounds is soothing for heartburn and hyperacidity, as well as ulcers.

This is not to decry aspirin, for like meadowsweet it offers a wonderful combination of pain-relieving and anti-inflammatory benefits. The plant, however, has a broader range of activity, including gentle

Harvesting meadowsweet

Pick **meadowsweet flowers** and **leaves** on a dry sunny day. Spread them on paper or a screen outside for a while to let all the little black beetles escape, then dry indoors. Once dry, crumble or cut into smaller pieces and store in brown paper bags or in jars, in a cool dark place.

Meadowsweet tea

Use a rounded teaspoonful of the **dried meadowsweet** per mug of **boiling water**, and allow to infuse for 5 minutes. It's best made in a teapot or covered mug to keep the aroma in. Drink a cup before meals if you suffer from acid indigestion or stomach problems, or one to three cups a day for arthritic and rheumatic aches and pains.

Meadowsweet glycerite

Pick **meadowsweet flowers** on a dry sunny day. Spread them on a cloth outside and let any insects escape, then pack the flowers into a jar large enough to hold them. Make a mix of 60% **vegetable glycerine** with 40% **water** (ie for 10 fl oz, you would use 6 fl oz glycerine and 4 fl oz water), and pour this mixture onto the meadowsweet until the jar is full. Stir to release any trapped air bubbles and top up if necessary.

Put the jar on a sunny windowsill, pushing the flowers back under the liquid every few days if necessary, or employ a plastic "preserving plunger" used in jam-making to keep it down. It's a good idea to put a saucer under your jar, as sometimes the glycerine will ooze out at the top. After two weeks, strain off the liquid, bottle, and label it.

Dose: 1 teaspoonful three times a day for stomach problems. A teaspoonful can also just be taken just when it's needed for heartburn and indigestion, with a second dose after an hour if necessary.

Meadowsweet electuary

For a particularly irritated digestive tract, mix **slippery elm powder** into your **meadowsweet glycerite** to make a runny paste or electuary.
Dose: 1 teaspoonful three times a day as needed.

Meadowsweet ghee

This is a lovely warming, pain-relieving rub, which goes on smoothly and smells of summer sweetness. To make the ghee, melt a packet of **butter** in a small saucepan. Simmer for about 20 minutes, skim off and discard the foam on top, then slowly pour the clear golden liquid into a clean saucepan leaving behind the whitish residue at the bottom. Put 5 or 6 heads of **meadowsweet flowers** in the ghee and heat gently for about 10 minutes. Strain and pour into jars to set.

Meadowsweet tea
- indigestion
- heartburn
- excess stomach acid
- gastritis
- hiatus hernia
- stomach ulcer
- arthritis
- rheumatism

Meadowsweet glycerite
- indigestion
- heartburn
- excess stomach acid
- gastritis
- hiatus hernia
- stomach ulcer
- arthritis
- rheumatism

Meadowsweet electuary
- heartburn
- diverticulitis
- bowel inflammation

Meadowsweet ghee
- muscle aches & pains
- sciatica
- backache
- painful joints
- arthritis

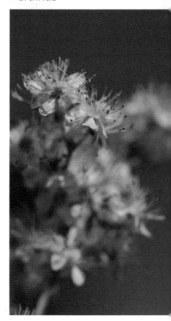

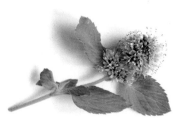

Mint *Mentha* spp.

Mint is wonderful for the digestion, as a tea, in food and medicinally. It also relieves nausea, spasms and gas, and offers the benefits of being both warming and cooling to the body.

Lamiaceae (Labiatae) Deadnettle family

Description: Aromatic perennials with dense whorls of lilac flowers.

Habitat: Most species prefer stream sides and damp places in woods or grassland.

Distribution: Native and naturalized mints are found around the world.

Species: Peppermint (*Mentha* x *piperita*) and field or wild mint (*M. arvensis*) are native and widespread in North America and Europe. Other European species such as water mint (*M. aquatica*), pennyroyal (*M. pulegium*), spearmint (*M. spicata*), and apple or round-leaved mint (*M. suaveolens*) are naturalized in North America. They hybridize freely with each other and with garden mints. Any of them can be used, but avoid pennyroyal if you are pregnant.

Parts used: Leaves and flowers, harvested in spring and summer.

A hot, hazy, sultry afternoon in high summer, under a high blue sky with scudding white clouds. We are visiting a wet part of the wood behind our house. Water mint and peppermint abound, at their washed-out purple peak, along with the almost identical colors of hemp agrimony and the commoner thistles.

This is an example of collective taking of turns as plants of similar colour ripen together. The pale purple flowers are active this week along with attendant pollinators. Butterflies, bees, flies, and smaller insects are pulled to the mints, and red admirals, peacocks, meadow browns, commas, and whites feast on the flowers. Photographing them is another matter, but eventually a meadow brown stays still.

It's one of those days when wild herbal medicine is at its most pleasant and mellow, with the sweet tang of bruised mint and lazy buzz of insects giving us a feeling we call content-mint.

But what do we mean by "mint"? There are at least two dozen different species and hundreds of cultivars, if you add the wild and garden mints together. Moreover, the mints hybridize willingly and produce subtle new forms. As a ninth-century treatise on plants put it, "if one were to enumerate completely all the virtues, varieties and names of mint, one would be able to say how many fish are swimming in the Red Sea…"

We must simplify, though, and suggest you can use any garden or wild mint. Mints are chemically divided by smell and taste into peppermint and spearmint types, with many variations.

What we usually mean by "mint" is probably peppermint (*M. piperita*), which has flourished in gardens and in the wild since the seventeenth century. It is considered to be a hybrid of watermint and spearmint, but has a stronger proportion of aromatic oils than either. These oils, particularly menthol, account for the greater "mintiness" of peppermint and for its commercial use.

Modern commercial uses of mint build on older and proven herbal applications, but to our mind the focus on taste has all but negated the original herbal virtues.

Use mint for...

Finding that mint cleaned the breath and settled the digestion, Romans of classical times valued it; they didn't have chocolate, but they did have after-dinner mint! They also brought mint to Britain. Perhaps, indeed, chewing mint leaves is superior, given that our chocolate "mint" doesn't contain any of the herb, and precious little of its oil. It's also moot whether it'd be better for us to clean our teeth on freshly picked mint than use a spurious "mint" toothpaste.

Peppermint's higher levels of aromatic oils come with necessary

The savor or smell of the water Mint rejoyceth the heart of man, for which cause they use to strew it in chambers and places of recreation, pleasure, and repose, and where feasts and banquets are made.
– Gerard (1597)

"Altogether," says Dr. Braddon, "the oil of Peppermint forms the best, safest, and most agreeable of known antiseptics."
– William Thomas Fernie (1897)

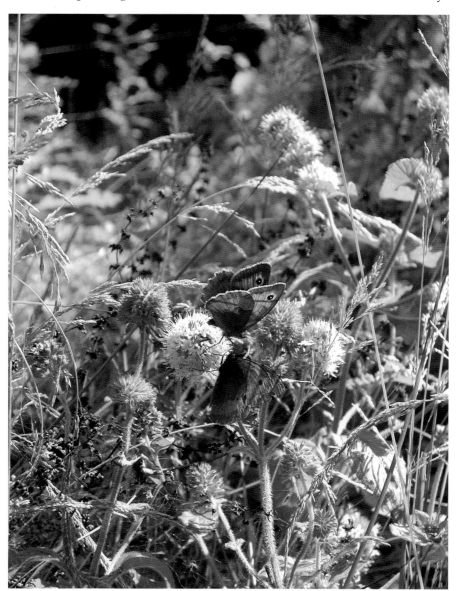

The essence of summer: flowering mint, meadow grasses, sultry sunshine and feeding hedge browns. Norfolk, England, July

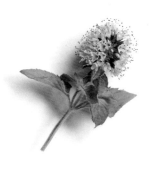

cautions, especially if you use peppermint essential oil. For example, while a mint tea of any species is soothing to the stomach, taking peppermint essential oil internally can lead to stomach spasms; it has been implicated in miscarriages. A drop or two of the essential oil, diluted with a carrier oil and applied to the brow, can relieve a migraine but larger quantities can cause bad headaches.

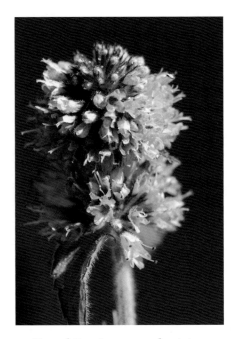

The vertues of the wild Mints are more especially to dissolve winde in the stomack, to help the chollick and those that are short-winded, and are an especiall remedy for those that have venerous dreames and pollutions in the night, used both inwardly, and the juyce being applyed outwardly to the testicles or cods.
– Parkinson (1640)

Using any of the wild mints is considered safe, although pennyroyal should not be taken in pregnancy. Peppermint is the strongest and most cooling mint and is the "official" mint. Mints with more of a spearmint taste are gentler and warmer, and are better for children's fevers, lack of appetite and weak digestive systems.

Medicinally, mint is classified as both cooling and heating, depending on use, species and form taken. This dual energetic pattern, tellingly, is recognized in traditional Chinese, Ayurvedic, and western herbal traditions. You can feel the effect when taking mint tea: it warms, then cools the palate and digestion, even the skin; it is stimulating and then soothing.

The heating effect is seen in the way mint is used as a heart tonic, which relieves palpitations, sending blood to the skin's surface, in the form of sweating. Hot mint tea is an excellent recourse for disturbed digestion, relieving spasm and relaxing the stomach

walls, while also anaesthetizing them. It is a proven and peerless remedy for such socially embarrassing conditions as bad breath, flatulence, and hiccups; it also works for indigestion, bloating, griping, colic, nausea, and vomiting (including morning and travel sickness).

Mint is also antiseptic and mildy antiviral and antifungal. It combats mouth ulcers caused by *Herpes simplex* virus. It is good for coughs, colds, and fever, alone or with elderberry. It also has a traditional use in treating gallstones and for hives, sinusitis and emphysema, earache, and toothache, all in addition to its culinary versatility. And, who knows, as Parkinson writes (see left), mint may still be used to reduce "venerous dreames and pollutions in the night," if that is needed.

Caution: Avoid taking pennyroyal if you are pregnant.

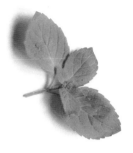

Mint tea

Fresh mint is better than dried to use for tea. Put a couple of sprigs in a teapot and pour in a cupful of **boiling water**. Cover and let infuse for a few minutes before straining and drinking.

But when you do not have fresh mint available, dried is still good. Dry the leaves on a screen outdoors or in a warm cupboard, until they crumble in the fingers. Use a teaspoonful per cup. Dried mint is a very useful addition to other medicinal herb teas, to make them taste better.

Mint and raspberry water

Water can be deliciously and subtly flavoured by adding a few sprigs of **mint** and some **raspberries**, and left to stand in a cool place for a couple of hours. Either still or sparkling water can be used. This cold infusion is a lovely cooling and refreshing summer drink.

If you want a stronger flavour, add a little cool mint tea to the jug.

Sekanjabin: A Persian oxymel of mint and vinegar

Boil **1 cup of water** with **4 tsp of white sugar**, till the sugar dissolves. Add **1/2 cup of vinegar** (we like to use raspberry vinegar). Simmer 20 minutes, stirring occasionally.

Remove from heat and add some sprigs of **fresh mint**, which adds its flavour to the oxymel (any mixture of honey and vinegar) as it cools. Serve diluted in ice-cold water, as you would a cordial. Alternatively, freeze in the form of ice cubes and store for future use.

Mint in white wine

Put a few sprigs of **mint** and a bottle of **white wine** in a jug, cover with a cloth and leave overnight. Remove the mint. This is a refreshing summer drink that can be served chilled, to keep you cool and improve your digestion.

For a more medicinal apéritif, add a few heads of meadowsweet blossom and a couple of sprigs of mugwort to your wine as well as the mint. This can be done at the same time or added later.

Mint foot bath

Make a big pot of **mint tea**, strain it and pour it into a foot bath or a basin large enough for your feet. When it is the right temperature, put your feet in the liquid and soak for ten to twenty minutes. Use it hot for tired, achy feet or cold if your feet are really hot and sweaty.

Mint tea
- indigestion
- colds and flu
- hot conditions
- flatulence
- nausea
- travel sickness
- headache
- stomach pains

Sekanjabin
- hot conditions
- lack of appetite
- weak digestion
- indigestion

Mint in white wine
- lack of appetite
- weak digestion
- indigestion

Mint foot bath
- tired, achy feet
- hot, sweaty feet

God's wrath is His vinegar, mercy His honey.
These two are the basis of every oxymel.
If vinegar over-powers honey, a remedy is spoiled.
The people of the earth poured vinegar on Noah;
the Ocean of Divine Bounty poured sugar.
The Ocean replenished his sugar,
and overpowered the vinegar of the whole world.
– Rumi (13th-century Persia)

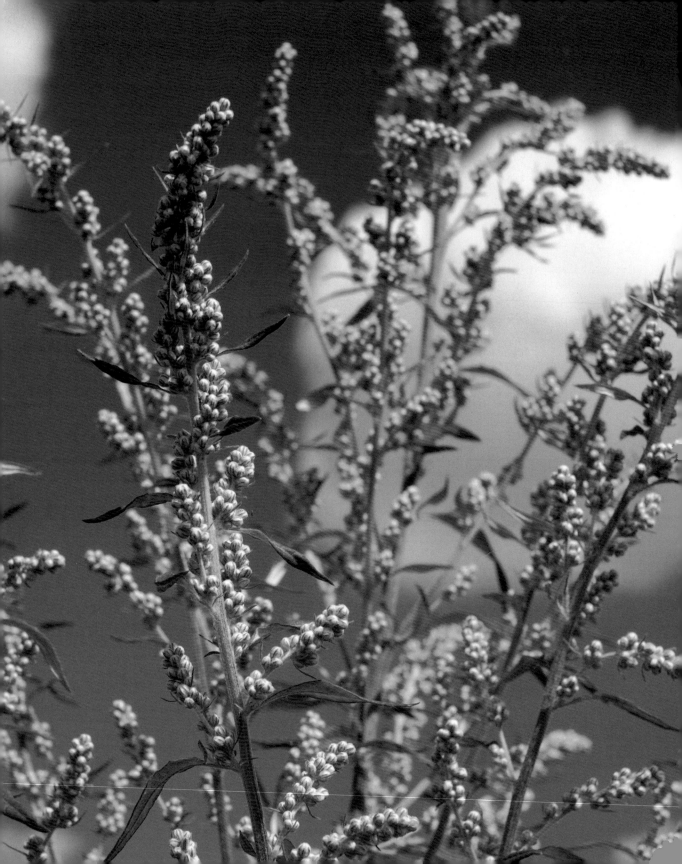

Mugwort *Artemisia vulgaris*

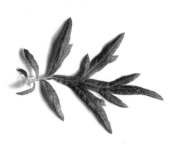

Mugwort is a stately, self-assured perennial, a tall summer presence at six feet or more high, found in country and town alike. It is, however, far more than a roadside curiosity.

It is an ancient herb of healing, magic, and divination throughout the world, a protector of women and travelers, renowned for its value in feminine disorders, and as a strong warming tonic. Mugwort was used in making ale in Europe before hops.

The first clue to mugwort's significance might be found in its scientific name. *Artemis* was the Greek moon goddess and patron of women, especially at critical phases of their life cycle – at the onset of menstruation, in childbirth, and at menopause.

Vulgaris can mean "of the people," or, a little more condescendingly, "common" and by extension "abundant." A frequently found herb that is available to assist women everywhere for critical times could hardly have a more apt name than *Artemesia vulgaris*.

Such qualities have been recognized far and wide. Mugwort has been called "the mother of herbs" in several cultures. Ayurvedic practitioners in India use it in treating female reproductive disorders; a related species has the same function in southern Africa, and it has long been known in China for regulating the menses and "calming a restless fetus."

Culpeper placed mugwort under the power of Venus; the Pennsylvania Dutch knew the plant as *Aldy Fraw*, or "old woman," underlining ancestral wisdom and feminine qualities; and a modern western herbalist calls it "the feminine remedy *par excellence*."

A saying from the North of England and Scotland underlines the traditional value placed on female spring tonics: "If nettles were used in March and muggings [mugwort] in May, many a bra' [brave] lass wouldna turn t'clay."

Another dimension to mugwort's popularity is its capacity to influence dreams, a powerful attribute in traditional cultures. A bundle of leaves and flower heads placed under the pillow, or made into a "dream pillow," can calm sleep and protect from nightmares. It might also yield lucid dreams in certain people. In this sense mugwort is shamanistic, underlining its use in divination.

Asteraceae (Compositae) Daisy family

Description: A tall, slightly aromatic perennial with silvery flower spikes, growing to 6 ft or more. Leaves are pinnate, dark green and smooth above, silver beneath.

Habitat: Waysides, roadsides, waste ground.

Distribution: Found across Europe to Asia and North America.

Related species: Worldwide, there are hundreds of species of *Artemesia*, including tarragon herb (*A. dracunculus*), the North American sagebrushes, Chinese mugwort (*A. verlotiorum*) and wormwood (*A. absinthium*). Many of them are used medicinally.

Parts used: Flowering tops and leaves.

A close-up of mugwort buds and flowers

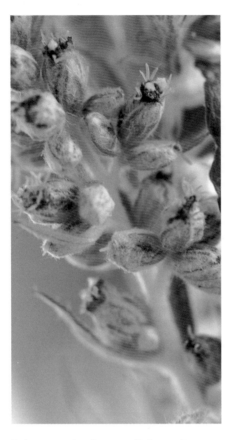

The leaves and tops of the young shoots and flowers in this plant are all full of virtue, they are aromatic to the taste with a little sharpness. The herb has been famous from the earliest times, and Providence has placed it everywhere about our doors so that reason, and authority, as well as the notice of the senses, point it out for use, but chemistry has banished natural medicines.
– Hill (1756)

It is a continuing tradition of a number of Native American groups to burn bundles of cured and dried sagebrush (*A. tridentata*), a close relative of mugwort, as "smudge sticks." These bundles burn slowly, like an incense stick, producing smoke that is used to cleanse the energy of houses and sacred spaces (see page 125).

Burning a mugwort smudge stick certainly worked in calming the frantic energy when our teenage son had a big boozy party at our home. It also helps shift old, stuck energy – we found ourselves therapeutically clearing out the garden sheds next morning.

Use mugwort for...

Burning mugwort can dispel midges and other summer biting insects, a quality sometimes suggested as a source of its name (Old Saxon *muggia wort* or midge plant). A case is made too for the Saxon *moughte*, a moth or maggot, referring to mugwort's ability to keep away moths from clothes.

The thirteenth-century Physicians of Myddfai in central Wales knew mugwort as a useful insecticide: "to destroy flies, let the mugwort be put in a place where they are frequent and they will die."

Our own favorite explanation for the name mugwort is its former use as a herbal flavouring for ale. It could have literally been the "mug-wort," the measure of a brew, from a time before hops came in during and after the Middle Ages, and the Briton's drink gradually switched from ale to beer. Mugwort, along with yarrow, myrtle and heather, was a common ingredient in *gruit* or *grut*, a strong herbal ale. This is currently enjoying a revival in the modern microbrewery movement.

An infusion of mugwort in cold drinks, whether beer or fruit in origin, adds a sharp summer tang and aromatic smell that you can enjoy in safety. These make for a more homely and less risky prospect than absinthe, the liqueur derived from the closely related wormwood (*A. absinthium*). As the world knows, this was the tipple of the *fin de siècle* French literary and art world. Containing a toxic essential oil that mugwort lacks, absinthe could be fatally addictive. It was banned in Europe for most of the twentieth century.

Mugwort, it will be clear by now, has had something of a dangerous past, at the hazy margin of sacred and secular culture – indeed, from a time when there was no distinction made between the two.

American herbalist Maida Silverman believes that "Folklore and superstition are bound up with the Mugwort plant to an extent hardly matched by any other herb." She instances as the oldest superstition the first-century AD Roman naturalist Pliny, who recommended that travellers carry mugwort as an amulet for psychic protection. This belief lasted through and beyond the Middle Ages, though it was roundly condemned by "rational" herbalists like Gerard (1597) and Parkinson (1640).

Mugwort was a key Anglo-Saxon sacred herb: the *Leech Book of Bald* from tenth-century Wessex extols it as "eldest of worts / Thou has might for three / And against thirty." Again the great age and protective power of mugwort are emphasized.

In medieval times mugwort passed from the patronage of the pagan Artemis to the Christian care of St. John the Baptist, who was said to have carried it into the wilderness to ward off evil. From this came "St. John's girdle" and the wearing of a mugwort garland on St. John's day, June 24, while dancing around the traditional fire. Throwing the garland into the fire would ensure protection for the following year, another pagan survival that so annoyed John Parkinson. He would be aghast to learn that a mugwort ceremony still marks midsummer in the Isle of Man (see box on page 124).

Wider afield, mugwort was known to Chinese medicine as a house protector and in the practice of moxibustion. This is an integral part of acupuncture, and many readers will have experienced the cone of dried mugwort leaves, moxa, being placed on the skin and burnt to stimulate an acupuncture point. The particular application of moxa is for treating abdominal pain from the cold, and it is mugwort's warming quality that makes it effective.

One other aspect of mugwort and fire can be mentioned briefly. Other names for the plant, gypsy's tobacco and muggar, record its persistent use as a smoking leaf, often inside strips of newspaper.

Burnt or not, mugwort has valuable warming qualities. It is known herbally as an aromatic bitter, which warms the digestion and stimulates a sluggish liver. Taking it in some form encourages the secretion of digestive juices and its oils help reduce gas and griping.

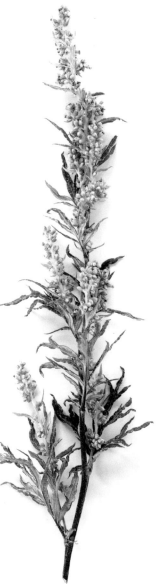

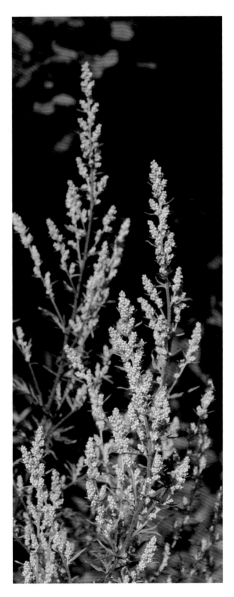

On a hot summer day, when the noxious fumes and stagnant air in the city seem even more oppressive than usual, it really is a "comfort" to crush a few leaves of the plant in one's hand and inhale the clean, pungent aroma. Mugwort lives up to its reputation and certainly has the power to revive the spirits and refresh the senses.

– Silverman (1997)

Herbalists value mugwort as a general calmer of the nervous system, helping to relieve stress and nervous tension. Mugwort pillows can help soothe disturbed sleep as well as promote dreaming. In general the plant has an uplifting effect on mood and is valuable in treating forms of mild depression linked with digestive weakness.

Taken as a tincture, mugwort can help in normalizing menstrual flow, and is particularly useful for bringing on delayed or suppressed periods where they have been absent for some time. It is a good herb for young women at puberty, helping to establish a regular cycle. Because it stimulates the uterus, it is not normally used in western herbalism during pregnancy, though in China it is an accepted treatment in preventing miscarriage.

Mugwort has some antimalarial activity, though much milder than Sweet Annie (*Artemisia annua*). It is also effective against threadworms and roundworms, like its stronger relative wormwood, and is an effective wash for treating fungal infections.

Manx mugwort magic

Mugwort is the symbolic plant of the Isle of Man and sprigs of it are worn on Manx national day, July 5. This is St. John's day in the old Julian calendar (it has been 24 June in England and Scotland since 1752, but the old date is kept on Man). On St. John's eve mugwort would be gathered and made into wreaths to be worn by cattle and men alike. Hedge and gorse fires were lit and cattle forced through while men and boys jumped over the flames. This combination of mugwort and fire would protect beast and people from evil spirits for the coming year. The next day was then safe for the many civic ceremonies of Midsummer Court, including the promulgation of laws from Tynwald Hill. As an invited guest, even Queen Elizabeth II on her visit in 2003 duly wore her spray of mugwort or *bollan bane* (white herb), as it is known locally.

Harvesting mugwort

Pick mugwort in summer, collecting the flower spikes when they are flowering or just before the flowers open when the buds are still silvery. The leaves can be collected too.

Mugwort tincture

Because mugwort becomes more aromatic as it dries, the tincture is best made with **dried mugwort**, although you can use fresh. Fill a jar with mugwort, then top up with **vodka**, shaking it to remove air bubbles. Put the jar in a cool dark place for 2 to 4 weeks, then strain and bottle.

Dose: half a teaspoon, three times a day.

Mugwort punch

Pour **a cupful of red wine** into a saucepan.

Add **a stick of cinnamon**, **5 cloves** and **a handful of mugwort tops**. Bring to a boil, then turn down the heat and simmer gently with a lid on for half an hour.

Strain out the herbs and spices. Sweeten with **honey**. It can be taken hot or cold before a meal to stimulate appetite and digestion. Either drink it fresh or keep in a bottle for several weeks.

Mugwort pillow

Pick **mugwort flowers and leaves** and dry them. Make a small bag for the pillow out of **cloth**, leaving one end open – any size you like, but 8" x 10" works well. Fill the bag loosely with the dried mugwort so that the finished pillow will be about 1" thick, then stitch up the open end. Place this under your regular pillow. Smaller cloth bags of mugwort can be stored among clothing to discourage clothes moths.

Mugwort smudge stick

Pick the silvery top 8" or so of **mugwort** when the flowers are in bud or first open. Leave them in a cool airy place to dry for a few days. Before they dry completely, and while they are still flexible, make small bundles up to about 1" thick, with the stem ends together. Starting at the stem end, wind a piece of **cotton thread** in a spiral around the bundle to the end and then back again, tying off securely. Leave the bundles to dry completely.

To use, hold the smudge stick by the stem end and light the other end with a match. You may need to blow on it at first to keep it burning. Wave the stick around with a circular motion as you move through a room or around a person – the movement helps keep the stick burning as well as spreading the smoke through the air.

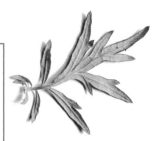

The underside of a mugwort leaf is covered with silvery, downy hairs.

Mugwort tincture
- irregular periods
- suppressed periods
- gas and griping
- stress and anxiety

Mugwort punch
- poor appetite
- sluggish digestion
- gas and griping
- stress and anxiety

Mugwort pillow
- protection from bad dreams
- promotes lucid dreams
- stress and anxiety

Smudge stick
- clears negative and old stuck energy
- calms and protects
- warms and dries

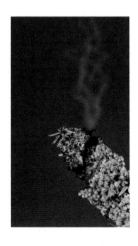

Scrophulariaceae
Figwort family

Description: Biennial plants, growing in their first year as a rosette of downy leaves, and sending up a tall spike with yellow flowers in their second summer.

Habitat: Sides of fields, roadsides, dry ground.

Species used: Great mullein is the species generally discussed in herbals, but any of the tall, yellow-flowered mulleins can be used, as can white mullein (*Verbascum album*).

Distribution: Great mullein (*V. thapsus*) is native to Europe, northern Africa and Asia, and naturalized in parts of North America, Africa and Australia.

Related species: There are about 300 species of *Verbascum*.

Parts used: Leaves and flowers, sometimes the root.

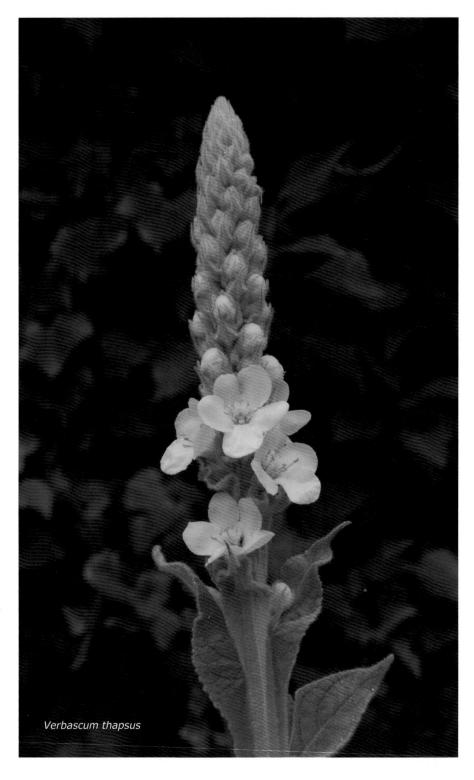

Verbascum thapsus

Mullein *Verbascum* spp.

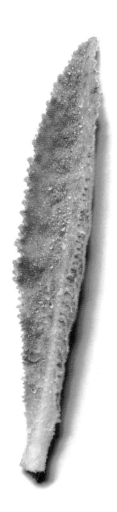

Mullein is unmistakable when it is in flower, with its spires of yellow flowers on a spike reaching six feet tall. It likes disturbed ground and dry soil, often growing on roadsides.

The flowers, infused in oil, are a remedy for earache and other nerve pain. The leaves and flowers taken as a tea relieve dry, irritable coughs. Mullein, so supple and strong itself, has an affinity for the spine and helps in setting bones.

Mullein has a long history of use in Europe, and has been attributed magical powers in several **my-thologies**. Almost three thousand years ago, according to Homer, Odysseus used the root of moly, which was probably the white mullein, as a protection against the enchantments of Circe. Odysseus was lucky to have the help of Hermes, for, in Homer's words, "it was an awkward plant to dig up, at any rate for a mere man. But the gods, after all, can do anything."

There are records of the long stalk of mullein being dipped in tallow and used as a taper by Roman legionaries and in medieval funerals. It also has a reputed association with witches' covens, recalled in the common name hag's taper.

Mullein leaves have made a natural toilet paper, diapers, food wrappers, and soothing insoles for shoes – all possible emergency uses today. Despite their softness, however, mullein leaves can be irritating when dry because of all their little hairs. It is this attribute that gave the plant the name of Quaker rouge, as Quaker girls were said to redden their cheeks by rubbing the leaves on them.

A cure for hoarseness, with mullein and fennel in equal parts, cooked in wine, goes back to Hildegard of Bingen in the 1100s.

John Parkinson (1640) recommends a decoction of the leaves with sage, marjoram, and chamomile (applied externally) for cramps. He mentions that country men gave a broth of mullein to cattle that had coughs and used a poultice of the leaves for horses' hooves injured in shoeing.

A Victorian doctor, Dr. Quinlan, publicized a traditional Irish TB treatment in which one handful of fresh mullein leaves was boiled with two pints of milk, strained and sweetened with honey; the mix was to be drunk twice a day.

Mullein is an herb for the lungs and throat and can be consumed in any rational quantity needed, being basically free of toxicity.
– Moore (1979)

Use mullein for...

Mullein's soft fuzzy leaves give a hint of its soothing qualities for internal use. Its particular affinity is for the respiratory system, but it also calms and strengthens the nerves, digestion, and urinary system. It is good for swollen glands, and helps relieve pain in general.

Think of mullein tea for easing throat and chest problems, especially dry and irritable coughs. It can quickly soothe an irritating tickle at the back of the throat.

Mullein flower oil is the best natural remedy for earache. Our son's ear infections when he was little were always quickly relieved (except for once when the oil was old and had lost its potency). The oil can be used externally for any kind of swelling and irritation.

Following up on ancient precedent, a useful remedy to ease the foot pain of plantar fasciitis is to put a fresh mullein leaf in your shoe, replacing with a new one when the first one has dried out.

Mullein poultices for external use are excellent to draw out splinters and boils, but, like the tea, also work at deeper bodily levels for backaches, lymphatic swellings, and even broken bones. The poultices are effective in soothing swollen glands and for mumps.

Mullein is the only herb known to man that has remarkable narcotic properties without being poisonous and harmful.
– Dr. Christopher (1976)

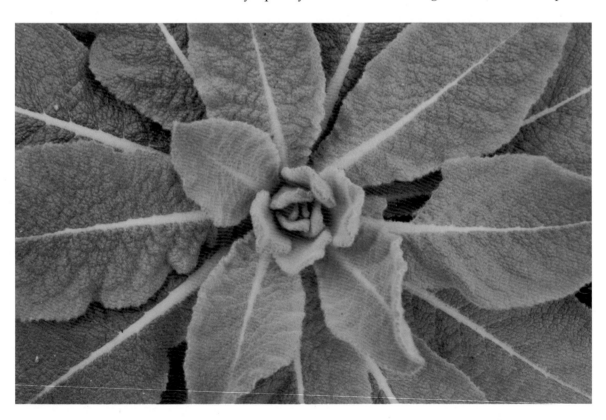

Harvesting mullein

The leaves are best picked before the plant sends up its flower spike. Dry the leaves whole and then crumble them for storage.

The flowers are quite soft, so pick them carefully to avoid bruising. Spread in a single layer on a sheet of paper or a mesh screen to dry.

Mullein tea

The leaves can be used on their own, or you can add flowers. To make the tea, use a good rounded tablespoonful of the **dried herb**, slightly more of the fresh, according to taste. Pour a mugful of **boiling water** over it, cover, and steep for 15 minutes. Strain through muslin or a fine sieve to remove any loose leaf hairs if you are using the dried leaf. Drink freely for dry coughs or any irritation of throat and chest.

Mullein flower oil

Pick the **flowers** on a dry sunny day, and lay them on a sheet of paper to dry a little overnight. Put them in a small jar and pour enough **extra virgin olive oil** over them to cover the flowers completely. Close the jar with a piece of cloth held on with a rubber band rather than using a lid – this allows any moisture to escape.

Put the jar on a sunny windowsill for two weeks, stirring every day to keep the flowers submerged in the oil. This is important, as the flowers will tend to float and may go moldy if left exposed.

When the flowers have faded and become quite transparent, the oil is ready to be strained and bottled. Pour through a fine sieve into another jar. There will probably be a layer of water at the bottom of the jar, so the oil needs to be poured slowly and carefully into a third jar, leaving the watery layer behind. Store in a cool dark place for up to a year.

For earache, put 1 to 3 drops of oil in the affected ear as needed for pain.

Mullein poultice

To make a poultice, lay a few **mullein leaves** in a dish (for a splinter you'll only need part of a leaf) and pour a little **boiling water** on them to soften them. Leave until they are cool enough to handle, then place them on the affected part. The poultice can be held on with a bandage, and you can keep it warm by holding a hot water bottle against it.

This is an excellent treatment for removing splinters, to draw boils, to soothe an aching back and for any lymphatic swellings. It can also be used to help heal broken bones, such as ribs or toes, that cannot be set.

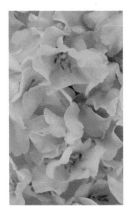

Mullein tea
- dry irritable coughs
- bronchitis
- laryngitis
- pleurisy
- swollen glands

Mullein flower oil
- earache
- nerve pain
- hemorrhoids & piles
- chest rub
- chilblains

Tip: Don't use a bottle with a pipette top for long-term storage of mullein oil. We have found that volatile oils from the mullein destroy the rubber bulb after a while, and the oil loses its potency.

Mullein poultice
- splinters
- boils
- backache
- mumps
- swollen glands
- broken bones

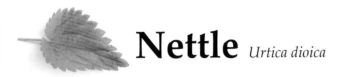

Nettle *Urtica dioica*

Urticaceae
Nettle family

Description: A wind-pollinated perennial with dark green, hairy, stinging leaves and stems, and tough, tangled yellow roots.

Habitat: Woods, river banks, farms, road-sides, field edges and wherever the nitrogen content of the soil is high.

Distribution: Native across North America, Asia, and Europe, and found in most of the temperate world.

Related species: The dwarf or small nettle (*U. urens),* an annual, is similar in use and appearance; it is the species used in homeopathy.

Parts used: Leaves, tops, seeds, rhizomes, and roots.

Nettles are one of the most useful of plants, despite their protective sting. The young tops are delicious and nutritious, a natural vitamin and mineral supplement. Medicinally, the leaves, seeds, and roots are used to treat a wide range of conditions including anemia, arthritis, asthma, burns, eczema, infections, inflammations, kidney stones, prostate enlargement, rheumatism, and urinary problems.

Nettles can also be used to make rope, nets, a linen-like cloth and paper, a dye, insect repellant, and green manure.

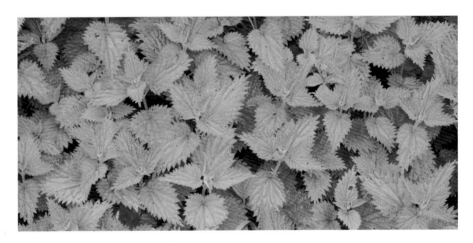

Stinging nettles are one of the best plants for human health, both as food and medicine. They are a complete, ready-packaged natural vitamin and mineral supplement, grow everywhere, and are free – an ultimate wild herb medicine.

Nettle was the Anglo-Saxon sacred herb, *wergulu,* and in medieval times nettle beer was drunk for rheumatism. Nettle tops helped milk to sour, as a rennet substitute in cheese-making. Nettle leaves brought fruit to ripening, and were used to pack plums; the whole plant is still useful as an excellent compost or green manure.

Nettle's high vitamin C content made it a valuable spring tonic for our ancestors after a winter of living on grain and salted meat, with hardly any green vegetables. Nettle soup and porridge were popular spring tonic purifiers, but a pasta or pesto from the leaves is a worthily nutritious modern alternative. We find all but the youngest shoots rather fibrous, and prefer a purée, as in a nettle form of the Indian dish *sag paneer*.

Nettle soup is described by one modern writer as "Springtime herbalism at one of its finest moments." This soup is the Scottish *kail*. Tibetans believe that their sage and poet Milarepa (AD 1052–1135) lived solely on nettle soup for many years, until he himself turned green: a literal green man.

Use nettle for...
Modern lifestyles need the kind of nutrition that nettle can offer. It is now known that the mineral content of intensively farmed foods has decreased dramatically over the past half-century, so even people eating a healthy diet may be mineral-deficient. Mineral deficiency contributes to a wide range of chronic health problems, including diabetes and cardiac disease, so nettles can improve diverse conditions purely through their mineral content.

Nettles have an antihistamine effect, valuable for treating hayfever and other allergies. They can help reduce the severity of asthma attacks. For treating hayfever, they combine well with elderflower.

Nettles enhance natural immunity, helping protect us from infections. Nettle tea drunk often at the start of a feverish illness is beneficial. It can be combined with elderflower, lime blossom, yarrow, or mint.

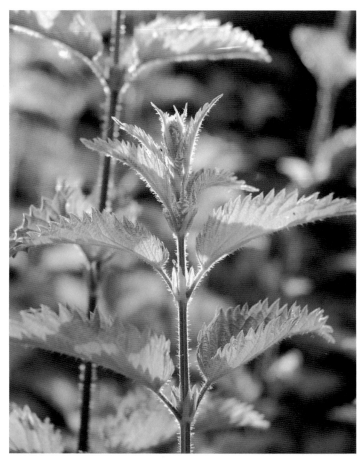

Nettles reduce blood sugar levels and stimulate the circulation, which supports treatment of diabetes. They also dilate the peripheral blood vessels and promote elimination of urine, which helps lower high blood pressure.

Taking nettles has an amphoteric effect on breast milk production, meaning that mothers make more milk if the flow is scanty or less if the flow is excessive.

Nettles have long been considered a blood tonic and are a wonderful treatment for anemia, as they are

The sting from nettles comes from the hairs, which are like tiny glass syringes that inject a stinging acid fluid

It is more appropriate that nature has given this plant the protection of [a] stinging exterior. Without it, we should probably never have the opportunity to benefit from its healing power. Animals, with their instinctive knowledge of what is good for them, would not leave us even one leaf.
– Dr. Vogel (1989)

Stinging nettle and one of the insects using it as a food plant, the peacock butterfly and larva, by Maria Merian, 1717

high in both iron and chlorophyll. The iron in nettles is very easily absorbed and assimilated.

The root is a leading herbal treatment for enlarged prostate, taken on its own as a tincture or with saw palmetto (*Serenoa repens*).

Stinging nettles help clear the blood of urates and toxins, partly through stimulating the kidneys. Nettle tops make a tea for treating gout and arthritis. Another old arthritis remedy is to whip the

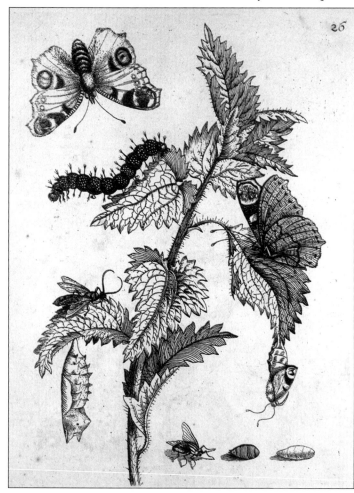

affected joints with fresh nettles (*Urtica urens* has a stronger effect than *U. dioica*). This creates a temporary nettle rash but alleviates pain and stiffness.

If you think this is odd behaviour, consider sado-botany, in which sexual partners beat each other with nettles for stimulation and pain/pleasure. The Romans and Greeks of old took nettle seed as an aphrodisiac.

What cooks will tell you is that two minutes of boiling nettle leaves will neutralize both the silica "syringes" of the stinging cells and the histamine or formic acid-like fluid that is so painful.

But if you are brave you can try munching raw leaves. Pinch the top shoot on a young nettle, roll into a tight ball and eat – delicious. This, incidentally, is the technique used in the world nettle-eating championship, held annually in Dorset (eat all the nettles you can in an hour, washed down by beer – the event is sponsored by a pub).

Sir John Harington (1607) had just the remedy for these competitors:

Tho Nettles ſtinke, yet make they recompence,/ If your belly by the Collicke paine endures,/ Againſt the Collicke Nettle-ſeed and hony/ Is Phyſick: better none is had for money./ It breedeth ſleepe, ſtaies vomits, ſleams [blood-letting instruments] doth ſoften,/ It helpes him of the Gowte that eates it often.

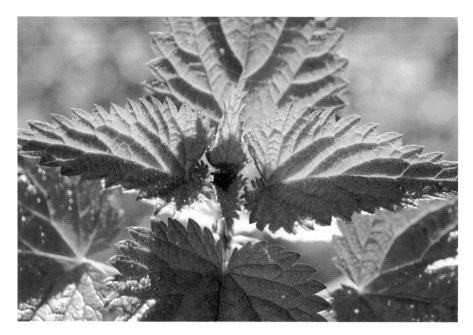

Harvesting nettle tops

Nettle tops are best in the spring, but if the nettles are repeatedly cut back they will send up fresh shoots, which can be harvested through summer and into autumn. Harvest the top 6", wearing rubber gloves to pick them, or use a pair of scissors to cut and lift them into a bag or basket.

Rinse them if they need it. Young spring nettles can be frozen for use later in the year. Blanch them in boiling water for two minutes, then drain and cool. Chop up or leave whole, and store in freezer bags.

Nettle tea

Use a couple of fresh **nettle tops** in a teapot per cup of **boiling water**, and allow to infuse for 15 to 20 minutes. This tastes so much better than any nettle tea you can buy. Drink as often as you like. Can also be used as a hair rinse and massaged into the scalp to promote hair growth.

Nettle juice powder

Juice fresh **nettle tops**, then mix the juice with enough nettle leaf powder (made by reducing **dried nettle tops** in a coffee grinder, then putting the powder through a sieve) to the thickness of double cream. Spread on fruit leather trays in a dehydrator or on non-stick baking trays in a warm oven until dry. Crumble and store in airtight jars.

Dose: Half to one teaspoonful daily.

NETTLE TOPS
Tea
- spring tonic
- anemia
- bleeding
- diarrhea
- gout
- fluid retention
- low blood pressure
- high blood pressure
- coughs
- allergies
- regulates breast milk production
- skin problems
- high blood sugar

Externally
- cuts and wounds
- hair tonic

Juice powder
- spring tonic
- anemia
- gout
- fluid retention
- low blood pressure
- high blood pressure
- allergies
- regulates breast milk production
- skin problems
- high blood sugar

Nettle top decocted tincture

By boiling nettles, you get the minerals that are not extracted well by alcohol. Chop up your **nettle tops**, and divide into two even batches. Put one half in a blender with enough 40% **vodka** to blend, and liquidize. Put the other half in a saucepan with just enough **water** to cover, bring to the boil and simmer for 15 minutes. Allow to cool.

Strain and measure both liquids, then combine, making sure the volume of alcohol is equal to or greater than the volume of water. (If your water volume is greater, return it to the saucepan and simmer down until it is a little less.) Bottle and label.

Dose: 1 teaspoonful three times a day. For burns, hold the burn under cold running water for a few minutes first if possible, then wet a cotton wool ball with the tincture and hold it on the burn until the pain eases.

Nettle soup

Sauté 1 or 2 chopped **onions** in a little **ghee, butter or olive oil** until the onions are lightly browned. Add about a pint and a half of **water or vegetable stock,** and several handfuls of **fresh nettle tops**. Simmer gently for 10 or 15 minutes, then purée with a hand blender and serve. You can add nutmeg, pepper or other spices to taste. Then add cream, potatoes, sorrel or whatever you like – the possible variations are endless.

Nettle flowers are soon followed by the seeds

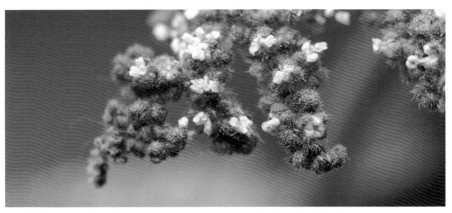

Nettle seed electuary

Cut nettle tops when the **seed** is almost ripe and lay them outdoors on brown paper. This allows any small insects that live on them the time to escape. When dry, strip the seeds off the stems. Grind the seeds in a coffee grinder and mix the powder into a paste with **runny honey**. Store in wide-mouthed jars.

Dose: 1 or 2 teaspoonfuls daily.

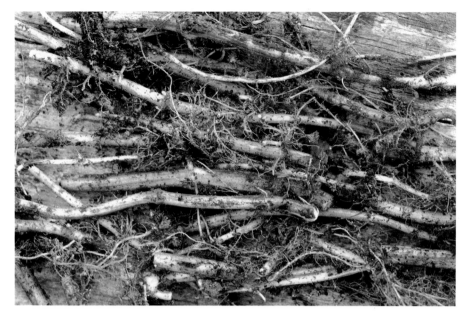

Researchers gave a few teaspoons of the [nettle] extract daily to 67 men over age 60 with BPH [benign prostatic hyperplasia or hypertrophy] and found that the herb significantly reduced their need to get up at night to urinate. ... German medical herbalists recommend two to three teaspoons of extract a day to treat BPH.
– Duke (1997)

Harvesting nettle roots

Nettle roots can be dug up whenever they are needed, but are probably at their best in the fall. You will need a stout fork and a pair of close-fitting gloves. The yellow roots are tenacious and tangled.

Wash them thoroughly and cut into pieces an inch or two long. To dry, spread on a cake rack or a screen; put in a warm, dry place until brittle.

Nettle root decoction

Simmer a handful of dried or fresh **nettle root** in a pint and a half of **water** for 20 minutes, then strain.

Dose: Drink a cupful two or three times daily, storing the rest in the fridge until you need it and then reheating.

Nettle root decocted tincture

Put fresh or dried **nettle roots** in a saucepan with enough **water** to cover them, and simmer for 20 minutes. When cool, pour off and measure the liquid, but keep the roots. Add an equal amount of 40% **vodka** to the liquid and pour it in a large jar or jars with the roots. Add a few handfuls of fresh chopped roots. Put the jars in a cupboard and leave for 3 to 4 weeks, shaking occasionally. Strain off and bottle the liquid.

Dose: 1 teaspoonful daily to maintain prostate health, or three times daily for more acute problems.

NETTLE ROOT
Decoction
• prostate enlargement
• infections
• inflammation
• bacterial and fungal infections

Decocted tincture
• prostate enlargement
• infections
• inflammation
• bacterial and fungal infections

Caution: Do not take nettle root during pregnancy.

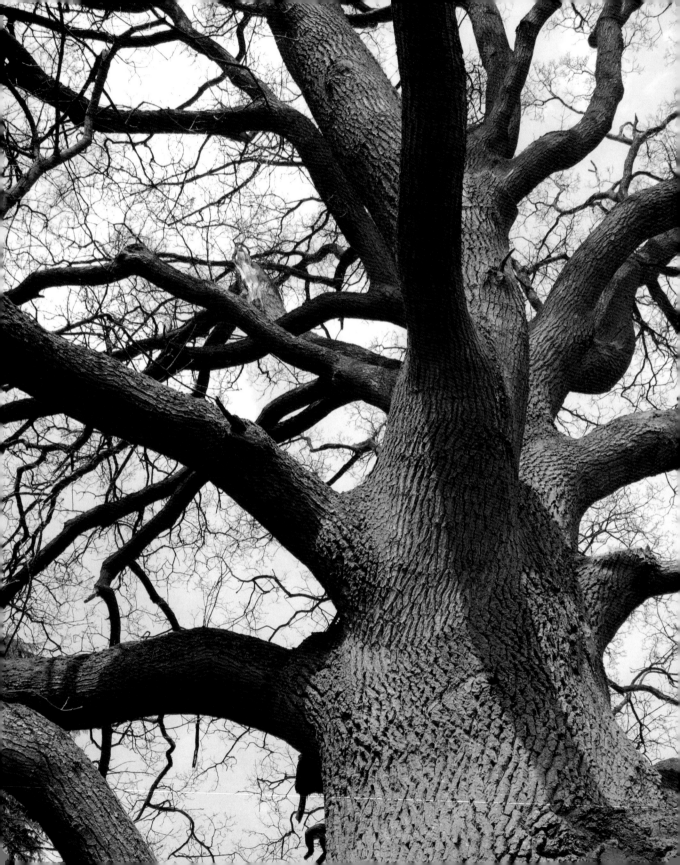

Oak *Quercus robur, Q. petraea, Q. alba*

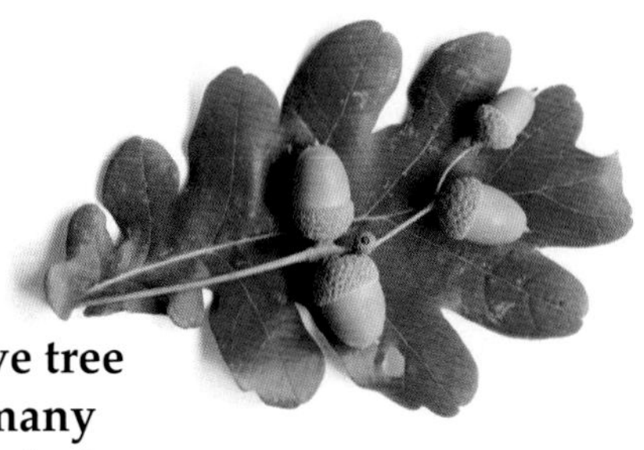

Oak has been a sacred and an economically productive tree for millennia, the symbol of Britain's secure power (many other countries rightly claim it too). But it has been a victim of its own success, with most of its old forests now gone.

In terms of wild herbal medicine it still has uses, mainly of the bark, leaves, and acorns rather than the galls of earlier times. Oak is also one of Dr. Bach's original flower essences, so its subtle authority lives on.

We have chosen the picture on the left from among many we've taken of oak in order to convey something of the massive presence and protecting influence of this most stalwart of trees.

There is insufficient space to relate the myths, sacred and secular, the uses, and the central role of oak in the British consciousness. Geoffrey Grigson points out that it has been too necessary and familiar a tree to allow any other general names than its own: oak it is.

Suffice it to say that oak's timber built houses, cathedrals, and ships, made furniture, barrels, and pews; its bark tanned leather for shoes and saddles, and provided dyes; its acorns fed pigs and was a famine food or coffee substitute; its galls (oak apples) gave ink; its wood supplied fuel and charcoal; the tree was a space for mistletoe, ivy, and ferns; it sheltered insects, birds, animals – and outlaws (Robin Hood) and kings (Charles II).

There was once a saying that oak was so important that a person came in contact with it every day of their life, from newborn's cradle to old man's coffin. Such a universal and steadying presence has been lost in modern times, but the tree still offers uses for an enthusiast of wild herbal medicine.

Use oak for...
The **bark** is the "official" botanical drug, used as an astringent. The *British Herbal Pharmacopoeia* specifies dried bark from younger stems and branches of *Quercus robur*, though herbalists in practice find that other oak species can be used interchangeably and that acorns, leaves, and galls, also rich in tannins, have equivalent benefits (nobody uses oak root!).

Tannins were first isolated chemically from oak bark, and it is thought that "tannin" came from a Celtic term for oak. Oak, tannins, and leather tanning have always been synonymous.

Fagaceae
Beech family

Description: A well-loved tree, which grows to 120 ft tall and can live for a thousand years. The lobed leaves are mainly deciduous, and the flowers are catkins borne in spring. Acorns in little cups are diagnostic for all oaks.

Habitat: Forests, woods, parkland.

Distribution: The English or pedunculate oak (*Quercus robur*) is native to most of Europe, and is found naturalized in parts of North America. The sessile or Durmast oak (*Q. petraea*) is a European species. White oak (*Q. alba*) is found across eastern North America.

Species: White oak (*Q. alba*) is the main North American species used medicinally. The American oaks with rounded leaves generally have edible acorns, while those with pointy leaves have acorns that are high in tannin and very bitter.

Parts used: Bark, leaves, acorns, galls.

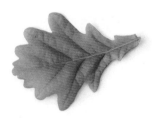

Oak should be placed first on any list of native remedies for hikers and backpackers. It is common, easily identifiable, easy to use, and effective for most of the potential problems faced in the wilderness.
– Moore (1979)

For the first time in history we can manage without oak. The reputation remains, but the worshipful and powerful tree has declined into a patriarch on half-pay.
– Grigson (1958)

Astringents are the body's tighteners and driers, being effective in binding and toning tissue and reducing excess discharges. The conditions treated by astringent herbs include diarrhea, dysentery, eye, mouth, and throat inflammations, disturbed mucous membranes of the digestive tract, and bleeding, burns, and sores.

Astringents are also antimicrobial and antiseptic, helping to create a barrier against infection. Herbalist David Hoffmann explains this by saying "astringents produce a kind of temporary leather coat on the surface of tissue."

Oak bark is most often taken as a decoction, small strips of bark from young branches being boiled in water for 10–15 minutes and drunk. It is strong and bitter from the 15% to 20% of tannins it contains, and is the primary treatment for acute diarrhea, taken in small but plentiful doses. If self-medication for diarrhea is not successful after three or four days, the usual advice is to consult a professional.

The same preparation is good as a mouthwash for gargling in sore throats, tonsillitis, and laryngitis, as a douche for leucorrhoea and as an enema for hemorrhoids.

In Germany the "official" uses for oak bark decoction include inflammation of gums and throat, sweating of the feet, chilblains, and anal fissures (the last three in a bath at room temperature). The dried young bark is also powdered in a grinder as a tooth powder, as in our recipe on the next page.

The **leaves** of oak in spring have been used hot as a tea to relieve diarrhea, and after cooling as a soothing compress for sore eyes. Culpeper writes that the distilled water of oak leaves is "one of the best remedies I know of for the whites [leucorrhoea] in women." In the field, chewing the leaves and applying them to bites, open wounds, or ulcers eases inflammation and promotes healing.

Acorns are the signature of oaks worldwide, and well chosen as a symbol for Britain's National Trust. While enjoyed raw by pigs and squirrels, humans find acorns palatable only when cooked after repeated boiling and renewing of the water, the tannins being gradually leached out. Acorns were a famine food for the Anglo-Saxons, but some North American oaks have more palatable acorns, and Native Americans living in forested areas had acorn flour as a staple part of their diet.

During World War I an ersatz coffee was made in Germany from roasted and ground acorns. The drink is still available today. It is tasty, good for those with poor digestion, and has little caffeine.

Acorns were once a herbal specific for alcoholism, a use reflected in a modern homeopathic remedy formulated to control craving.

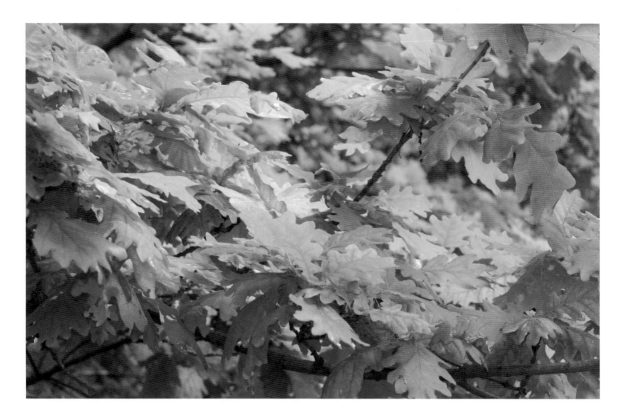

Oak twig toothbrush

Oak twigs can be used as a natural toothbrush with built-in antiseptic and anti-inflammatory benefits. Simply pick a small twig and chew the end to fray it, then use this to massage your gums and clean your teeth.

Harvesting oak bark

Select young branches about an inch in diameter, and use a sharp knife to remove small strips of bark, cutting along the length of the branch. The bark is thicker than you might expect, brown on the outside but white underneath. Dry the bark strips in a warm place.

Tooth powder

Break up the dried oak bark into small bits and grind finely in a sturdy coffee grinder. Sieve to remove larger pieces. The fennel seed in the recipe can also be ground in this way.

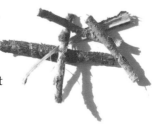

Mix 3 parts **oak bark powder** with 1 part **cinnamon powder**,
1 part **fennel seed powder** and 1 part **bicarbonate of soda**, or to suit your own taste.
Store in a small jar, and use to brush your teeth every day.

Oak twig toothbrush
- gum problems

Tooth powder
- gum disease
- weak gums
- bleeding gums
- mouth ulcers

Description: A red-stemmed perennial with tiny white flowers, growing mainly on walls, to about 2 ft high. Forms dense patches locally.

Habitat: Walls, stony places, hedgebanks, and gardens.

Distribution: Native to Europe and north Africa, introduced to North America and Australia.

Related species: Stinging nettles are in the same family. Pennsylvania pellitory (*Parietaria pensylvanica*) is native to North America.

Parts used: Above-ground parts.

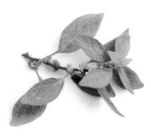

The dried herbe Paritary made up with hony into an Electuarie, or the juice of the herbe, or the decoction thereof made up with Sugar or Hony, is a singular remedy for any old continuall or dry cough, the shortnesse of breath and wheezings in the throate.
– Parkinson (1640)

Pellitory of the wall

Parietaria judaica syn. *P. diffusa, P. officinalis*

This overlooked wild plant is a noted tonic for the kidneys and bladder. It is soothing and increases the flow of urine, while also reducing inflammation and helping dissolve kidney stones. Herbalists use the tea for a range of urinary problems.

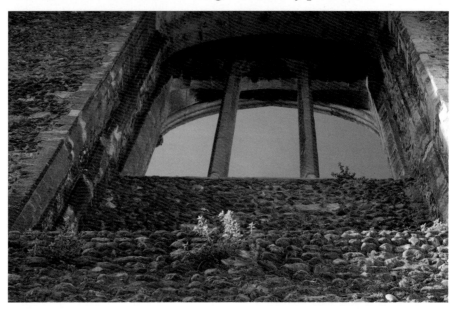

Pellitory, named from the Latin *paries* or house wall, was once given a variety of "virtues" or uses, but herbalists today regard it as a specialized urinary tract herb. It is an excellent gentle tonic for cystitis, nephritis, pyelitis, kidney stones, renal colic, and urinary problems linked with prostate enlargement. It will relieve edema and urine retention, and is soothing as well as urine-producing.

In the seventeenth century, John Parkinson and Nicholas Culpeper wrote of using pellitory internally for coughs and uterine pain, and externally for skin problems, burns, and hot conditions. Parkinson said the juice put in the ears "'eases the noise and hummings in them" and that the herb "applied to the fundament" opens piles and soothes their pain.

Culpeper had such faith in a syrup made of pellitory juice and honey that he promised free treatment to anyone who took a teaspoonful daily or even just once a week and still got dropsy (edema or fluid retention).

This was a popular remedy at the time. We came across it again in a Norfolk gentleman's notebook:

For a Dropsie
Given mee 18th Novem: 1664 by
Mr.Sheepeside
Take ye juice of Pellitorie of ye wall &
boyle it up to a syruppe with honey
& so keepe it in a Glasse. Take one
spoonefull of this every Morninge.

Our own preference is to make an infusion as a tea, but a pellitory syrup or even the ale tincture that was once current would be equally effective today.

Pellitory is used in Europe to treat *Herpes zoster* infections, and has possible wider applications in combating viral infections. There is ongoing research into its effects on FIV, the feline form of HIV.

Pellitory causes hayfever in some people, and is called asthma weed in parts of Australia. It is declared a noxious weed there, which must be destroyed. Even in Britain, it is best avoided if you suffer allergies.

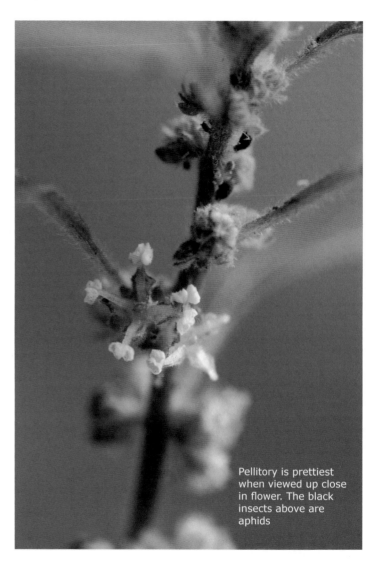

Pellitory is prettiest when viewed up close in flower. The black insects above are aphids

Pellitory tea
Harvest pellitory in the summer while it is flowering, breaking off a stem about halfway up (it snaps easily), leaving the rest to grow back. The fresh herb is considered to be the most effective, but it works well dried too.

Pour a cup of **boiling water** onto 2 teaspoons of the **chopped fresh** or 1 teaspoon of the **dried herb** and leave to infuse for 10–15 minutes. Add honey to taste (the tea is somewhat astringent).

Dose: Drink a cupful three times a day.

Its action upon the urinary calculus is perhaps more marked than any other simple agent at present employed.
– Mrs. Grieve (1931)

Pellitory tea
- cystitis
- bladder irritation
- urinary gravel
- painful urination
- fluid retention

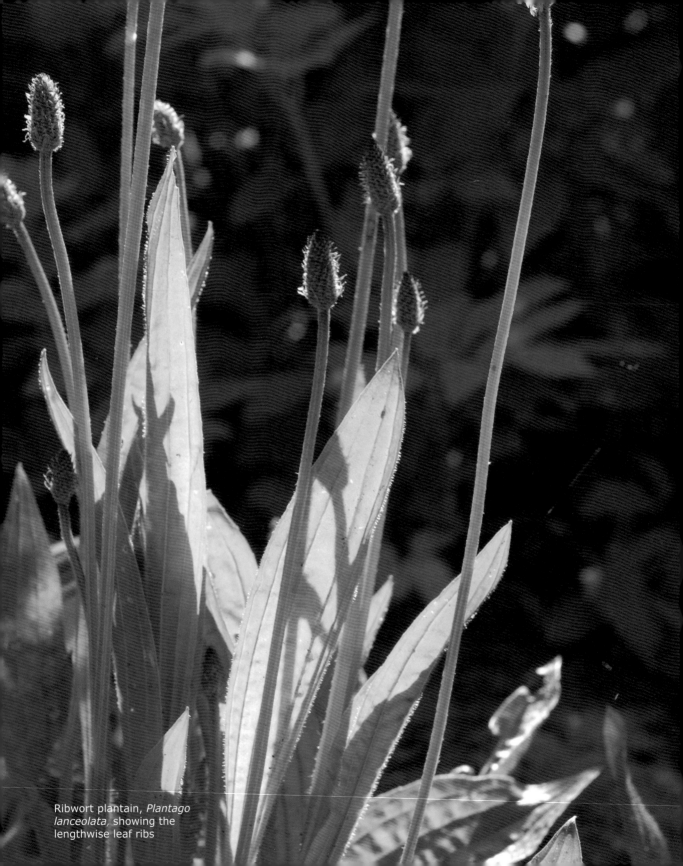

Ribwort plantain, *Plantago lanceolata*, showing the lengthwise leaf ribs

Plantain *Plantago major, P. lanceolata*

Common weeds of footpaths and lawns, the plantains were once celebrated as magical herbs in pre-Christian times, and have followed European settlers around the world.

Plantain is the best first-aid remedy for insect stings, and quickly deals with bites, cuts, and ulcers. It is widely available, safe to use, and effective for common ailments including old coughs, bronchitis, sore throats and irritable digestive tracts.

Plantain is a plant now regarded primarily as a weed except by herbalists, but it had an illustrious past, being one of nine sacred herbs of the Anglo-Saxons, a "mother of worts." It had a reputation for clearing poisons, from bites as well as infections.

Plantains are found almost anywhere there is human habitation, though they have never had an economic value. Greater plantain in particular grows by preference on the compacted soils of paths and tracks, and seems to thrive on being downtrodden.

To Native Americans this plant became "white man's footprint," one that sprang up in the footsteps of the settlers. The plant's name *Plantago* itself comes from *planta* or sole of the foot.

The Anglo-Saxon name of plantain was *waybroed* or *waybrode*, later "waybread," because it grew by the way or path rather than because it made wonderful eating.

Plantains are familiar "weeds" in any lawn, and will return, even when cut often and short. The young leaves have a slightly bitter flavour from tannins, and though quite tough can be eaten in salads or as a spinach. They become bitter and more fibrous as they age. Buckshorn plantain is grown as a perennial salad crop in Italy and other parts of Europe.

Children all over the world use the flower heads of ribwort, as seen in the photo on the opposite page, as a sort of natural pop gun in the game "soldiers" or "kemps."

In Europe a piece of plantain root used to be carried in the pocket to protect against snakebite, but was no doubt more effective when actually applied to the wound as well as being ingested. The North American name snakeweed is an echo of that time.

Use plantain for...
Ribwort is the number one field remedy for insect stings and bites.

**Plantaginaceae
Plantain family**

Description: Perennial plants with a rosette of ribbed leaves and wind-pollinated flowers on erect stalks.

Habitat: Footpaths, roadsides, waste ground, meadows, and lawns.

Species used: Greater plantain (*P. major*) and ribwort or narrowleaf plantain (*P. lanceolata*) are the main species used medicinally.

Distribution: Ribwort and greater plantain are found virtually everywhere with a temperate climate.

Related species: Buckshorn plantain (*P. coronopus*) is grown in Italy as a salad crop. There are around 250 species in the *Plantago* genus worldwide, many of them with similar medicinal properties.

Parts used: Leaves, seeds, sometimes root.

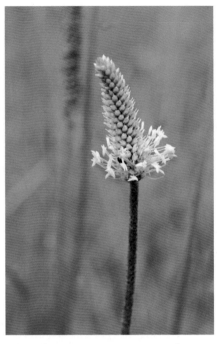

A crushed leaf rubbed onto the painful area will bring relief at once – it's almost miraculous.

Greater plantain also works for pain relief, but the leaves are tougher and not as juicy, so choose ribwort first if it is available. We find that any plantain, applied immediately, is effective for nettle stings and prefer it to dock leaf.

Plantain's antihistamine effect is also beneficial for hayfever and other allergies, and combines well as a tea with elderflower and mint. Plantain has long been a trusted plant for healing wounds (a vulnerary), and Shakespeare mentions it twice as a healer of broken shins. We haven't tried it on broken bones, but have found it to be very efficient at clearing heat and inflammation.

Pliny records in the first century AD that "Themison, a famous physician, sets forthe a whole booke of the hearbe waibred or plantaine, wherein he highly praiseth it; and challengeth it to him-self the honour of first finding it out, notwith-standing it be a triviall and common hearbe trodden under everie man's foot."
– quoted in Gordon (1980)

Running sore in ye Legge
Plantine water & oat-meal flour made into a plaster on the sore, wetting again with Plantine water and use plantine water to wash it.
– Archdale Palmer's recipes 1659–72

Indian bandaid.
– a Cherokee elder's view of plantain

A patient of Julie's had deep red and painful shins from a radiation burn, and came every few days for several weeks for a dressing of fresh plantain juice mixed with slippery elm powder. Other fresh herbs such as chickweed and yarrow were added to the juice at times, but ribwort was the main-stay. The patient's legs healed and have not needed further treatment.

Julie also uses plantain poultices for the heat and swelling of vari-cose veins and varicose eczema.

Plantains are great purifiers, with an ability to draw dirt, pus, and venom out of wounds. They have even been used to treat blood poisoning and gangrene. A poul-tice of crushed plantain leaves is the perfect remedy for the skinned knees of childhood, drawing out dirt while soothing and healing.

Abbé Kneipp (1821–97) character-ised plantain's healing action thus:

plantain closes the gaping wound with a seam of gold thread; for, just as gold will not admit of rust, so the plantain will not admit of rotting and gangrenous flesh.

These same qualities make plan-tain useful for treating infections of the teeth and gums. Simply place a wad of plantain leaf against the affected area and back it up by plantain tea or tincture as a mouthwash. Plantain can be used to help relieve toothache until you can get to the dentist.

Plantain has a soothing effect on the mucous membranes of the digestive tract, and has been used successfully for stomach ulcers and irritable bowel complaints. The leaves stop the bleeding too, so are good for ulcerative colitis. The seeds are even more soothing than the leaf, but probably do not stop the bleeding as well.

The seeds can be eaten raw or cooked, and are very rich in vitamin B1. Ground into a meal and mixed with flour they can make a form of bread. The whole seeds can be boiled like sago, and have a pleasant mild flavour, but this is a bit fiddly and time-consuming.

The seed husks swell up and are very absorbent, providing a source of dietary fibre for constipation and other digestive disorders. It is not surprising that the mucilaginous and binding herb psyllium (or isaphagula) is from *Plantago ovata*, a close relative of our plantains and native to the Middle East and India. As well as being anti-diarrheal the mucilage in plantain is good for starching clothes.

Ribwort is the best of the plantains for treating coughs, and is recommended for chronic bronchitis as well as other persistent irritable coughs. It helps to bring up old stuck phlegm, and is particularly good for hot, dry coughs.

Greater or hoary plantain, having broader leaves, is better for hot, tired feet or plantar fasciitis. Do as the Native Americans did and put the leaves in your shoes; keep there until the leaves dry out and then replace by fresh ones.

Plantain's long history has been benign. One exception came in a case of witchcraft in Scotland. In 1623 Bessie Smith confessed to treating "heart fevers" by giving "wayburn leaves" to take for nine mornings, with a charm. But was this worse than using plantain on St. John's eve, as everyone did?

It is the best herb for blood poisoning: reducing the swelling and completely healing a limb where poisoning has made amputation imminent.
– Dr. Christopher (1976)

Plantago major
by Maria Merian (1717)

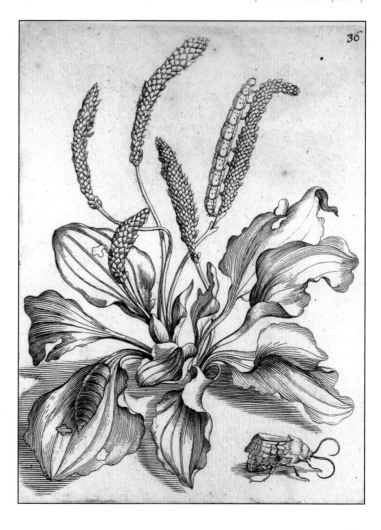

LEAF
Leaf in shoe
- plantar fasciitis
- tired feet

Crushed leaf
- insect bites & stings
- allergic rashes
- cuts and wounds
- infected cuts
- bleeding
- mouth ulcers
- boils and ulcers
- burns
- acne rosacea
- shingles

Plantain tea and tincture
- coughs
- mild bronchitis
- irritable bowel
- hemorrhoids
- hay fever & allergies

Plantain succus
- coughs
- sore throats
- mild bronchitis
- irritable bowel
- stomach ulcers

SEED
- constipation
- irritable bowel

Harvesting plantain

For first-aid use, plantain leaves can be picked and used whenever needed as they remain green through the year. Crush or chew, then apply. If you live in an area with harsh winters, you can freeze the leaves for winter use. For making a medicine to preserve, gather the leaves during the summer. To dry the leaves, spread them on brown paper or a drying screen in a warm dry place, turning the leaves daily until they are crisp. Discard if they go black.

Harvest the seeds when they are ripe, picking the heads and spreading them on brown paper to dry completely before stripping the seeds off for storage in brown paper bags or in jars.

Plantain tea

Use a heaped teaspoonful of **crumbled dry leaf** or a **fresh leaf of plantain** per mugful of boiling water, and leave to infuse for ten minutes.

Dose: Drink a mugful three times a day.

Plantain tincture

Pick **fresh plantain leaves** and put them in a blender with enough **vodka** to cover them. Blend to a green mush, and pour into a jar. Put in a cool dark place for a few days, then strain and bottle.

Dose: Half to one teaspoonful three times a day.

Plantain succus

Juice **fresh plantain leaves** and mix the juice with an equal amount of **honey**. Pour into sterilized bottles and store in a cool place.

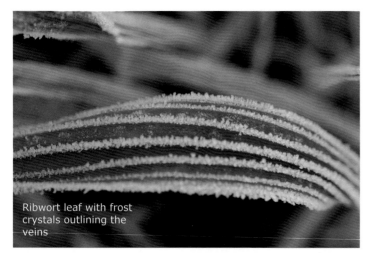

Ribwort leaf with frost crystals outlining the veins

Dose: 1 teaspoonful as needed for coughs (ribwort is best); 1 teaspoonful 3 times daily for stomach ulcers. Use externally as a dressing for ulcers and other sores.

Plantain seed

The seeds and husks can be ground in a coffee grinder before use, or used whole.

Dose: 1 teaspoonful sprinkled on food, once to three times daily.

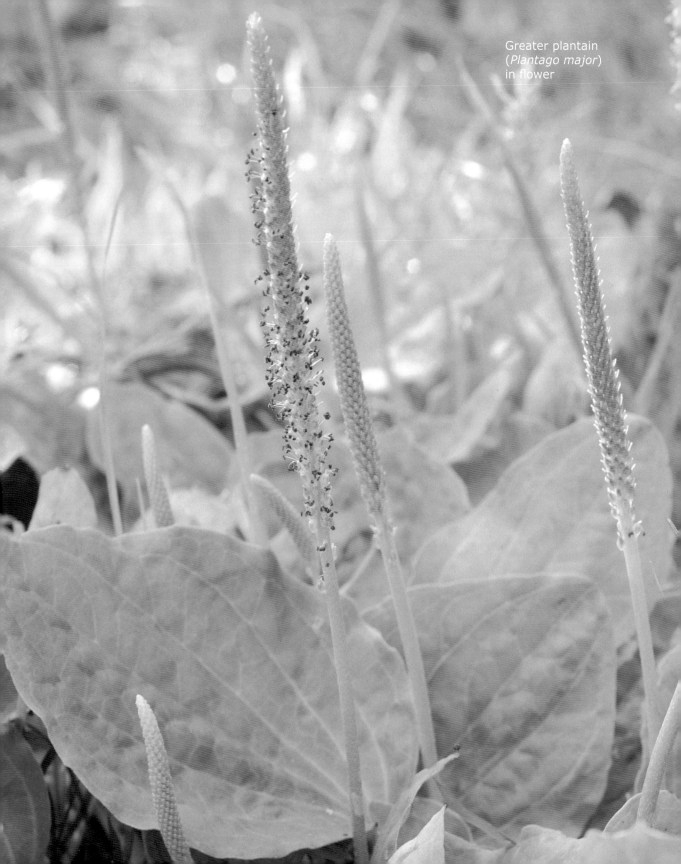

Greater plantain
(*Plantago major*)
in flower

Ramsons, Bear garlic *Allium ursinum*

Finding a swathe of ramsons (bear garlic) in a dark wood is one of the joys of early spring, with the bright green leaves and strong garlic smell tempting you to gather for the pot.

This is also a wonderful medicine for the digestive tract, and helps keep the heart and circulation healthy. Ramsons cleanses the body, balancing the gut flora, and is effective in removing infections.

**Amaryllidaceae
Amaryllis family**
(formerly in the Alliaceae)

Description: A bulb producing a carpet of greenery in damp wooded areas in spring, followed by beautiful white starry flowers in early summer. Up to 15" tall.

Habitat: Woodland, stream banks, and moist field sides.

Distribution: Widely distributed in the British Isles, Europe and Asia. A garden plant in North America.

Related species: There are a number of *Allium* species found in North America that have similar uses to ramsons, including wild garlic (*A. canandense*) and the introduced field garlic (*A. vineale*). Use smell as your guide: if it smells strongly of onion or garlic, it is edible.

Parts used: Leaves, flowers, and sometimes bulbs.

Let food be thy medicine and medicine be thy food.
– Hippocrates (460–377 BC)

Ramsons has been a folk medicine favourite in Europe since the ancient Greeks, its uses in both kitchen and medicine cabinet matching those of its cultivated garlic cousin. Its unusual common name probably comes from an Old English word, *hramson*, which unsurprisingly meant wild garlic; its second Latin name of *ursinum*, or bear, perhaps relating to the smell, seems to have little relation to British experience (though see Mrs. Grieve's gripes on the next page!).

You don't find this wonderful herb for sale in a herb or health shop, so you have to harvest your own. Luckily, it is usually abundant where it grows, carpeting woods and dells with its pungent greenery in the early spring.

Ramsons has similar medicinal properties to garlic, with the added benefit of being tolerated well by people who have problems with onions or garlic. We hope you find it as delicious as we do.

Gourmet cooks and posh restaurants extol the piquant flavour of fresh ramsons leaves, but it is also there for you to forage. The leaves can be eaten raw or cooked. Try them chopped and sprinkled on a variety of foods. A bright green garlic butter made from the leaves would be at home on a science fiction set, but is actually really tasty.

The bright white flowers can be used too, and are attractive and flavoursome sprinkled on salads. But note that once the flowers open, the palatability of the leaves decreases as they become harsher-tasting and less full-bodied.

Use ramsons for…
Fresh ramsons eaten in spring is a gentle tonic for the whole body. By "cleansing the blood" it also helps with skin problems. Like ordinary garlic, ramsons improves the circulation and helps protect

Ramsons growing near High Force, Teesside, England, May

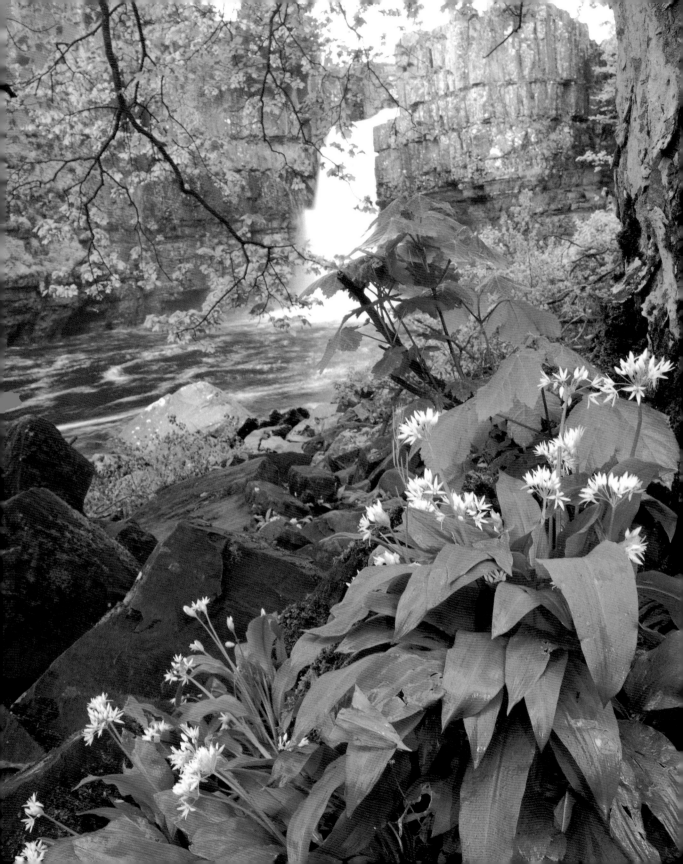

the heart. Better circulation assists memory and eyesight, and will generally lift the health.

You can make a poultice for boils and minor cuts by mashing a fresh ramsons leaf to place on them, holding it in place with a sticking plaster. Reapply a couple of times a day until healed. Ramsons is a good antibacterial and antifungal agent, though not as strong as ordinary garlic.

Ramsons is one of the best medicines for bowel problems. Julie has found in patients that it can settle a digestive tract that has never been quite right since a gut infection. Also, ramsons balances the gut flora, and is beneficial for ulcerative colitis, Crohn's disease, irritable bowel syndrome, chronic gastroenteritis, colic, and flatulence – in fact, it helps relieve most forms of intestinal unhappiness.

Ramsons is best used as a fresh seasonal food and medicine but can be preserved for later use. Garlic tincture doesn't sound very appealing, however! Many herbalists recommend taking ramsons juice, which is effective, but we'd much rather have a few tablespoons of ramsons pesto or sauce and enjoy taking our medicine as food (recipes below).

Fresh ramsons leaf
• spring tonic
• skin problems
• irritable bowel
• gas and bloating
• chronic colitis
• ulcerative colitis
• Crohn's disease

Fresh leaf poultice
• boils
• cuts

Ramsons pesto and sauce
• spring tonic
• skin problems
• irritable bowel
• gas and bloating
• chronic colitis
• ulcerative colitis
• Crohn's disease

Harvesting ramsons

Ramsons leaves can be harvested as soon as they appear in spring, and are at their best before the flowers open. The flowers are tasty, sprinkled on salads and other food. The bulbs can also be eaten, but we prefer to leave them to grow again the next year. Ramsons are locally abundant, so you should be able to harvest and preserve plenty of leaves without needing to disturb the bulbs.

Ramsons pesto

Put **ramsons leaves** and enough **olive oil** to cover them in a blender. Blend until smooth. This vivid green sauce can be eaten fresh with pasta just like the more familiar Italian pesto made with basil and garlic. You can alter the taste by adding chopped pine nuts or sunflower seeds and freshly grated pecorino cheese. It is delicious spooned onto savory foods and can be added to salad dressings. This pesto can be frozen in small batches for use throughout the year.

Ramsons sauce

Another way to preserve **ramsons** is to blend as above, but use 1 part **cider** or **white wine vinegar** to 3 parts **olive oil** as the liquid. The vinegar helps preserve the ramsons, and a jar of this will keep well in the fridge for months if it doesn't get eaten before then.

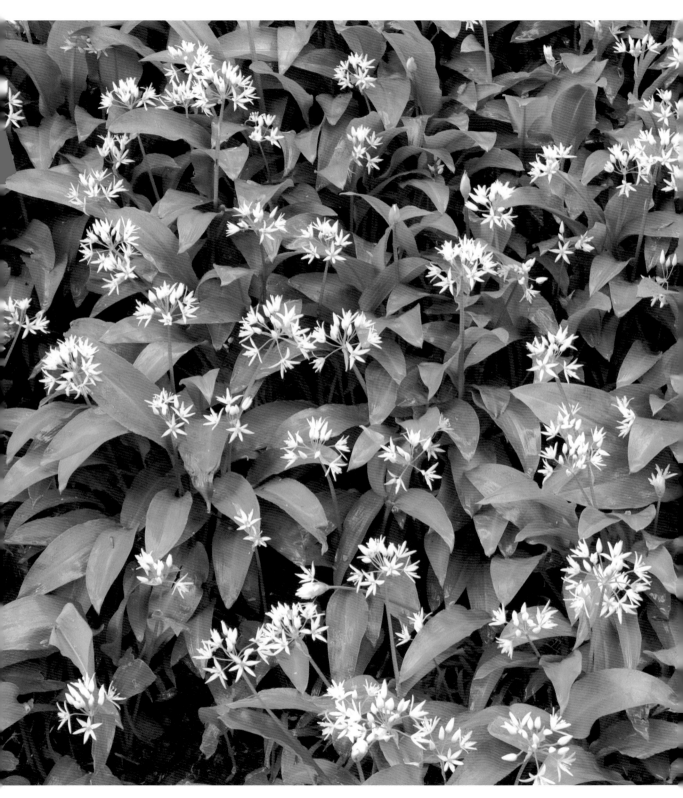

Raspberry *Rubus idaeus*

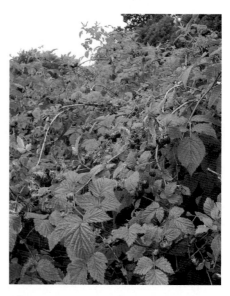

Raspberry leaf tea is well known for strengthening the uterus prior to childbirth, and for relieving painful periods. It is also an effective and soothing remedy for flu and fevers, helping reduce the aches and pains that go with them.

This tea is a good source of readily assimilated calcium and other minerals, making it a health-enhancing alternative to regular tea. Raspberries, especially wild ones, are very high in salvestrols, a class of cancer-fighting chemicals.

**Rosaceae
Rose family**

Description: A slender shrub, up to 6 ft high, with arching stems; less spiny and more delicate than black-berry canes. The leaves are a light green, and silvery underneath. The stems are bare in winter.

Habitat: Wild raspberries are often found growing with blackberries along the edges of woods.

Distribution: Found throughout North America, northern Europe and northern Asia.

Related species: The North American grayleaf red raspberry (*R. idaeus* spp. *strigosus*) is used interchangeably with the European species. In China, Korean bramble (*R. coreanus*) fruit is used as a kidney and liver tonic.

Parts used: Leaves and berries.

Raspberry is a member of the rose family, a plant of the Old World, spreading out to the temperate regions from the Mediterranean. The second part of its name, "idaeus," refers to this ancient origin.

The Greek version of the raspberry legend concerns Ida, daughter of the King of Crete. One day she was looking after her infant, Jupiter, while picking berries on a mountainside. The lusty babe made so much noise that Ida was distracted. When she pricked herself her blood caused what were white berries to turn red. They have remained so ever since – and still grow on the slopes of Mt Ida in modern Crete.

Raspberry was given the common name "raspis," meaning rough or hairy fruit (by contrast with the blackberry), and also "hindberry" because female deer would feed on the leaves, and thereby assist in their own birthing.

The noted animal herbalist Juliette de Baïracli Levy long advocated dog breeders using raspberry leaf tea, with impressive whelping results throughout the world. She quoted a Romany source: "Let all creatures with young, human and animal, take freely of raspberry herb. They will have very easy 'times' and will be saved a tremendous amount of suffering."

Use raspberry for...

The best way to enjoy wild raspberries is to eat them straight off the bush. They may not be as large as the commercial and garden varieties, but the deep, satisfying flavour is special. As the English herbalist John Parkinson wrote in 1629: "The berries are eaten in the Summertime, as an afternoones dish, to please the taste of the sicke as well as the sound."

But it is the leaves rather than the berries that have the most benefit medicinally. The best time to pick them is on a sunny morning after the dew has dried off. Most herbals say drying the leaves is best, but we find the fresh and dried alternatives equally good.

If you are drying the leaves to use later, hang up bunches of the canes tied together with string, or spread the leaves on a drying rack – a linen cupboard is an ideal place. When they are crisp, they can be packed away in brown paper bags or bottles for storage.

Raspberry leaf is astringent, which means it tightens and tones tissue. It is high in nutrients, including iron, manganese, and calcium.

The leaf tea is mainly used in pregnancy to help ease delivery and reduce pain in labor. Julie drank it when she was pregnant, and while she wouldn't say labor was easy (the very name means work, after all!) it was not painful. Raspberry leaf continues its work

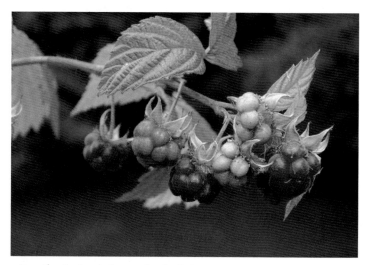

after the baby is born, by helping the uterus return to normal and promoting milk production.

You may find disagreement in various books about how long to use raspberry leaf in pregnancy. Some authors advise taking it throughout while others restrict it to the last two or three months only. It partly depends on the dose, and we suggest you follow what your midwife or herbalist says is best for you personally.

Many herbals recommend using an ounce of dried leaf per pint of water, but this is a very strong brew and isn't too pleasant to drink. Unless you are trying to stop diarrhea, this strength isn't necessary. We think a weaker tea taken more often is a better idea.

As well as pregnancy and for periods, raspberry tea and vinegar can be used to counter aemia, and to relieve colds, 'flu, and diarrhea. See the recipes overleaf.

Raspberries are high in vitamin C and other antioxidants. They are also high in a newly discovered class of chemicals called **salvestrols**, which have proven anti-cancer activity.

Professor Gerry Potter, Head of Medicinal Chemistry at De Montfort University, UK and Director of the Cancer Drug Discovery Group, recommends a diet of foods that are naturally high in salvestrols, which includes raspberries and other red and blue berries.

Recent research has found that agrochemicals inhibit plants from producing salvestrols, so wild or organically grown plants have higher levels. Here's another reason to enjoy your wild raspberries!

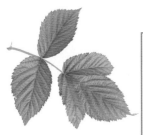

Raspberry leaf tea

Pour a cupful of **boiling water** onto 1 rounded tablespoonful of dried **raspberry leaf** or a handful of fresh leaves. Let it brew for 15 minutes, then strain and drink, either hot or cold.

Dosages: For general use, drink 1 cupful one to three times a day.

In the last two/three months of pregnancy and for several weeks after giving birth, drink two cups daily, or as instructed by your herbal practitioner or midwife. To normalize heavy periods, drink 3 cups a day during your period, and 1 cup a day the rest of the month. At the first sign of a cold or flu, stop eating for a day or two and drink lots of raspberry leaf tea.

For diarrhea, make a stronger infusion with 2 to 3 teaspoonfuls of dried leaf per cup of boiling water. Drink 1 cupful three times a day. Children can have a wineglassful, and babies given a teaspoonful.

Raspberry vinegar

Fill a jam jar with freshly picked **raspberries** and pour in enough **cider vinegar** to cover them. Cover the jar and put it in a warm place such as a sunny windowsill, shaking it every few days.

After two weeks the vinegar should be a lovely deep pink. Strain through a jelly bag or fine sieve. If you want a clear vinegar, don't press the pulp – just let the liquid drip out – otherwise squeeze to get the most flavour out of your raspberries, and pour into a sterile bottle and label.

Dosage: Take 1 teaspoonful every few hours for colds and flu.

This rich, sweet-sour vinegar can also be used to bring a touch of summer sunshine to winter salad dressings. It has a wonderful flavor, enjoyed in the best gourmet restaurants – and your own home.

Raspberry oxymel

Mix equal parts of **honey** and **raspberry vinegar**.

Dosage: For sore throats, use 1 tablespoon as a gargle before swallowing. For a sluggish digestive system, add 1 tablespoon of the oxymel to a mug of hot water, and drink before meals.

Raspberry leaf tea
- childbirth
- lactation
- heavy menstruation
- anemia
- flu
- muscle cramps
- osteoporosis
- diarrhea
- nausea

Other uses for raspberry leaf tea
- as a mouthwash for mouth ulcers and gum problems
- as a gargle for sore throats
- when cool as a soothing eyewash for sore and irritated eyes
- as a healing wash for cuts and abrasions

Raspberry vinegar
- colds & flu
- sore throats
- digestion
- arthritis
- salad dressing

Raspberry oxymel
- sore throats
- colds & flu
- sluggish digestion
- arthritis

Red clover *Trifolium pratense*

An important nitrogen-fixing forage crop, red clover is also a significant medicinal plant with a long history as a blood cleanser. It is used for chronic constipation, skin complaints, chronic degenerative diseases, and bronchitis. It has been included in many anti-cancer formulae, and helps balance hormone levels during the menopause, relieving symptoms such as hot flashes.

Fabaceae (Leguminosae) Pea family

Description: A common perennial with purplish-red flowers and a single pale chevron on the leaves.

Habitat: Grassland, roadsides.

Distribution: Native and also cultivated throughout Europe; naturalized in the Americas, Australia, and many other places.

Related species: The other common species is white clover (*T. repens*), with medicinal uses similar to those of red clover. There are over 200 species of clover worldwide.

Parts used: Flower heads with upper leaves, collected in early summer.

Clover or trefoil (three leaves) has a sacred past. It had significance for the Druids, and St Patrick was said to have used a clover in the meadow to explain the Trinity to Irish pagans. As befitted a plant of such fortunate lineage clover was worthy, with other holy herbs, to protect the virtuous against dark forces. One old rhyme went (in Sir Walter Scott's 1815 version):

Trefoil, vervain, St. John's wort, dill,/ Hinder witches of their will.

The oldest form of the name "clover" we have is Anglo-Saxon *cloeferwort*, the last syllable being a marker of its herbal value (a "wort" is a medicinal herb). The name may have from the Latin *clava* or club, probably the three-knotted club of Hercules; from the fourteenth century clover was the symbol of the card suit "clubs."

In Tudor times the plant was called *claver*, which later became *clover*. The Irish national flower, the shamrock, means "small clover," though it's really an *Oxalis*.

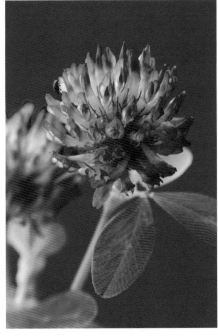

In the Middle Ages legumes, like peas, beans, and vetches, were grown as fodder and food crops. From the mid-seventeenth century farmers added red and white clover; only much later did scientists learn why it was so useful: clover fixed organic nitrogen in the soil in its root nodules. Clover remains an excellent hay (to be "in clover" still means to have abundance).

Red clover is wonderful for scrofulous and skin diseases, as an antidote to cancer, and for bronchitis and spasmodic affections.
– Dr. Christopher (1976)

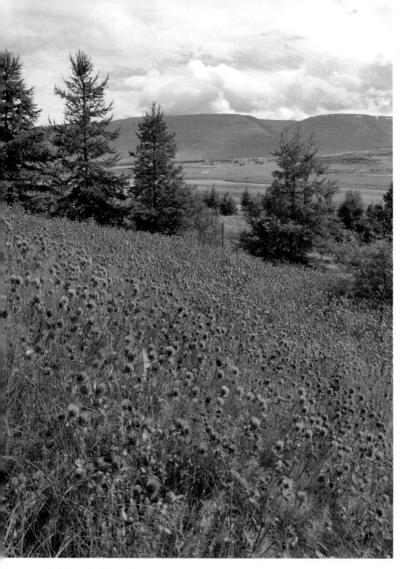

A field of wild red clover in Iceland, June

Red clover seldom cures cancer, but it fairly reliably will cause a membrane to grow around the tumor and contain it, which is helpful, especially if followed by surgery. This has especially been observed in breast cancer.
– Wood (2008)

Also, clover is beloved of bees and yields wonderful honey (the white clover is superior), and the white form, with a mass of roots, gives a fine lawn – though clover lawns are currently unfashionable.

In terms of culinary uses, clover leaves and flowers can be eaten in salads, and the seeds soaked and sprouted. Clover wine is well-liked. The dried flowers are mixed with coltsfoot leaves as a herbal tobacco or used as a snuff.

Use red clover for...

The best-known use of all for clover is of course the luck of finding a rare four-leafed one. In some folk traditions, the three leaves represented faith, hope, and charity (love), and the fourth was God's grace; in everyday terms, it meant luck. Nowadays you can order a plastic-sealed lucky four-leaved clover online (some sites offer organically grown ones). Who gets the luck, one wonders – probably the seller.

Your luck may be more certain if you use clover herbally. Red clover works gently to improve elimination over a wide front, helping the body rid itself of toxins – it can help increase the flow of urine, move mucus out of the lungs, increase the flow of bile, and act as a gentle laxative.

This slow and steady action plus its high content of trace minerals means that red clover is effective for a wide range of health problems, and is gentle enough for children. Clover is most effective when taken consistently for several months for chronic conditions such as skin problems.

Clover's ability to remove waste products, along with a capacity to prevent the formation of abnormal cells, underlies its popular reputation for treating cancers, including breast, prostate, and lymphatic forms. As with any claims for treating cancer, this has been controversial. One US pioneer of plant-based cancer remedies, Harry Hoxsey, had red clover as the main herb in his formula, and it has been used in many others.

Red clover's soothing expectorant effect is beneficial in treatments for coughs and bronchitis, and it remains "official" in the *British Herbal Pharmacopoeia* as an anti-inflammatory.

Red clover's ability to alleviate menopausal symptoms is related to its flavonoid content. Flavonoids are estrogen-like plant chemicals (or phyto-estrogens) that help maintain normal estrogen levels during menopause, providing relief for hot flashes. However, red clover is safe to use and beneficial in cases of breast cancer through reduction of high estrogen levels (see box on right).

Red clover itself does not have a blood-thinning effect but the coumarin it contains can convert to dicoumarol, which is a blood thinner, if the plants ferment on drying. If dried quickly, this will not occur, but clover should not be used in quantity by anyone taking blood-thinning medication.

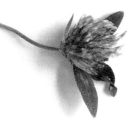

Phyto-estrogens
Phyto-estrogens can exert an estrogenic effect in the body, which is useful in the menopause when estrogen levels are low. What is less well known is the fact that they can also exert an anti-estrogenic effect in the body.

This is because phyto-estrogens have a weaker estrogenic effect than estrogens produced by the body, and both bind to estrogen receptor sites. If estrogen levels are high, the weaker plant estrogens reduce the overall estrogenic effect, which is one reason why red clover is beneficial in breast cancer treatment.

Harvesting red clover
Pick the flowers and top leaves in early summer (the flowers growing in autumn are not as sweet) when the morning dew has dried off. Choose newly opened pink flowers. Dry thoroughly, spreading them out on paper or trays, no more than one flowerhead deep, in a warm dry place away from direct sunlight. When fully dried they are crumbly to the touch. Store in glass bottles away from the light to maintain the red colour.

Red clover tea
Use 1 or 2 heaped teaspoons of dried red clover flowers per cup or mug of boiling water and allow to infuse for ten minutes. Strain and drink.

Dose: 3 or 4 cups a day. Can be taken by children. For chronic toxicity, constipation, and skin problems this tea needs to be taken consistently over a period of five or six weeks, as the effect is cumulative. To help with hot flashes, it is best drunk cold at the first onset of a flash.

Red clover and curled dock tincture
Put roughly equal amounts of **red clover blossom** and chopped **curled dock root** in a jar, and pour in enough **vodka** to cover the herbs. Leave in a dark place for two weeks, then strain. Pour the liquid into clean bottles and label.

Dose: Half a teaspoon 2 to 3 times daily.

Red clover tea
- chronic constipation
- acne
- eczema
- psoriasis
- swollen glands
- hot flashes
- coughs
- bronchitis

Red clover & curled dock tincture
- chronic constipation
- toxicity
- acne
- eczema
- psoriasis
- swollen glands

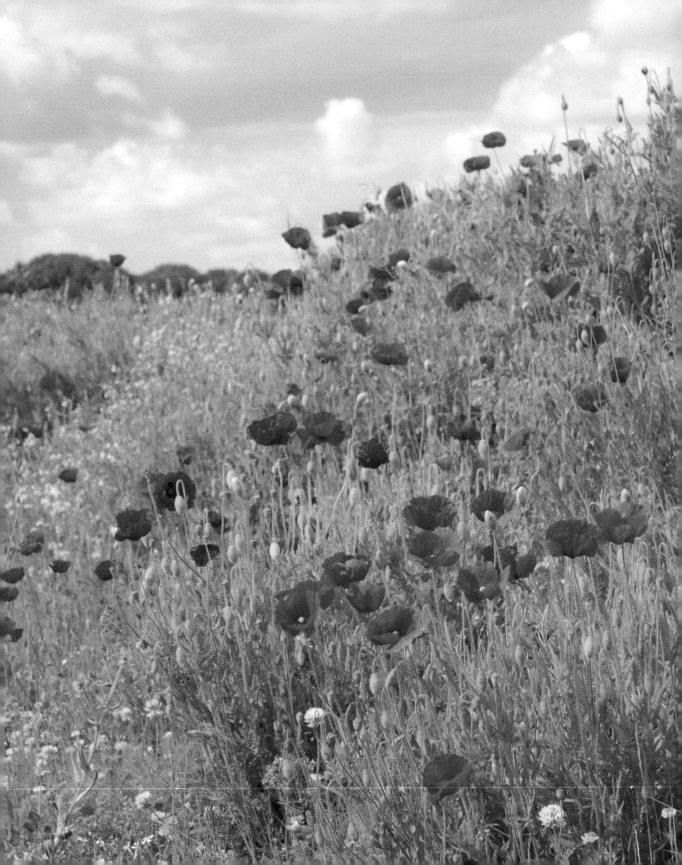

Red poppy *Papaver rhoeas*

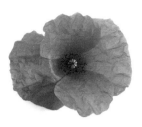

Red poppy is an archetypal weed of summer, flowering in profusion on disturbed soil and among unsprayed crops. Unwanted by farmers, it has long been a useful country herbal remedy. Red poppy is soothing and sedative, relieves pain and helps sleep, but without the narcotic effects of its relative, the opium poppy.

Papaveraceae
Poppy family

Description: An annual with bright red flowers, growing to about 2 ft. Lasts most of the summer.

Habitat: Farmland and other disturbed ground.

Distribution: Native to Europe, naturalized in much of North America.

Related species: Long-headed poppy (*P. dubium*) is very similar but has paler petals and long seed capsules. Opium poppy (*P. somniferum*) has gray–green leaves and the flowers are usually pale lilac with darker centers.

Parts used: Flowers and seeds, harvested in summer.

The poppy has always had a powerful hold on human imagination, and not just in opium dreams. Everybody in Britain knows "poppy day," held in memory of the sacrifice made by millions in World War I and since. Yet poppy is also symbolically the plant of forgetfulness and sleep. In some cultures it has been a plant of fertility, with its vast production of seeds and vivid red petals a reminder of the blood of life and of war, as also of renewal and rebirth.

As befits a plant of life, death, blood, dream and sleep, poppy coincides with man's many civilizations, and its own history is intertwined in them. It is as old as agriculture itself, growing in and alongside the earliest grain crops.

Yet British fields have not always been scarlet with poppies as the grain ripens through a hot summer. It's well within memory that the fields and hedgerows lacked virtually any poppies and other once common wild plants. Why? Because we have endured a fertilizer, herbicide and insecticide bombardment of heroic propor-

tions. The pace has only dropped in the past twenty to thirty years. Policy-makers have now rediscovered the value of leaving land fallow and of field margins, and have paid farmers to do it. Presto! the poppies have duly come back, especially where fields have been left unsprayed.

One of poppy's characteristics is that it looks and feels fragile, its stem being thin and wobbly, its gossamer-fine petals falling off to the touch, whereas in reality it is tailor-made for survival. Its flowering season is long, through the summer. Calculations have shown that each mature plant produces some 17,000 tiny seeds a year, which can sit in a state of dormancy for fifty and more years, awaiting the right conditions.

A change such as new ploughing or deep trenches being dug will release forgotten poppy seeds and give them the disturbed ground they need to flourish *en masse*. Hence the shock when poppies suddenly flowered amid the killing fields of the Great War. This stark contrast led to a Canadian

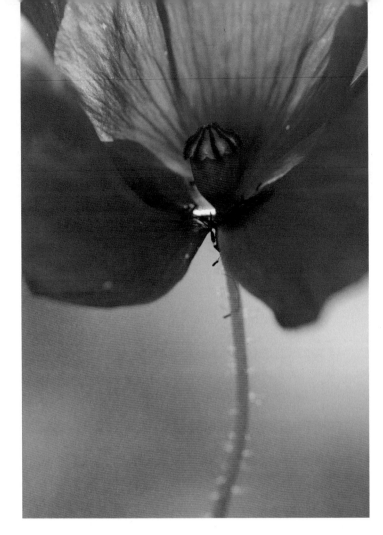

November, solemn services are held for the fallen of all wars. Participants and many besides all wear red poppies made of paper.

It is worth underlining here that our focus is on the red poppy and not the opium poppy. Opium poppies have been grown domestically in England for millennia, and 150 years ago went into laudanum (a tincture in alcohol) and paregoric elixir (a camphorated extract). Modern pain-relieving medications including morphine and codeine are derived from opium poppy, but are prescription-only.

Use red poppy for...

Red poppy doesn't have the dangerous reputation of its infamous cousin. Taking red poppy herbally is non-addictive and generally safe: its weak opiates work well medicinally but are not in strong enough concentration to do harm.

Red poppy has long been familiar in British country traditions. For example, the petals were collected as a colouring agent for wines and other herbal remedies. Indeed, the petals are still used to add colour to sweets and some herbal teas.

Red poppy petals can be added to summer salads for brightness, and the seeds collected as a topping for bread and to use in cooking. The seeds have mild sedative qualities.

Our glycerite recipe is effective for coughs, nervous digestion, anxiety, and insomnia. It is gentle and

Boil poppy heads in ale; let the patient drink it, and he will sleep.
– The Physicians of Myddfai (13th century)

The Flowers cool, and asswage Pain, and dispose to Sleep. ...
– Pechey (1707)

medical orderly, John McCrae, finding time between his terrible duties at Ypres in 1915 to write the poem "In Flanders Fields." He posted it to a magazine in London. It was printed and became immensely popular worldwide.

The poem and its powerful link to an archetypal plant of war inspired the British Legion (now the Royal British Legion) after the armistice to take up the call of remembrance. Since then, on Remembrance Day each 11th of

safe for over-excited children who cannot sleep. The petals can also be made into a tincture that will tackle similar conditions.

In general, red poppy acts as a mild sedative that also promotes perspiration, soothes respiratory passages, and calms the system. Being slightly astringent, it helps remove excess mucus and improves the digestion. It soothes itchy or sore throats and hacking coughs. For insomnia, it combines well with lime blossom, wood betony, and vervain, and can also be used with hops and wild lettuce.

Red poppy is a great plant of myth and archetype, with medicinal virtues on a more humble scale for the home medicine cabinet.

Red poppy glycerite

Fill a jar three-quarters full of a mixture of 60% **vegetable glycerine** and 40% **water**. Add **poppy petals** to fill the jar, stirring so that the petals are covered in the glycerine mixture. Put the lid on the jar and place it in a sunny spot in the garden or on a window sill.

One of the little plastic inserts used by jam makers to keep the material pushed down under the surface of the liquid is handy, but if you don't have one just shake the jar or stir the contents every day. This will keep the petals from floating on the top. Once the petals have faded to white, usually after only a few days, they can be removed and fresh ones added over the summer until your liquid is a rich deep red colour. It can then be strained, bottled, and labeled. Your glycerite should keep well in a cool dark place until next year when you can make a fresh batch.

The glycerite is particularly good for children, as it cpntains no alcohol and they will like the sweet taste. It is also good for coughs and irritable or nervous digestive tracts.

Red poppy tincture

Fill a jar with **fresh poppy petals**, then top it up with **vodka**. Put the lid on and shake well, adding a little more vodka if needed to fill the jar. Place the jar in a cool dark place – a cupboard is perfect – for two weeks, then strain and bottle.

The alcohol in a tincture makes it more warming and dispersing. While the uses are much the same as for the glycerite, the tincture is probably better for pain as it is more rapidly absorbed and has a quicker effect.

You can also combine your tincture and glycerite half and half, reducing the sweetness of the glycerite and making the tincture taste better.

Red poppy glycerite
- insomnia
- irritable cough
- nervous digestion
- irritable bowel
- headache
- over-excitability
- anxiety
- nervousness

Red poppy tincture
- insomnia
- nervous digestion
- irritable bowel
- headache
- over-excitability
- anxiety
- nervousness

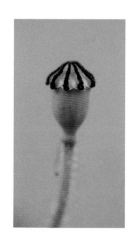

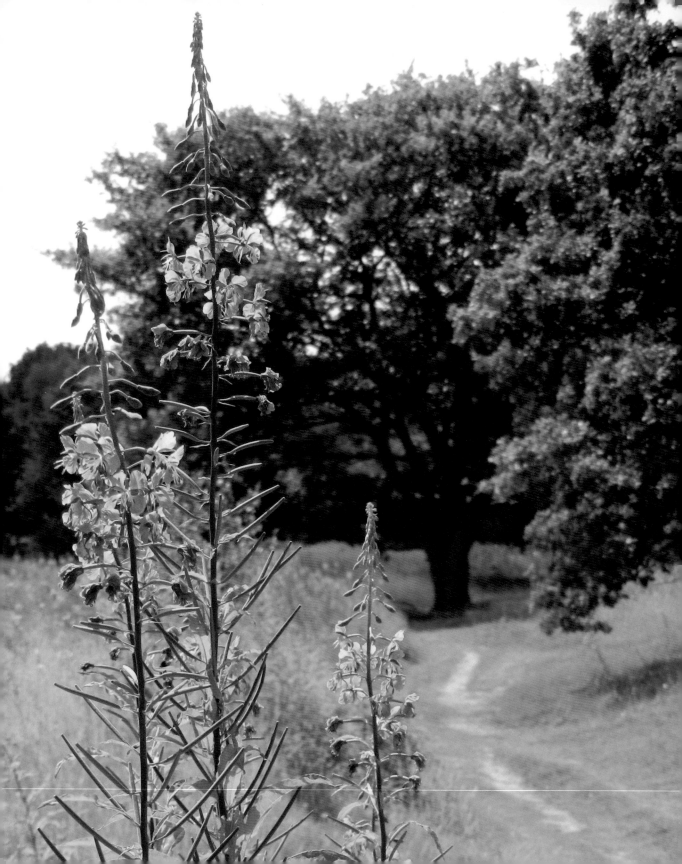

Rosebay willowherb, Fireweed

Chamerion angustifolium syn. *Epilobium angustifolium, Chamaenerion angustifolium*

This beautiful native plant is stunning enough to be grown in any garden and yet is considered a weed. A tea of rosebay has a modern use in treating prostate cancer, and the American Eclectic physicians favoured it for alleviating diarrhoea and typhoid. Its soothing, astringent and tonic action is wonderful for all sorts of intestinal irritation, and it makes a good mouthwash.

**Onagraceae
Willowherb family**

Rosebay willowherb is one of our largest and most beautiful wildflowers. In North America, it is called fireweed because of its tendency to spring up as an early pioneer on burnt land. It is rarely grown in gardens these days, except for the rare white form.

Julie remembers the excitement of seeing her first fireweed as she and her parents drove north on the Alaska Highway, when she was eleven. We've heard of one American herbalist who cheers every time she sees fireweed by the roadside, sometimes drawing strange looks. It's a plant that brings joy just by being there.

Rosebay willowherb is one of the first plants to appear whenever the earth is scarred. In World War II Britain, it sprang up on bomb sites in London and elsewhere, rising like a phoenix from the ashes and rubble (its seeds last for years in a dormant state). In Clydebank, Scotland, it colonized the bombed Singer sewing machine factory site and was nicknamed Singerweed.

The "narrow leaves" (the English version of *angustifolium*) of the plant do resemble willow enough to earn its common name, but there is no real connection, medicinal or otherwise.

Rosebay is a traditional drink and domestic medicine in northern and eastern Europe. In Russia, its fermented leaves are known as Kapor or Ivan tea, while in Alaska the flowers are a valuable source of nectar for honey, and are made into jellies and syrups. This honey is said to be the most northerly available anywhere.

Various groups of native North Americans have used rosebay as a food plant. Supposedly the young shoots boiled in the spring taste like asparagus, but we haven't tried it, and "wild food" expert Roger Phillips is not a fan, as the attached quotation suggests.

Use rosebay for...

The plant's astringency, however, works well in our syrup recipe, which is good for diarrhea and a

Description: A tall 4 to 5 ft perennial, with stunning magenta flower spikes in summer and into fall.

Habitat: Heaths, mountains, forest clearings, waste ground, and railroad embankments.

Distribution: Across northern Europe, Asia and North America; also parts of north Africa.

Related species: Rosebay willowherb is closely related to other willowherbs in the *Epilobium* genus: see page 204.

Parts used: Flower spikes and leaves, harvested in summer.

Despite all the exotic tales of eating rosebay willow-herb I have been unable to make it palatable. It is far too bitter to enjoy as any kind of vegetable.
– Phillips (1983)

pleasant remedy for children (and adults) suffering digestive upsets.

America's Eclectic doctors of a century and more ago favored rosebay willowherb for all kinds of diarrhea and enteritis, cholera infantum or typhoid dysentery. *King's American Dispensatory* (1898) said of one of the leading Eclectics: "With Prof. Scudder, infusion of epilobium was a favorite remedy to correct and restrain the diarrhea of typhoid or enteric fever."

That it has not attained prominence as a remedy is not the fault of the plant, for in certain cases of summer bowel troubles it is without an equal.
– King's American Dispensatory (1898)

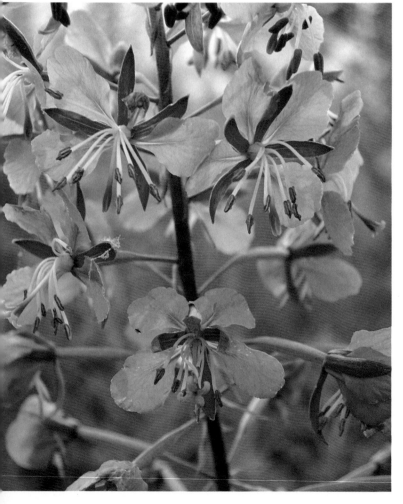

The Eclectics also used the leaf infusion for uterine bleeding and heavy periods, and the fresh leaves as a poultice for "foul and indolent ulcers." We have found it works well for mouth ulcers.

Modern American herbalist David Winston uses rosebay leaves to treat candida overgrowth.

Research on rosebay in recent years has focused on its role in treating BPH (benign prostatic hyperplasia), including a 2013 in vitro study described as "promising." The ellagitannin known as oenotherin B contained in rosebay leaves and flowers (both have been shown to be equally effective) is now accepted as the significant factor in inhibiting prostate cancer cell growth in animals and by inference in humans.

Other recorded uses of rosebay include the leaves as a smudge stick (the Upper Tanana Indians of Alaska) and from Scotland boiling down roots to treat minor wounds of horses, such as saddle burrs.

Several flower essence makers produce a fireweed essence, for connecting us to the healing energies of nature and the earth. They believe it helps in resolving problems concerning change and in shifting stagnant energy patterns. It is used both for a "burnt-out" feeling and for shock and trauma. If you'd like to try making your own rosebay essence, follow the instructions given on page 170.

Rosebay willowherb leaf poultice

The fresh leaves can be crushed and applied as a poultice to help minor wounds heal. Hold the leaves on with a plaster, and change for fresh crushed leaves a couple of times a day until healed. The early American Eclectic doctors found it effective for old ulcers.

Rosebay willowherb tea

The leaves can be harvested in the spring or while the plant is in flower in the summer, and dried for use throughout the year. To dry, spread the leaves on paper in a shady place, turning them occasionally until crisp.

Use 3 or 4 **leaves** per cup of **boiling water** and infuse for about 5 minutes. Drink frequently for diarrhea, or use as a substitute for ordinary tea.

Can be used as a mouthwash for mouth ulcers and a gargle for sore throats.

Fermented rosebay willowherb tea

The **fresh leaves** are placed in a jar with the lid on and left in a sunny place until they have sweated and darkened. This will only take a few days, but we forgot a jar once and it was still OK six months later. The leaves can be used straightaway or be dried and used as above as a tea. The flavor is slightly sour and less astringent than the unfermented tea.

Rosebay willowherb syrup

20 flower heads
2 cups water

Bring to the boil and simmer until the colour leaves the blossoms, in about 5–10 minutes. Strain the juice, return to the pot.

Add **4 oz sugar** to the reduced fluid, and **juice of a lemon.**

This turns the pale colour a bright pink, almost like the blossoms you start with. Boil for 5 minutes, allow to cool a little, then bottle and label.

It will keep in the fridge for a few months.

This is a pleasant remedy for childhood diarrh ea, and can be used for any case of intestinal irritation associated with loose bowels.

Dose: A dessertspoonful for children and a tablespoonful for adults, every few hours as needed.

Rosebay poultice
- ulcers
- minor wounds

Rosebay leaf tea
- digestion
- diarrhea
- irritable bowel
- heavy periods
- mouth ulcers
- sore throats
- prostate problems

Rosebay syrup
- diarrhea
- loose bowels
- childhood diarrhea

[Rosebay essence]
Cleanses old patterns from the body and stimulates renewal of energies on all levels of being; attracts restorative healing energy from our surroundings.
– Rudd (1998)

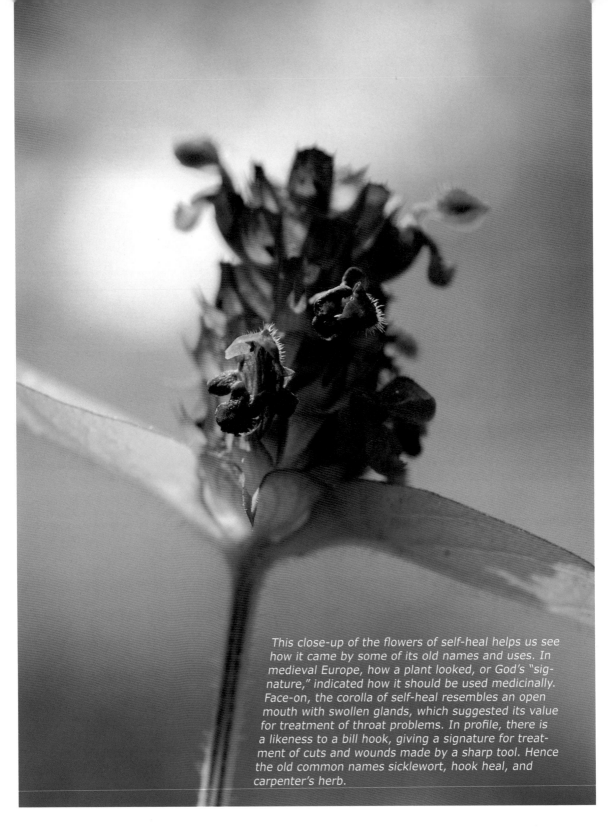

This close-up of the flowers of self-heal helps us see how it came by some of its old names and uses. In medieval Europe, how a plant looked, or God's "signature," indicated how it should be used medicinally. Face-on, the corolla of self-heal resembles an open mouth with swollen glands, which suggested its value for treatment of throat problems. In profile, there is a likeness to a bill hook, giving a signature for treatment of cuts and wounds made by a sharp tool. Hence the old common names sicklewort, hook heal, and carpenter's herb.

Self-heal *Prunella vulgaris*

Also called all-heal, self-heal was mentioned in Chinese medical literature of the Han dynasty (206 BC to AD 23), and is still used in Traditional Chinese Medicine. It was popular for centuries in Europe as a wound herb and for throat problems.

Self-heal has gained recent respect for its antiviral qualities. Effective for combatting feverish colds and flu, it has been proposed for treating herpes and AIDS, and is an underrated liver, gallbladder, and thyroid remedy.

As you would expect from a plant known as all-heal, self-heal has a wide range of medicinal actions. It is, however, underused in contemporary western herbal medicine.

Self-heal has a long history of western folk use. One name it acquired was "touch and heal," indicating its value as first aid for cuts and wounds. It was also found to staunch bleeding and help knit a wound together. Taken internally as a tea, it treated fevers, diarrhea, and internal bleeding.

The Latin name *Prunella* was given by Linnaeus to *Brunella*, the German name of the plant. This reflected its use for "die Braüne" or quinsy, meaning a throat abscess. A self-heal tea was taken internally, and a self-heal mouthwash and gargle used to treat a wide range of mouth and throat problems.

In the European tradition the plant is picked just before or while flowering, but in China the flower tops are collected in late summer when they are starting to wither. This variation in time of harvesting, along with regional variations in the plant's chemistry, could explain the different uses of self-heal in the two traditions.

In Chinese medicine, self-heal is given for ascending liver fire and liver deficiency. It clears liver congestion and stagnation and brightens the eyes, which are regarded as linked to the liver. In common with European use, it is said to lessen heat and dissipate nodules, particularly in the neck, such as scrofula, lipoma, swollen glands, and goiter.

Use self-heal for...

Julie has always used self-heal in her practice, mainly for treating flu and hot flashes. We knew we needed to take a deeper look at this plant when it seeded itself with exuberance all over our garden while we were writing this book – it seemed to be trying to

Lamiaceae (Labiatae) Deadnettle family

Description: A creeping perennial with downy leaves and violet flowers, reaching up to a foot tall.

Habitat: Lawns, meadows, and woods.

Distribution: Found virtually worldwide in temperate areas. Widespread in North America.

Related species: Cut-leaved self-heal (*P. laciniata*) has creamy white flowers and is found on dry lime soils.

Parts used: Flowers and leaves, dry flower spikes.

tell us something. The more we thought about and used self-heal, the more impressed we became.

Recent studies have shown self-heal to be an effective remedy for herpes. If we look back at the old herbals, we see this is not new. In 1640, John Parkinson wrote that self-heal "juice mixed with a little Hony of Roses, clenseth and healeth all ulcers and sores in the mouth and throate, and those also in the secret parts." We know today that both roses and self-heal have antiviral properties.

Self-heal is a good remedy for flu and fevers because it combines cooling, immune-stimulating, and antiviral qualities. It has been found to be effective against a broad range of bacteria, including *Mycobacterium tuberculi*, which causes tuberculosis.

The old use for goiter ties in with American herbalist James Duke's research on self-heal. He found it to be among the most effective herbs for hypothyroidism (underactive thyroid), which often leads to a goiter formation. He has also confirmed that self-heal treats Graves' disease and other hyperactive thyroid conditions. This means its effect is amphoteric, that is, it normalizes function by stimulating an underactive gland or reducing overactivity.

Self-heal is high on Duke's list of plants with marked antioxidant activity. Studies show that self-heal has strong immune-stimulatory effects, and calms inflammatory and allergic responses. In preventing viruses from replicating, it shows promise in the treatment of AIDS. It is also used for diabetes and high blood pressure.

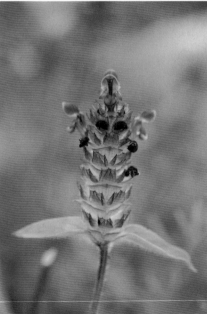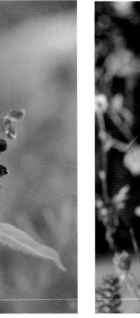

Self-heal ready for picking: the fresh flower in western medicine (left); the dried flower in Chinese medicine (right).

Self-heal tea

For tea, we prefer to harvest the flower spikes when they mature and are turning brown, drying naturally on the plant. You can shake out any ripe seeds to sow, ensuring a supply of plants for the years ahead.

Use about two **flower spikes** per mug of **boiling water** and infuse for 5 to 10 minutes. Drink freely. For hot flashes, it is best drunk cool. It can be used as a mouthwash and gargle for mouth ulcers and sore throats.

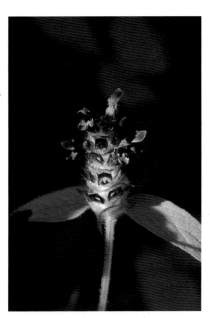

Self-heal infused oil

Fill a jar with **fresh self-heal blossoms and leaves**. Pour **olive oil** in to fill the jar, stirring as you do so to allow air bubbles to escape. Cover the jar with a piece of cloth held on with a rubber band – this will allow any moisture to evaporate. Place the jar on a sunny window sill.

Check the jar every few days, and if necessary push the plant material back down under the surface of the oil. After two to four weeks the colour will have drained out of the plants. Strain off the oil. Allow it to settle, so that any water will sink to the bottom, then pour the oil carefully into bottles and label. This oil will keep for several years, but it is best to make a fresh batch every summer if you can.

Self-heal cream

To make a cream, you will be using some of the **self-heal oil** you have made, and combining it with a strong **self-heal tea**. This cream recipe can be used for other herbs or combinations of herbs too.

2 fl oz self-heal oil
3/4 oz beeswax
2 fl oz self-heal tea

Put the oil and beeswax in one bowl and the tea in another, and stand them both in a large pan of hot water. Heat until the beeswax melts. It is important that they are both the same temperature. Slowly pour the tea into the oil mixture while beating with an electric mixer set at the slowest speed. If you want, you can add a few drops of **self-heal stock essence** (instructions on next page). Once all the oil is mixed in and the mixture has emulsified and thickened, pour the cream into clean jars. Once set, label, and store in a cool place or in the fridge.

Self-heal tea
- general well-being
- fevers
- flu & viral infections
- mouth ulcers
- thyroid disorders
- throat problems

Self-heal cold infusion
- hot flashes

Self-heal oil and cream
- cuts
- sores
- wounds
- aches and pains
- swellings in the throat

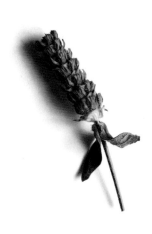

Self-heal flower essence

To make the flower essence, find a patch of self-heal growing in a peaceful sunny spot. Just sit near the plants for a while until you feel relaxed and at peace with the plants and the place. Because flower essences are based on the vibrational energy of a plant rather than its chemistry, your intention is important.

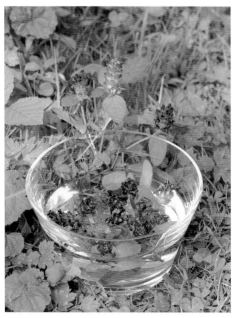

When you are ready, place a small clear glass bowl on the ground near the plants. Fill it with about a cupful of **rain water or spring water**, then pick enough **flowers** from nearby to cover the surface of the water. Leave them there for an hour or two – you can relax nearby or go for a walk while they infuse. The water will still look clear, but the flowers may have wilted. Use a twig to lift them carefully out of the water, and then pour the water into a bottle that is half full of **brandy.** This is called your **mother essence**. You can use any size of bottle you like, but a half pint blue glass bottle works well, and it may be easier to fill if you make use of a funnel. If there is any water left over, you can drink it.

Flower essence
- self-healing
- motivation
- inner direction
- transformation

To use your essence, put three drops of mother essence in a small (1 fl oz) dropper bottle filled with brandy. Using this **stock bottle**, you can:
- put 20 drops in the bath, then soak in it for at least twenty minutes.
- rub directly on the skin, or mix into creams.
- put a few drops in a glass or bottle of water and sip during the day.
- make a **dosage bottle** to carry around with you, by putting three drops of stock essence into a dropper bottle containing a 50/50 brandy and water mix or pure distilled rosewater. Use several drops directly under the tongue as often as you feel you need it, or at least twice daily.

Self-heal essence reminds us that all healing is self-healing, and is valuable if you are ill and don't know where to turn for help. It will help you choose the therapies that will be beneficial, and enkindle your own innate healing energy. It can be used alongside any other form of treatment to enhance its effectiveness and benefits without risk of negative interaction. Self-heal doesn't just work on a physical level, but will support the mental and emotional aspects of healing. It also serves to calm and center the spirit, benefitting meditation and prayer.

Shepherd's purse _Capsella bursa-pastoris_

Shepherd's purse stops bleeding of all sorts from nosebleeds to blood in the urine. It was used in World War I battles to staunch bleeding from wounds when ergot, an effective but more dangerous remedy, was not available.

Shepherd's purse also has an amazing ability to correct prolapses, especially of the uterus but also of the bladder, moving the organs back into their correct position.

This common little herb, which most people know as a weed if at all, has an ancient history of herbal use, suggested in its beautiful Latin name. The plant's seed cases are said to resemble the heart-shaped satchels once worn on men's belts, whether shepherds or not.

Use shepherd's purse for...
The aerial parts of shepherd's purse are all used herbally. Externally, it has been found excellent and safe in treating rheumatic aches and pains, and for ecchymosis, i.e., bleeding beneath the skin. Taken internally for kidney and bladder irritation, it is particularly good for mucus in the urine.

Less well known is its ability to treat prolapses. Julie had first-hand experience when she suffered a uterine prolapse. Within an hour of taking shepherd's purse tincture she could feel the uterus moving back into place, and three hours later the discomfort was mostly gone. She was back to normal in three days with the tincture, helped by yoga and reflexology.

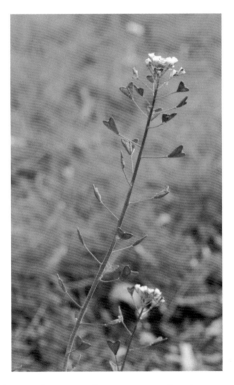

Brassicaceae (Cruciferae) Cabbage family

Description: Most easily recognized by its heart-shaped seed pods, this is a small annual with a rosette of slightly hairy, lobed leaves and tiny white flowers.

Habitat: Cultivated and disturbed ground.

Distribution: Native to Europe and Asia but widely naturalized in North America and other temperate regions.

Related species: There are several other plants in the genus. Pink shepherd's purse (_C. rubella_) has pink flowers and is occasionally found in the British Isles.

Parts used: Above-ground parts.

Another case history involved a patient who had great discomfort and a bulging on the side of her vulva. She went to the nurse at the doctor's surgery, who examined her and said she had a uterine prolapse. The patient started taking shepherd's purse, and felt a fairly rapid improvement. Six days later,

Contra-indications
Avoid taking shepherd's purse internally during pregnancy because it can stimulate uterine contractions.

Fresh shepherd's purse plant
- cuts
- nosebleeds
- rheumatism
- bleeding under skin

Shepherd's purse tincture
- bleeding
- heavy periods
- prolapses
- blood in urine
- wounds
- hemorrhoids

Combined with hawthorn and lime blossom
- high blood pressure

Perhaps the most important cruciferous plant with medicinal use, it has been known as a haemostatic for centuries and evidence of its use has been found at Neolithic sites, probably as condiment and vegetable as much as medication.
– Barker (2001)

her doctor examined her again and said the nurse must have made a mistake because the patient didn't have a prolapse at all.

Shepherd's purse also works for bladder prolapse. A woman had been diagnosed with this condition, which was causing her pain and discomfort. She didn't want surgery, so came to see Julie.

The formula Julie gave was shepherd's purse and a bladder tea of uva ursi, couch grass, buchu, cornsilk, and horsetail. To support this, the patient began Pilates and did Kegel, i.e., pelvic floor, exercises. After a month she felt much better, and her doctor was amazed. Her urine had cleared. Two months later there were no signs of any problem and she felt fantastic.

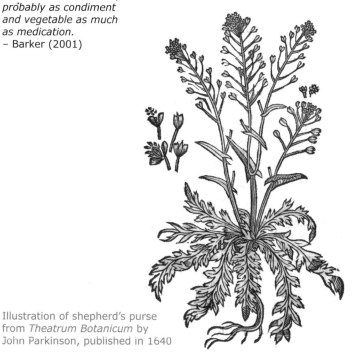

Illustration of shepherd's purse from *Theatrum Botanicum* by John Parkinson, published in 1640

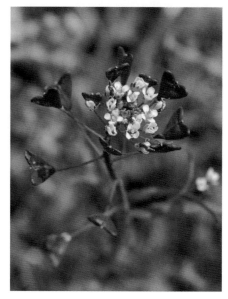

Shepherd's purse has small white flowers, which are quickly followed by the plant's signature heart-shaped pods

Shepherd's purse has been used during childbirth to stimulate uterine contractions and reduce postpartum bleeding.

For high blood pressure, shepherd's purse combines well with hawthorn and lime blossom. Mix the tinctures together, using 5 parts hawthorn, 3 parts lime blossom and 2 parts shepherd's purse. Take 20 drops in a little water or juice twice a day.

During World War I in Germany shepherd's purse was used as a less toxic substitute for ergot to stop bleeding.

One of Julie's patients complained of blood in his urine. The man's doctor had found that the blood was coming from weak blood vessels in his prostate. Shepherd's purse soon stopped the bleeding, and he then took bilberry to strengthen the blood vessels. He occasionally needed to take shepherd's purse over the next year, but had no later bleeding problem.

Shepherd's purse puts out flowers and seeds virtually all year round. It is best picked in the summer for making a tincture, but can be used fresh at any time. The leaves are tastiest before the flowers appear and can be eaten in salads; they are rich in vitamins A, B, and C. The seedpods can be used chopped up in soups and stews for their peppery taste. In Japan, shepherd's purse is grown as a vegetable and to flavor rice.

Because the flowering plant has a rather unpleasant taste, we prefer the tincture form (where a small dose is sufficient) rather than as an infusion or decoction, although these will work perfectly well too.

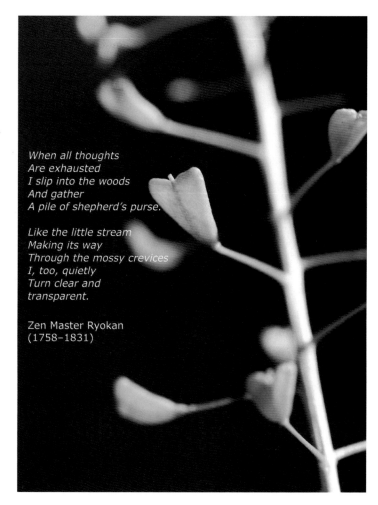

When all thoughts
Are exhausted
I slip into the woods
And gather
A pile of shepherd's purse.

Like the little stream
Making its way
Through the mossy crevices
I, too, quietly
Turn clear and
transparent.

Zen Master Ryokan
(1758–1831)

Shepherd's purse tincture

Pick **shepherd's purse** while it is flowering, preferably in the summer. Fill a jar with the herb, then pour on **vodka** until it is covered. Put the jar away in a cool dark cupboard for a month, shaking the jar daily or as frequently as you can remember to do it. Strain off the liquid, pour it into a bottle, and label.

Dose: For bleeding, take half a teaspoonful three times a day until the bleeding stops and then discontinue. For prolapse, 5 drops three times a day in a little water is usually sufficient. Continue taking it for a few days after everything has moved back into place.

Formula for high blood pressure

Combine tinctures: 2 parts **shepherd's purse**, 3 parts **lime blossom** and 5 parts **hawthorn berry**.

Dose: 20 drops twice daily in water.

Sorrel *Rumex acetosa*

**Polygonaceae
Dock family**

Description: Slender perennial, 8" to 2 ft tall, with hollow stems; lower leaves have downward-pointing lobes, upper leaves clasp the stem; flowers reddish, in massed whorls.

Habitat: Meadows, pastures, mountains, and seashore.

Distribution: Widespread across Eurasia; introduced to northern states of US/Canada.

Related species: One of 200-plus *Rumex* species, with curled dock (p58), buckwheat and rhubarb. Sheep's sorrel (*R. acetosella*) is as common as sorrel, and more so across North America; it is smaller, low-growing, with solid stems; likes poorer soils. French sorrel (*R. scutatus*) has broader, silvery "shield-like" leaves; a garden plant and once widely cultivated. Wood sorrel (*Oxalis acetosella*) is unrelated but has similar qualities and taste.

Parts used: Leaves and roots.

Caution: High intake of sorrel causes build-up of oxalic acids, and sometimes kidney stones. Avoid if prone to gout or rheumatism.

Wild sorrel is newly fashionable (e.g., sorrel sorbet or oil) and widely foraged; it is a French cookery classic (as in the famous soup). It has an old reputation as a refreshing palate-cleanser, but also an exaggerated respect as a plague herb and in modern times as part of a controversial herbal anti-cancer formula. There is a middle ground, where its cooling astringency can be beneficial.

Sorrel is sour and astringent, but refreshing to the taste, as reflected in such old English names as sour leaves, green sauce, and sour dabs. The Latin species name *acetosa* means vinegar-like.

Like the Egyptians before them, ancient Greeks and Romans would chew on baskets of sorrel leaves between courses of their meals. Country dwellers in England and their children appreciated wild sorrel leaves too; we now know these are high in vitamin C.

A Channel Islands folk saying, probably from the 17th century, ran: "Eate leekes with sorye [sorrel] in March, cresses in April, Ramsons in May, and all yeare after ye physitions may goe play."

This was everyday wisdom. A more elite view is that of John Evelyn at much the same time. Sorrel, in his 1699 work on salads (*Acetaria*), is "sharpning Appetite, asswages Heat, cools the Liver, strengthens the Heart; is an Anti-scorbutic, resisting Putrefaction."

For Evelyn sorrel was a citrus substitute; indeed, it has been called "the lemon of the North," used in place of rennet for curdling milk.

Sorrel is cooling, and was used to bring down fevers. John Parkinson (1640) claimed more: sorrel would "refresh overspent spirits with the violence of furious or fiery fits of agues." Before antibiotics, any strong-flavoured herb was called into use against the plague, but, regrettably, nothing really worked.

In a somewhat parallel way, in our own times the Canadian herbal formula Essiac (which includes sheep sorrel) has been acclaimed for treating cancers; a clinical trial of 510 Canadian women (2006), however, found no such effect.

On the other hand, another herbal formulation, Sinupret®, which also has sorrel as an ingredient, was shown (2011) to reduce symptoms of rhinosinusitis and common cold. Sorrel's antiviral potential should be further explored, e.g., for inflamed mucous membranes.

Sorrel juice alone, in ale or with milk (a posset) is a tart gargle, or can ease an upset stomach. French naturopath Maurice Mességué liked sorrel "for all urinary and digestive malfunctions."

Externally, sorrel leaves make an effective poultice. Parkinson wrote that leaves "roasted under the embers, and applied to an hard impostume [abscess], botch, bile or plague sore, both ripeneth and breaketh it." Acne and any hot skin condition will be eased by a sorrel juice poultice.

Another word of caution, to add to that on oxalic acid noted opposite. Use stainless steel pans for cooking sorrel; aluminium utensils can react with it to create harmful toxins.

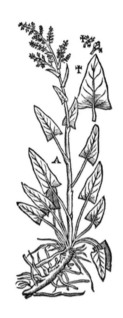

"Our ordinary Sorrell'," *Acetosa vulgaris*: a woodcut from Parkinson, *Theatrum Botanicum* (1640)

Sorrel zhug

Zhug is a Yemeni savory sauce. It is often fiery, but on a recent trip to Tel Aviv we were given a more moderate version that is now a family favorite. We replace the usual lemon juice with sorrel leaves here.

In your blender load two handfuls of **coriander leaves** to one handful each of **parsley** and **sorrel leaves**. Add a small **green chilli**, a teaspoon of **cardamom powder** (this harmonizes the ingredients) and a pinch of **salt**. Pour in enough **olive oil** to blend into a paste. It will keep for a week in the fridge, but actually is usually gobbled up within a day.

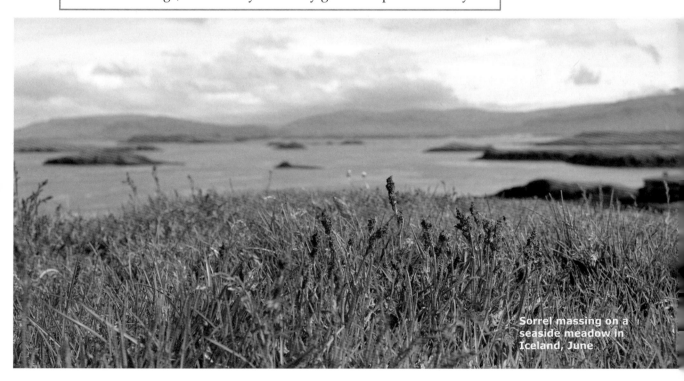

Sorrel massing on a seaside meadow in Iceland, June

St. John's wort *Hypericum perforatum*

Hypericaceae
St. John's wort family

Description: A midsized perennial with yellow flowers. It is distinguished from other species of *Hypericum* by the "perforations" in the leaf, which are actually oil glands.

Habitat: Roadsides, hedge banks, rough grassland, meadows, and open woodland.

Distribution: Native to Europe; an introduced weed in North America and Australasia.

Related species: There are several other species of St. John's wort, but they are not as good medicinally, so check for the "perforations" in the leaf by holding one up to the sun.

Parts used: Flowering tops.

St. John's wort has become well known as a herb for treating depression and SAD, but it is far more than that. An antiseptic wound herb of ancient repute, it was the main plant of St. John, the sun herb of midsummer and a protector against evil and unseen influences. In modern terms, it strengthens the nervous system and the digestion, protects the liver, is antiviral, and reduces pain; it is a plant for support through life-cycle changes.

The protecting power of St. John's wort derives from a powerful mix of observed herbal benefits and the plant's part in the Christian adaptation of older midsummer sun and fire "pagan" ceremonies.

Its Latin name *Hypericum* gives us clues about the takeover of one form of sun-magic by another. The *hyper-ikon* was a herb placed above St. John's image, or painted icon; by extension, it meant power over ghosts or invisible bad spirits. It was particularly important to invoke the plant's help on St. John's eve against witchcraft or diabolic influences (see panel on p179).

St. John's wort was a powerful sun herb to dispel darkness, and it had the "signatures" to prove it. The so-called "holes" in the leaves, the *perforata* of the Latin name, were emblematic of St. John's holy wounds and martyrdom, along with the red "blood" of the plant's extract. Scientists now know the holes to be resinous glands of hypericin and other active com-

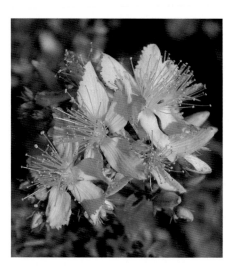

pounds. The cross formed by the leaves, seen from above, was also symbolic of the plant's power.

The sun is said to control the solar (sun) plexus in the body. In yogic systems this is a center of protective energy that is ruled by the yellow part of the spectrum. This affinity of St. John's wort with the solar plexus extends to the plant's use in treating the digestive and nervous systems. It is also taken for life-cycle conditions, e.g., bedwetting in the young, menstrual problems, and menopause. The solar plexus governs "gut instinct" and life's unseen influences – again leading us to protection.

This may sound rather esoteric, but we have certainly found for ourselves that the actual time of picking St. John's wort flowers does matter in a practical sense.

We once gathered it on impulse on a summer evening while driving to a party in north Norfolk. We knew we should harvest in the middle of the day, but thought we'd try anyway. We put our beautiful yellow flowers into olive oil on arriving home, and placed the jar on a south-facing window-sill to infuse. Nothing happened. That jar was in the sun for months, but never turned red.

On the other hand, some of the best St. John's wort oil we've ever made was on a visit to Italy. In Ostia Antica, the ancient harbor town for Rome, there were many interesting plants, including St. John's wort, which was growing only among the ruined temples.

It was actually St. John's day, June 24, and very hot. We picked enough flowers to make a small jar of oil and infused it on our friend's balcony in Rome. Within hours it was a wonderful deep red color.

Use St. John's wort for...
What we find interesting is that modern uses of the plant, as we will outline, differ so much from

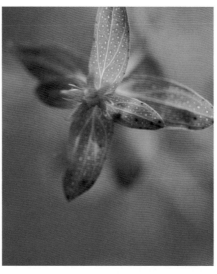

When the light shines through the leaves of perforate St. John's wort, the oil glands look like holes (hence *perforatum* in the name). There are ten times more glands in the flowers than the leaves or stems.

S. Iohns wort is as singular a wound herbe as any other whatsoever, eyther for inward wounds, hurts or bruises, to be boyled in wine and drunke, or prepared into oyle or oyntment, bathe or lotion out-wardly... it hath power to open obstructions, to dissolve tumours, to consolidate or soder the lips of wounds, and to strengthen the parts that are weake and feeble.
– Parkinson (1640)

the more traditional uses. Look at Parkinson's list of its benefits (right): few herbalists will now use St. John's wort to dissolve tumors. Mrs. Grieve, writing in 1931, says it is good for pulmonary complaints, bladder problems, diarrhea, jaundice, and nervous depression, among others.

No mention there of a modern and effective use of St. John's wort for what we now call seasonal affective disorder (SAD), where people feel low and depressed in the dark months of northern European winters. A spoonful of home-made St. John's wort tincture will light you up inside with a warm glow.

St. John's wort's reputation for helping lift the darkness of de-pression has grown considerably. This use of the herb has been well researched in the last forty years and has stimulated a surge in sales of St. John's wort products. It is known that hypericin interferes

Caution: Do not take St. John's wort along-side antidepressant medication without the supervision of a herbal or medical practitioner. Seek professional advice before taking the herb if you are on any medication, includ-ing the contraceptive pill, or are pregnant.

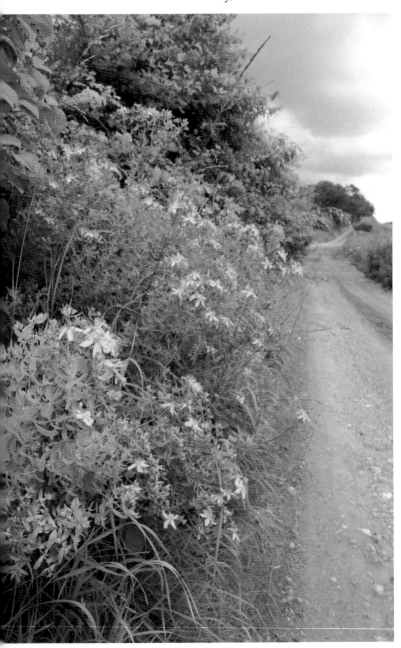

St. John's wort growing along a lane in Norfolk, England, St. John's day, June 24

with monoamine oxidase (MAO), which contributes to depression. Pharmaceutical products also act as MAO inhibitors, but St. John's wort is a slow treatment, and, crucially, has few side effects.

Taking the plant as a flower essence or tincture will help in improving sleep quality, an important issue in depression. We also give a sleep pillow recipe.

St. John's wort treatment has been officially recognized in Germany since 1984 as effective for mild to moderate depression. When the protocol was publicized, St. John's wort products soon outsold Prozac by a factor of seven to one.

A "modern" way of looking at depression has some interesting precursors. One example is an early nineteenth-century verse by Alfred Lear Huxford; this links a ceremonial use of St. John's wort leaves bound to the forehead and the relief of "dark thoughts":

So thus about her brow/ They bound Hypericum, *whose potent leaves/ Have sovereign powers o'er all the sullen fits/ And cheerless fancies that besiege the mind;/ Banishing ever, to their native night/ Dark thoughts, and causing to spring up within/ The heart distress'd, a glow of gladdening hope,/ And rainbow visions of kind destiny.*

If you change the world-view from religious to scientific, from old "superstition" to modern "rationalism," is it so far from fear of possession by evil spirits to modern clinical depression? Perhaps, like great literature, our major herbs adapt to the neuroses and psychic needs of the time; St. John's wort has done this beautifully.

However, it would not be true to say the herb has no side effects at all. One, which is sometimes experienced among the fair-skinned, is to make them more sensitive to the sun. Care is needed if you burn easily, and the herb should be avoided if you need to be out in the sun and in danger of burning.

This proneness to sunburn extends to cattle. They are liable to gorge on the plant and can die, which is why many state laws have proscribed as noxious *H. perforatum*, the introduced St. John's wort, known as Klamath weed.

It was also an unwelcome chance arrival in Australasia and South Africa in the nineteenth century. Spreading by seeds as well as active vegetative roots, it quickly overtakes native vegetation and becomes a problem for livestock.

In the doctrine of signatures yellow-colored herbs are often associated with the liver and an ability to treat jaundice. This can be unfounded, but St. John's wort is a case in point, working to relieve liver tension and harmonizing the action of the liver with other digestive organs.

Its action is gently decongesting, strengthening both liver and gallbladder. But because St. John's wort helps the liver break down and get rid of toxins, it can lower levels of certain drugs in the body, reducing their effectiveness. The best advice here is: do not use

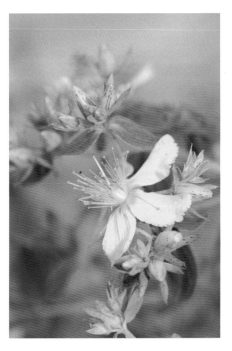

St. John's wort alongside any pharmaceutical medication without first seeking the advice of your herbal practitioner or doctor.

Taking St. John's wort improves your absorption of nutrients, and helps normalize stomach acid levels whether too high or too low. It is a well-known treatment for ulcers, heartburn, and bloating.

It is also one of the best herbs for treating shingles, being antiviral as well as pain-relieving and also speeding up tissue repair. Use the infused oil externally over the painful area, and take the tincture internally at the same time.

As a proven antiviral, St. John's wort may have future benefits for HIV and AIDS treatment, but more human research is needed.

Herbs of St. John
St. John's wort is one of the main herbs of St. John the Baptist, whose birthday was taken to be June 24. It is no coincidence that John, the precursor of Christ, was given a birthdate in midsummer and Christ himself in midwinter. This was one way the year's solstices were appropriated from older pagan festivals by the Christian Church.

St. John's wort, which blooms so brightly around midsummer, whether taken as solstice or saint's day, is the name-plant for this time. Other herbs of St. John were great plantain, mugwort, yarrow, and vervain (all in this book), and corn marigold, dwarf elder, ivy, and orpine (*Sedum telephium*).

The herbs of St. John were gathered on the morning of June 24, before sunrise. That evening fires were lit, the smoke purifying both herbs and the people (and cattle) who crossed over the fires. The plants were now sanctified by the saint's power, and went into amulets, were placed above doorways and in cattle stalls, and stored for later use.

The overall protection afforded is well summarized in the French phrase *avoir toutes les herbes de la St-Jean*, meaning ready and safeguarded for everything.

St. John's wort tincture
- seaonal affective disorder (SAD)
- mild depression
- liver congestion
- shingles
- nervous exhaustion
- menopausal moods
- viral infections
- jet lag

St. John's wort infused oil
- backache
- sore muscles
- neuropathy
- neuralgia
- shingles
- arthritis
- surgical scars
- bruises
- sprains

St. John's wort pillow
- nightmares
- bad dreams
- fear of the dark

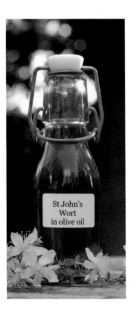

St John's Wort in olive oil

The oil also works well as a rub for backache, sore muscles, and gums, and being antiseptic will help heal wounds arising from injuries or surgery, as in older formulations.

From its former reputation as a "cure-all" is derived the name of the garden form of St. John's wort, tutsan, the name a corruption of the French name *La toute-sainte*.

Harvesting St. John's wort
St. John's wort really needs to be picked on a sunny day, when the sun is high in the sky. Pick the **flowering tops** of the plant, i.e., the flowers, buds, and leaves. The stems are quite wiry, so use a pair of scissors.

St. John's wort tincture
Put the **flowering tops** in a clear glass jar large enough to hold what you've picked, then pour on **vodka** until the herb is submerged. Put the lid on the jar, and shake to remove any air bubbles. Top up with a little more vodka if necessary.

Put the jar in a cupboard or other place away from the light for about a month, shaking occasionally. Your tincture is ready when the flowers have faded and the liquid is a reddish colour. Strain, bottle, and label.

Dose: Half to 1 teaspoonful three times daily.

St. John's wort infused oil
Put the **flowering tops** you have picked into a clear glass jar, then pour on **extra virgin olive oil** until the herb is completely covered. Put the lid on and shake the jar to remove any air bubbles, then place on a sunny window sill for a month.

Check every now and then to make the sure the herb is still submerged in the oil, and if necessary stir it back under. The oil should turn red.

Strain off the oil, bottle, and label.

Use externally as needed for backache, sore muscles, sciatica, neuralgia, arthritic joints, and to help heal wounds.

St. John's wort pillow
Dry St. John's wort flowering tops outside in the shade. Strip the leaves and flowers off the stalks and discard the stalks. Make a small cloth bag, leaving one end unstitched. Fill the bag loosely with the dried flowers and leaves, then stitch or tie the open end shut. Place the bag underneath your pillow.

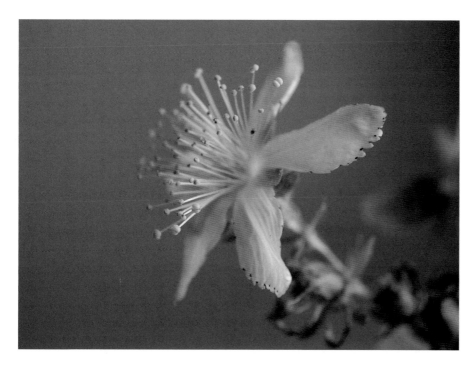

St. John's wort flower essence

Find a patch of St. John's wort growing in a peaceful spot. On a clear sunny day sit near the plants for a while until you feel relaxed and at peace. Because flower essences are based on the vibrational energy of a plant rather than its chemistry, your intention is important.

Place a small clear glass bowl on the ground near the plants. Fill it with about a cupful of **rain water or spring water**, then use a pair of scissors to pick enough **flowers** to cover the surface of the water. Leave them there for an hour or two. The water will still look clear, but the flowers may have wilted. Use your scissors to lift them carefully out of the water, then pour the water into a bottle that is half full of **brandy**. This is your **mother essence**. You can use any size of bottle you like, but a half pint blue glass bottle works well, and it may be easier to fill if you use a funnel. If there is any water left over, drink it.

To use your essence, put three drops of mother essence in a small (1 fl oz) dropper bottle filled with brandy. Using this **stock bottle**, you can:
• put 20 drops in the bath, then soak in it for at least twenty minutes.
• rub directly on the skin, or mix into creams.
• put a few drops in a glass or bottle of water and sip during the day.
• make a **dosage bottle** by putting three drops of stock essence into a dropper bottle containing a 50/50 brandy and water mix. Use several drops directly under the tongue as needed, or at least twice daily.

St. John's wort flower essence
• allergies
• environmental stress
• nightmares
• bedwetting
• seasonal affective disorder (SAD)
• protection

Sweet cicely *Myrrhis odorata*

**Apiaceae
(Umbelliferae)
Carrot family**

Description: An aromatic perennial with foamy umbels of creamy white flowers, up to 3 ft tall.

Habitat: Stream banks, roadsides, grassy places, and gardens.

Distribution: A European plant that has been introduced into North America.

Related species: In North America, aniseroot or sweetroot (*Osmorhiza berteroi*) is also known as sweet cicely. Both plants belong to a huge family, which includes many food plants but also a small number of poisonous species, such as hemlock, so take care with identification.

Parts used: Leaves, flowers, unripe seeds.

Sweet cicely is a common roadside plant in the dales of northern England, and is widely grown in gardens. The whole plant has a sweet aniseed flavour, giving it many culinary uses. It is traditionally cooked with acid fruit, reducing the amount of sugar needed, and can be used as a sugar substitute by diabetics.

Sweet cicely is an herbal tonic that restores energy, lifts the spirits, and settles the digestion.

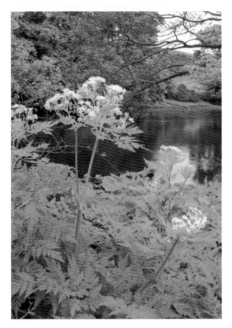

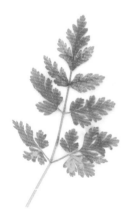

Like many herbs, sweet cicely was more widely used in the past than it is now. It was once valued as a protection against infection in the time of plague, and greatly appreciated in salads.

Gerard, writing in 1597, said: "The seeds eaten as a sallad whiles they are yet green, with oile, vinegar, and pepper, exceed all other sal-lads by many degrees, both in pleasantnesse of taste, sweetnesse of smell, and wholsomnesse for the cold and feeble stomacke." He also liked the leaves in salads, and found the boiled roots were tasty and good for old people.

Use sweet cicely for...

Sweet cicely still tastes just as good as it did all those years ago. It stimulates the appetite, relieves flatulence, griping and indigestion, and lifts the spirits. The whole plant is edible, and as Culpeper said: "It is so harmless, you cannot use it amiss."

Try the fresh young leaves, at their best before the plant flowers, chopped in salads. Use them as a flavoring in both sweet and savoury dishes. Add the flowers to salads and desserts, or use as a garnish. Nibble the green unripe seeds to stimulate the appetite or to settle indigestion or gas and griping. They have a stronger flavour than the leaves or flowers. The young stems can be eaten too.

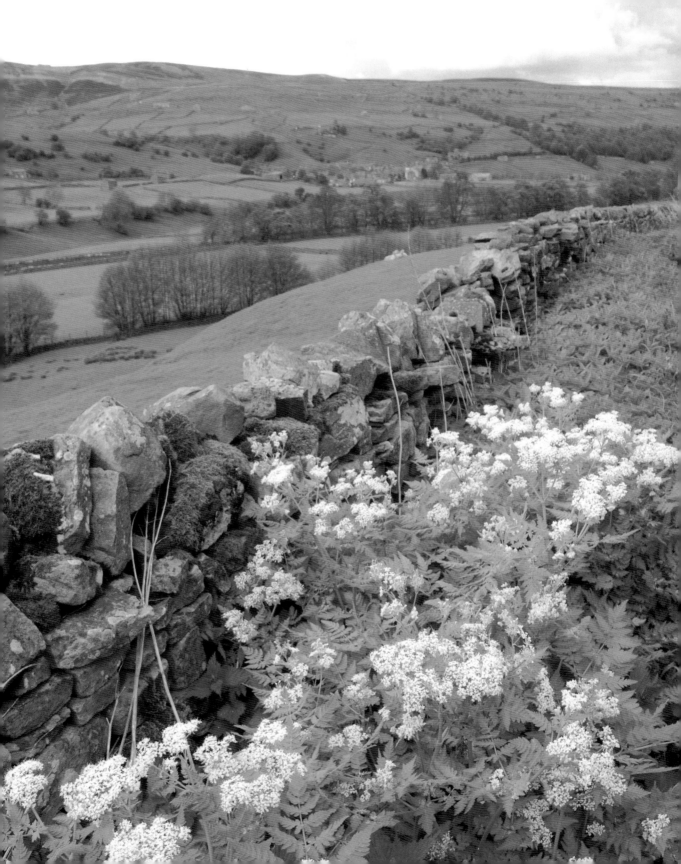

Sweet cicely is particularly good for older people who have lost their enthusiasm for life, as it lifts the spirits and enkindles the digestive fire. It enables them to enjoy their food with good appetite, warming the digestion and improving absorption of nutrients.

This plant is also beneficial for anyone who is weak or exhausted, perhaps after a chronic illness or through caring for someone else. It will help them get back their energy and *joie de vivre*, slowly rebuilding their strength and gently warming the whole system.

Sweet cicely apéritif
• poor appetite
• weak digestion
• flatulence
• indigestion

Sweet cicely apéritif

This can be drunk before meals to stimulate the appetite, or used as an after-dinner drink to settle the digestion. It can also be taken purely medicinally for flatulence, colic, or griping pains.

Use either a handful of green **sweet cicely seeds** or several handfuls of **leaves and stems.** Chop them up and put into a large, clean glass jar.

Add about a pint of **vodka**, and let steep in a dark place for two or three days. Taste it to check that the flavor of the herb has been absorbed by the alcohol, then strain and bottle in a clean glass bottle. The flavor improves if the bottle is left to age for two months in a dark place at room temperature before using.

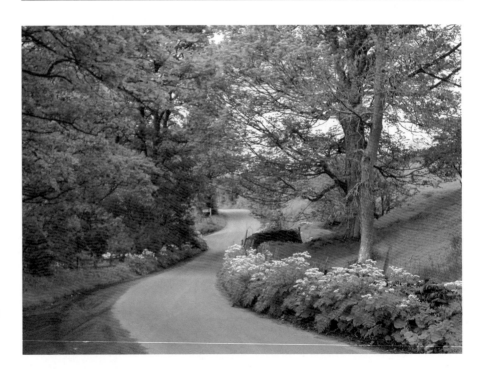

(*This and previous two pages*) Sweet cicely in the North Yorkshire dales, May

Teasel *Dipsacus fullonum* syn. *D. sylvestris*

Teasel is a stunning plant, tall and stately but also beautiful if observed in detail when flowering. Its medicinal uses have long been appreciated in China, but are only recently being rediscovered by western herbalists.

Teasel helps with joint and tendon injuries, muscle pain and inflammation, chronic arthritis, and lower back weakness. It is now being used for Lyme disease, ME, and fibromyalgia.

Teasel folklore has long referred to the way it collects rainwater in the cups where the leaves surround the stem, known from ancient times as the bath of Venus. This teasel water was said to be good for warts but particularly beneficial as an eyewash and as a wash for beautiful skin. We update this healing potential of teasel water with a home-made flower essence.

Teasel's famed commercial application is the use made of the dead flowerheads of the closely related fuller's teasel (*D. sativus*) in "teasing up" the nap on wool. *Taesan* is the Anglo-Saxon term for fulling or cleaning cloth. Common names for teasel like card weed, barber's brush, brushes, and gypsy's comb reflect this formerly important economic activity.

Fuller's teasel, with its hooked spines, was found to be uniquely effective both in manual and later in machine applications to raise the nap on fresh-made wool without breaking the cloth.

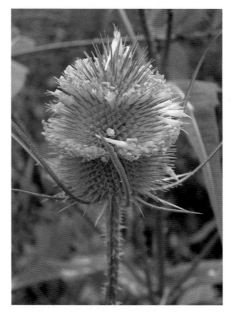

Use teasel for...

In Traditional Chinese Medicine, teasel root "tonifies the liver and kidneys," and works on painful lower backs and knees, weak legs, cartilage, and joints. It is also held to promote circulation and reduce inflammation. American herbalists William LeSassier and Matthew Wood have built on these uses and found in practice that the teasel

Caprifoliaceae Honeysuckle family (formerly in the Dipsacaceae)

Description: A tall biennial, up to 10 ft, with prickly rigid stems; small pale purple flowers in large conical flowerheads, opening from the middle; large and prickly basal leaves.

Habitat: Grassland, hedgerows, waste land and by freeways.

Distribution: Native to Europe, introduced to North America.

Related species: This species is sometimes called fuller's teasel, but the true fuller's teasel (*D. sativus*) has hooked spines there were once used to card wool; Japanese teasel (*D. japonicus)* is used in Traditional Chinese Medicine.

Parts used: Root, flowers used as an essence.

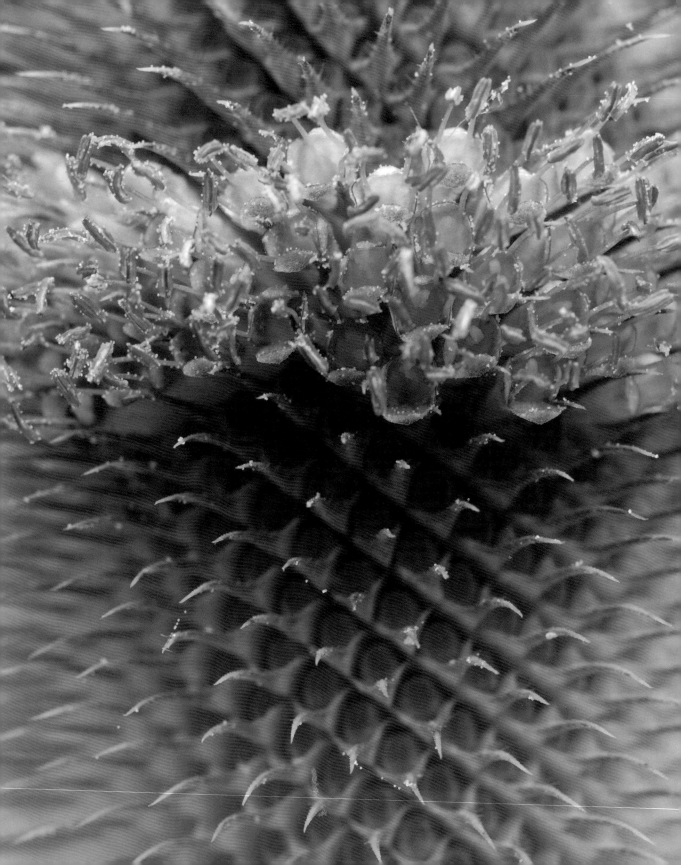

(introduced from Europe) is, in Wood's words, "invaluable" for joint injury and chronic inflammation of the muscles. It is indicated for fibromyalgia, chronic arthritis, and Lyme disease.

The acute infection of Lyme disease, as explained in an excellent monograph by herbalist Stephen Harrod Buhner (which any Lyme sufferer should buy), involves these same issues of joint pain, blood circulation, and tonifying of cartilage. Buhner finds results of using teasel root tincture for Lyme in the US are promising, though inconsistent in different regions.

Teasel flower essence has been found not only to bring relief in Lyme disease but also fibromy-

algia, chronic fatigue, and lupus. Treatment for these complex conditions should be in consultation with a herbalist and your doctor.

Because teasel root has to be dug in the first year when the plant is harder to identify, and as using the root kills the plant, we prefer a recipe for a flower essence.

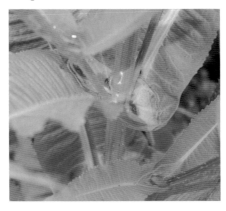

Teasel essence

Make this essence on a sunny day, using the **rainwater** collected for you by the teasel plant. Bend the plant over to pour some of this water from the leaf cups into a jug, then choose a flowerhead and bend it over into the jug so that it is immersed in the water for a minute or two. Alternatively, you can hold the flowerhead over a bowl and pour the rainwater from the jug over the blossoms into the bowl. If there is any debris in the water, filter it through a piece of muslin or a tea strainer as you pour it into a clean container to take home with you.

Measure the water and add an equal amount of **brandy** to preserve it. Bottle in a clean blue glass bottle, and label it.

To use, put three drops of this essence in a 1 flo ozl dropper bottle filled with brandy. Add 20 drops to bathwater, or as directed below.

Dose: Put three drops in a glass or bottle of water and drink during the day. Or put three drops into a small dropper bottle filled with half brandy and half water, and take by dropping a few drops directly under your tongue several times a day.

Teasel essence
- exhaustion
- chronic fatigue (ME)
- joint pain
- muscle aches

Vervain *Verbena officinalis*

An herb with a reputation for magic as well as medicine, vervain has a long history of use in Europe and Asia. It had so many reputed benefits that it gained a name as a cure-all; it was sacred for the Druids and used as an altar plant in ancient Rome.

It restores and calms the nervous system, is a digestive tonic and alleviates headaches. It can be used for premenstrual tension, menopausal hot flashes, fevers, gallstones, jaundice, asthma, anxiety, stress, tension, and insomnia. Vervain is a go-to restorative during convalescence from chronic or long-term illness.

**Verbenaceae
Verbena family**

Description: A slender perennial, to 2 ft, with square stalks and spikes of small white or pale lilac flowers in late summer.

Habitat: Roadsides and grassy places, especially on dry soil.

Distribution: Found across Europe and Asia to Japan, and as an introduced species in many states in the US.

Related species: The North American blue vervain (*V. hastata*) is used similarly. Lemon verbena (*Aloysia triphylla*) is often called vervain.

Parts used: Above-ground parts when in flower.

A prayer for picking vervain
*All hail, thou holy herb, vervin,
Growing on the ground;
On the Mount of Calvary
There wast thou found;
Thou helpest many a grief,
And staunchest many a wound.
In the name of sweet Jesu,
I lift thee from the ground.*

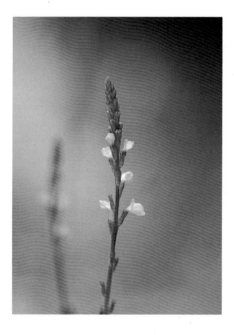

Vervain has a rich past, both magical and medicinal, sacred and secular. It was an important herb to the Druids and Romans. Picking was always accompanied, until recent times, by a prayer.

Once used to treat madness and epilepsy, vervain is a powerful nerve restorative, and is particularly good for nervous exhaustion following periods of prolonged physical activity or stress. It is excellent in convalescence for the weakness that follows viral infections. Julie has used it to treat ME/chronic fatigue syndrome.

Vervain is such a delicate plant that it is easy to overlook, but its medicinal power is belied by its humble appearance. Tincturing it is always surprising, as a few skinny stalks of pale lilac or white flowers yield a strong, dark, almost black, brew.

Vervain is a good herb to have on hand for the stress and hurried pace of modern lifestyles. It is particularly suited to people who are strong-willed, enthusiastic, work too hard, and cannot relax. It is one of Edward Bach's 38 original flower remedies, a specific for this type of intensity.

The physicians of Myddfai, in Wales in the thirteenth century, recommended vervain for scrofula, a tubercular infection of the lymph glands in the neck. Later, the great English herbalists had an uneasy relationship with the plant, Gerard decrying it and Culpeper favoring it. Parkinson (1640) chose the positive side by recommending vervain for "generally all the inward paines and torments of the body."

Use vervain for...

Because vervain works on the nervous system, liver, kidneys and digestion and also balances hormones, in addition to being a wound herb, it is still valid in an unusual array of conditions, and deserves to be more widely used.

A vulnerary treatment in classical Rome, the crushed or chewed fresh leaf can still be applied to cuts and scrapes to soothe and promote healing. It is effective where there is heat and irritation, so works well on bramble scratches, boils, and burns.

Vervain had a role in both love and war in Rome. It was aphrodisiac, being dedicated to Venus: a Roman bride would wear a sprig at her wedding. A *verbenarius* was a herald-at-arms who wore a chaplet of vervain as a flag of truce.

Coming to recent times, research in the US confirms that vervain, along with self-heal, is a top herb for normalizing levels of thyroid

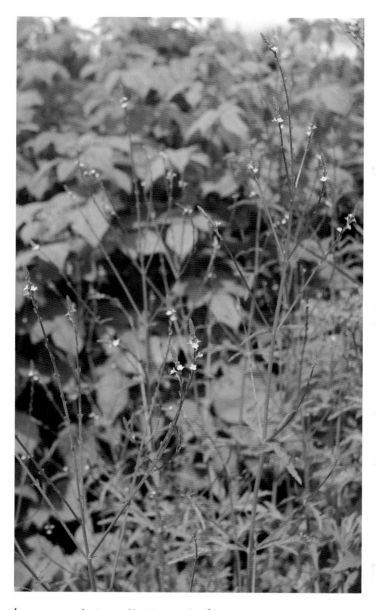

hormones, being effective in both the underactive and overactive conditions. Vervain appears to affect the amount of TSH (thyroid-stimulating hormone) released by the pituitary gland.

Drinking vervain tea very hot will make you sweat, which means it is

So many Virtues are attributed by Authors, to this Plant, that it would tire one to reckon them up.
– Pechey (1707)

Spenser called it "vein-healing verven." It had the old name of "simpler's joy."
– Pratt (1857)

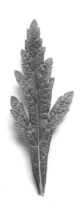

Vervain tea
- nervous tension
- anxiety
- colds and fevers
- premenstrual tension
- menstrual headaches
- poor absorption
- digestive problems
- inability to relax
- living on nerves
- hyperactivity
- thyroid imbalance
- muscular tension

Vervain tincture
- stress and tension
- anxiety
- premenstrual tension
- menstrual headaches
- nervous tension
- menopause
- hot flashes
- poor absorption
- digestive problems
- inability to relax
- living on nerves
- hyperactivity
- thyroid imbalance

a really effective treatment at the start of a cold or fever, when you are actively eliminating toxins. But it also relaxes and soothes, settling an upset digestion as well as a preoccupied, racing mind.

As a tincture, vervain is cooling for menopausal hot flashes. It is particularly valuable to have available where restlessness and nervous tension are part of the menopausal picture.

Vervain tea is good for childhood illnesses, where the child is restless and irritable. Instead of fidgeting, he or she will be helped to relax and recuperate. If there is a fever, vervain will encourage sweating and prevent the temperature from going too high. It combines well with lime blossom or elderflower for fevers.

While there have been regrettably few human clinical trials on vervain, the experience of the herbalists who use it largely support its old reputation as a "heal-all." It is a safe remedy, gentle enough for children and convalescents, and is tonic for older people.

Unfortunately, vervain seems to be becoming less common as a wild plant. If you can't find any near you, it is worth growing some in your own garden for medicinal use.

Harvesting vervain

Pick vervain when in flower, ideally towards the end of flowering. For use as a tea, dry the above-ground parts whole in a warm cupboard or in the open air on a piece of paper. When the plant is crisp, discard the larger stems and cut up or crumble the leaves into small pieces.

Vervain tea

Use a heaped teasoonful of the **dried herb** per mug of **boiling water**, and allow to steep for 5 minutes. Strain and drink hot.

Dose: 1 mug three times a day. For insomnia from restlessness, drink a cupful or two in the evening. For sprains and deep bruises, 2 or 3 cups a day for at least three or four days.

Combinations: Mixes well with lime blossom for flavour and therapeutic value; also effective with self-heal.

Vervain tincture

Chop up fresh **vervain** and put in a blender with enough **vodka** to cover. Blend briefly, then pour the mixture into jars and keep in a cool, dark place for a week. When blackish it is ready to strain and bottle.

Dose: 20 drops in a little water three times daily.

White deadnettle, Archangel

Lamium album

White deadnettle is a uterine tonic with an ability to stop loss of fluids from the body, whether excessive menstrual flow, abnormal vaginal discharge, diarrhea, or a runny nose.

The leaves and flowers can be eaten, raw or cooked. The flowers are full of nectar, enjoyed by insects and children alike, and the leaves can be used as a poultice for cuts and splinters.

Lamiaceae (Labiatae) Deadnettle family

Description: Perennial with leaves similar to stinging nettle, but paler green and without the sting. Grows to 2 ft and has whorls of creamy white flowers.

Habitat: Roadsides, gardens, and waste ground.

Distribution: Found across north and central Europe to Asia; naturalized in North America, Australasia.

Related species: There are several other common species in the genus, but none that can be confused with white deadnettle. The other species were used medicinally in the past.

Parts used: Flowering tops whenever flowering, which can be at almost any time of year.

The white deadnettle is so named because it resembles a stinging nettle, but has no stinging hairs. Other old names, such as deaf, dumb or blind nettle, also refer to the plant's benign nature. The white deadnettle is also known as bee nettle, with stores of honey at the base of its corolla attracting the humble bees that fertilize it. The same sweet taste has also made sucking the white flowers irresistible to generations of children.

It can be confusing in spring when both the stinging and non-stinging plants, which often grow together, are in leaf and there are no flowers to distinguish them. The secret lies in the stem, which is square and hollow in white deadnettle, but round and solid in stinging nettle.

The white deadnettle is perhaps too common for its own good, and has been unduly neglected both as an attractive plant with some border potential – and making an excellent mulch – and for its many medicinal qualities.

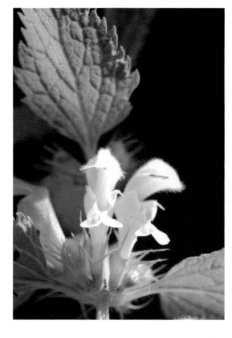

The plant's older name of archangel refers to Archangel Michael, whose day at one time correlated roughly with the first deadnettle flowers. We like the name for its protective connotations: it supports the female reproductive system and prevents the body from losing precious fluids through discharges of all sorts.

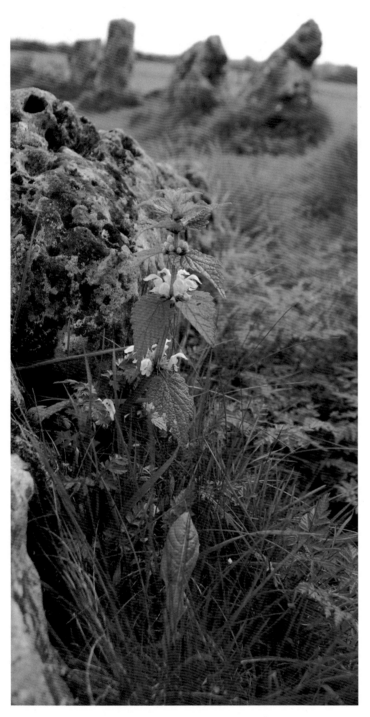

Use white deadnettle for...

The main use herbalists make of the plant is as a uterine tonic. Julie finds it effective in treating painful periods and bleeding between periods, in reducing excessively heavy menstrual flow, and for cystitis. It can be used for treating leucorrhoea or vaginal discharge (once called "whites"), in which case the tea treatment (three cups a day) is continued for at least three weeks. A douche, made from a strong deadnettle tea, is good for vaginal discharges.

The tea also forms part of a treatment regime for benign prostate hyperplasia (BPH), and to speed recovery after prostate surgery.

The tea's mild astringency is supportive in treating respiratory complaints, especially where there is phlegm and catarrh.

White deadnettle also helps to regulate the bowel, and works well for gastrointestinal disorders, constipation, flatulence and, in particular, diarrhea. It eases cramps and increases urination.

Externally, it has its uses in treatment as a poultice for cuts, bites, bruises, burns, splinters, varicose veins, and arthritic pain. For first aid, if you are out walking, the simplest method in the field is to chew deadnettle leaves and apply them to the sore point.

White deadnettle at the Rollright Stones, Oxfordshire, England, April

Harvesting white deadnettle

White deadnettle can be found blooming almost any time of year, even right through the winter in mild areas. It is most prolific in the spring, but can be harvested whenever found in flower. Break off the stem a few leaves below the flower spikes.

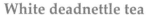

If you want to store it, dry the sprigs whole, either by spreading them on a drying rack or paper, or by hanging small bunches tied with string or thread from the rafters or a laundry airer. When they turn crisp and dry, crumble the leaves and flowers, and discard stems.

White deadnettle tea

Use a sprig of fresh flowering **white deadnettle**, or 1 to 2 teaspoons of the dried herb, per cup or mug of **boiling water**. Allow to infuse for about 10 minutes, then strain and drink.

Dose: 1 cup or mugful 3 times a day.

White deadnettle douche

Make a strong tea with a handful of **fresh or dried herb** to 1 pint of **boiling water**, and let it infuse until cool. Strain, and inject the liquid into the vagina using a douche bag. Repeat once a day until the discharge stops. If it continues for a week, consult your doctor or herbal practitioner.

Fresh white deadnettle leaf poultice

Pick the **fresh leaves** and either chew them or mash them with a mortar and pestle, then apply to the affected area and hold in place with a bandage or plaster. Change for a fresh poultice once or twice a day until healed, or, in the case of a splinter, until it is drawn out.

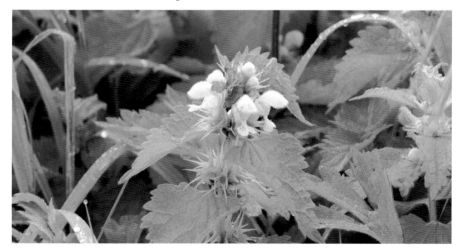

White deadnettle tea
- heavy menstruation
- painful periods
- vaginal discharge
- irritable bowel
- cystitis
- diarrhea
- respiratory catarrh

White deadnettle douche
- vaginal discharge

Fresh leaf poultice
- burns
- bruises
- splinters
- cuts

[the distilled water of deadnettle] *is used to make the heart merry, to make a good colour in the face, and to refresh the vitall spirits.*
– Gerard (1597)

It is without question a gentle but really useful remedy for troubles of the reproductive organs in women, especially leucorrhoea.
– Barker (2001)

Wild lettuce *Lactuca virosa, L. serriola*

**Asteraceae
(Compositae)
Daisy family**
two

Description: Prickly lettuce (*Lactuca serriola*) is a 3–4 ft tall biennial with broad grey–green leaves and arrays of small, pale yellow flowers. Great or greater prickly lettuce or lettuce opium (all *L. virosa*) is darker green, with purple, less spiny stems and similar small yellow flowers. Both species have distinctive spines along the underside of the midrib of the leaves.

Habitat: Roadsides, disturbed or waste ground.

Distribution: These two species are native to Europe, and introduced in North America. Prickly lettuce is generally more common than great lettuce.

Related species: Garden lettuce (*L. sativa*) can be used similarly, but is not as strong. Canadian lettuce (*L. canadensis*) is the most widespread North American wild lettuce.

Parts used: Leaves and latex, gathered when plant is in flower, in late summer.

If you grew up with Beatrix Potter, you know from *The Tale of the Flopsy Bunnies* **that eating flowering lettuces makes you sleepy. Our garden lettuces have been bred to reduce their bitterness, and hence herbal value, and as a result have less of a soporific effect than does wild lettuce.**

The lettuce we buy in the shop or grow in our garden is a distant and hybridized relative of wild lettuce, but much altered in appearance and flavor. The only thing they have left in common is a milky sap or latex (*lactuca*) found in the stems of some commercial varieties and all through the plant in wilder varieties.

Strangely, though, if you allow a lettuce in your garden to "bolt" (i.e., flower and then seed), it reverts to something like the wild form, recovering the healthy bitterness we try so hard to breed out of domesticated versions.

It is this bitter latex that is valued medicinally, and all lettuces have some of it. It is most abundant in great lettuce, less so in prickly lettuce and less again in garden forms. It can be harvested by cutting the flowering tops or leaves in summer and scraping off the juice. White when fresh, this juice oxidizes to brown in the air.

In this form it is known as lactucarium, and is chemically akin to opium, though unrelated

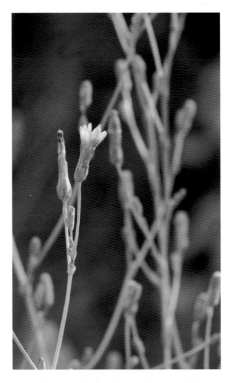

botanically. Introduced to medical practice in 1771, it was later named lettuce opium. It was much used to adulterate opium in cough mixtures and as a sedative.

Lactucarium could be bought in British pharmacies until the 1930s and was still "official." Nowadays the only "official" part of wild lettuce is the dried leaves. It is just as well, lactucarium being unreliable in content and action.

Taking lettuce for insomnia is old medicine. Galen, first-century AD physician to Roman emperor Marcus Aurelius, wrote: "I have found no better remedy for my trouble than eating lettuce of an evening."

But in one respect the reputation of lettuce has changed dramatically since ancient times. A form of cos lettuce, with its wild growth and white sap, was once held sacred to Min, the Egyptian god of fertility. But by the time of the ancient Greeks lettuce had become "the eunuch's plant."

Nowadays lettuce is a recognized anaphrodisiac, with a role in reducing sexual desire; externally, a cold lettuce tea is soothing and cooling for inflamed sexual organs. This effect works equally on both sexes (unlike hops). An old saying from Surrey went: "O'er much lettuce in the garden will stop a young wife's bearing."

Wild lettuce's sedative, cooling value extends to soothing the respiratory system, for dry, irritat-

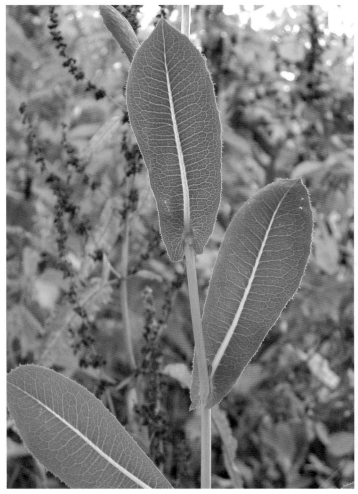

Prickly lettuce; flowers shown opposite

ing coughs and whooping cough. Relaxing spasm in the stomach and uterus, it relieves gripes and period pain. It is also beneficial for muscular and rheumatic pains.

Wild lettuce tincture

Harvest leaves and above-ground parts of wild lettuce while it is in flower in the summer. Chop it up and place in a blender with enough **vodka** to cover. Blend, then put the mixture into a jar and leave it in a cool dark place for two weeks. Strain, bottle, and label.

Dose: Half a teaspoonful 3 times a day to calm over-excitement, or 1 teaspoonful at bedtime to help with sleep.

Wild lettuce tincture
- insomnia
- overactivity
- excitability
- colicky pains
- irritable coughs

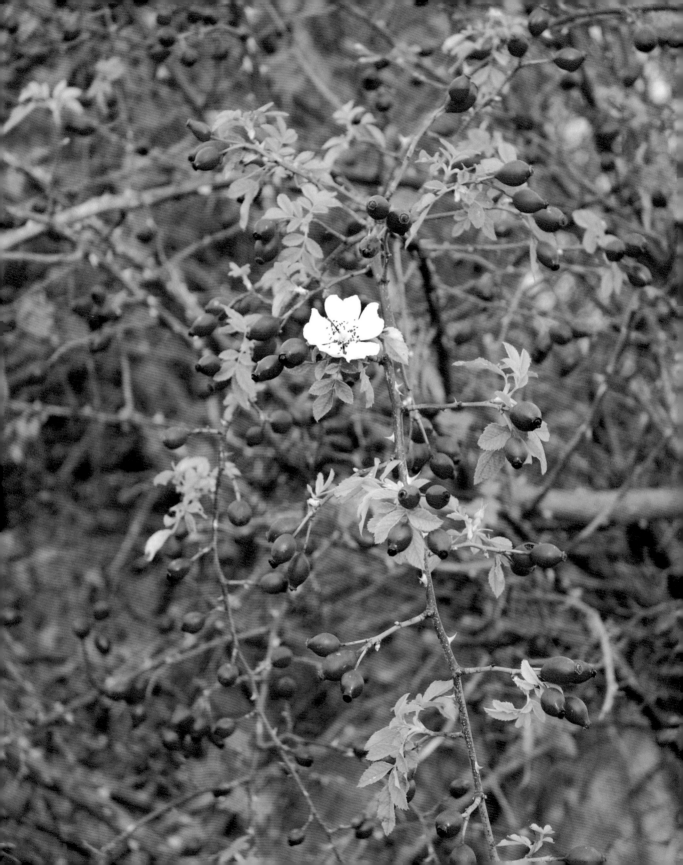

Wild rose *Rosa* spp.

For centuries the wild or dog rose was valued most for its galls, used to eliminate the stone. It was only in the 1930s that the value of the hips was proven, just in time for their use in a vitamin-rich syrup given to Britain's wartime children against infection.

Rose is the plant of love, the petals being the basis of the perfume industry. Herbally, it supports the immune system, is a good eliminator, and is cooling to the body.

Autumn brings mist and mellow fruitfulness, in Keats's famous words, but he overlooks the frosts and flus of the fall. Fortunately, our fields and woods are "loaded and blessed" with a bounty of **rose hips** to help us build up strength and resistance for the winter.

Everybody now knows that rose hips contain plentiful vitamins and minerals, but it was only in the 1930s that research established that home-grown hips had twenty, even forty times more vitamin C than imported oranges, plus good supplies of vitamins A, B, and K.

Oranges were to be an early casualty of World War II in Britain, and the Ministry of Food turned to the nation's school children to collect the domestic alternative. By 1945 amounts of 450 tons or so of rose hips were gathered each fall to make into syrup; collectors were paid threepenny a pound, a useful bit of pin money for youthful entrepreneurs.

Rose hip syrup was rationed and provided to mothers for their children through the war years and for some time thereafter. The syrup (made by Delrosa) was in the shops, although Matthew, a post-war baby, remembers better the joy of seeing and eating his first orange in the early 1950s.

Use wild rose for...

Rose hips and petals (the leaves are not used much) offer support to the body's immune system and help fight infection in the digestive tract; they are also diuretic, i.e., assist in elimination of wastes through the urinary system, as well as cooling to the body, bringing down fevers and reducing heat on the skin in the form of rashes and inflammations.

This threefold action – supporting immunity, helping elimination, and being cooling – makes rose a superb natural reliever of cold and flu symptoms, sore throats, runny noses, and blocked chests.

Rosaceae
Rose family

Description: Rambling deciduous shrubs with thorny stems and pink or white flowers, followed by bright scarlet hips in the fall.

Habitat: Field sides, scrub, and woods.

Distribution: Widespread around the world, mainly in temperate areas.

Species used: There are several species, and they can all be used medicinally. Choose fragrant varieties if you are using the petals. Dog rose (*R. canina*) is the most common in Europe, with fragrant pale pink or white flowers and scarlet hips. North American native species include prickly rose (*R. acicularis*), prairie rose (*R. arkansana*), smooth rose (*R. blanda*), climbing rose (*R. setigera*), Virginia rose (*R. virginiana*), and Wood's rose (*R. woodsii*).

Parts used: Flowers gathered in midsummer and hips harvested in the fall.

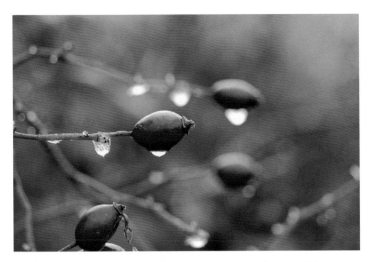

for support in life-cycle stages. Rose hips, petals and essential oil all buttress the nervous system, relieving insomnia, soothing the nerves and lifting depression, as well as evening out heart palpitations and arrhythmias.

The astringent effect, particularly of the petals, is a result of high tannin levels, which help make rose useful in staunching bleeding and unwanted discharges. There is an effect too on the digestive system, cutting over-acidity and over-activity in the stomach, as well as reducing the spasms involved in diarrhea, colitis, and dysentery.

The petals have good antiviral properties and combine well with St. John's wort, elder, and self-heal for treating viral infections. There are recent claims for anti-HIV qualities in *R. damascena*, the damask rose.

Additionally, the petals, whether in the form of a water infusion, a distilled rose water or, as in our recipe, a glycerite, make a fragrant skin toner and cleanser, which will take the heat out of boils, acne, spots, and rashes. Rose water is also a soft, safe eyewash, mouthwash and gargle, and a douche.

A story is told in *The Odyssey* of how good rose is for the skin, as well as winning the heart. Milto, a young girl and the daughter of a humble artisan, would put a fresh garland of roses each morning in

The effect is not only good for children, and rose hip tea as well as syrup are often given to convalescents and older people to improve their general resistance, as well as lighten their mood.

But there is one note of caution in this roll-call of autumnal virtue. The official wartime instructions emphasized that while the flesh of dog rose hips was so good for you the seeds, with their short hairs, were possibly dangerous if taken internally. However, the same hairs have provided "itching powder" fun for generations of boys.

Straining stewed hips to remove the irritant hairs was specified in the wartime recipe, and is still noted in instructions for the syrup.

Rose petals were favored by herbalists of old mainly for cooling and astringent qualities, and to strengthen the heart and spirits. Today's herbalists use them in hormone-balancing formulae and

the temple of Venus, the goddess of love. Milto was beautiful, but at one time a boil began to grow on her chin, and she became distraught.

In a dream the goddess came to Milto and told her to apply some of the roses to her face. She did so, and recovered her beauty and equanimity to such an extent that she later became the favorite wife of the Persian emperor Cyrus.

Rose petals make a wonderful cooling tonic for the whole female reproductive system, reducing uterine pain and the cramp of heavy periods, and supplementing other treatment of infertility and low libido. Rose's cooling and balancing qualities are particularly helpful during the menopause.

This is the ultimate feminine flower, found in practically every perfume, soap, and aphrodisiac, yet men often need it too, and rose can be used to treat impotence.

Rose has a softening action on the heart on an emotional level, and it is no accident that a dozen red roses are a conventional expression of the lover's feelings. Rose is prescribed by herbalists if the emotional aspect of "heart" is affected or there is a need for love. Rose helps us to love ourselves and be open to the love of others.

So, given all this, does the wild rose deserve its name "dog"? This might derive from derogatory comments on its commonness – Pliny the Elder (AD 23–79), for example, thought Britain was named Albion because it was covered with white roses (*alba* meant white).

But rose's defenders prefer an origin from an Anglo-Saxon term meaning "dagger," for the thorn, or perhaps the branch out of which dagger handles were made. Another version of the name is that rose root was once thought to cure rabies, hence dog rose.

Take three roses, white, pink and red. Wear them next to your heart for three days. Steep them in wine for three days more, then give to your lover. When he drinks, he will be yours forever.
– traditional love-charm, Germany

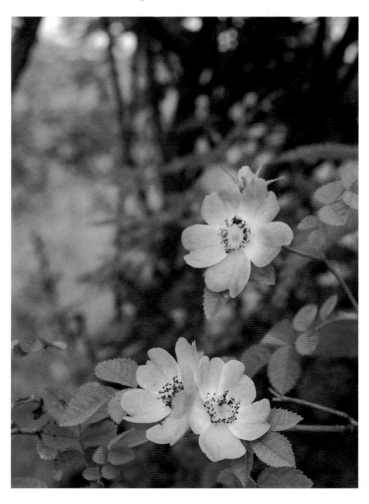

What may be less known today is that for centuries the main use of wild rose was for its gall or "briar balls," known as Robin's pincushions or bedeguars. Apothecaries ground them into a powder and sold them to treat kidney or bladder stone and as a diuretic. This use is long obsolete.

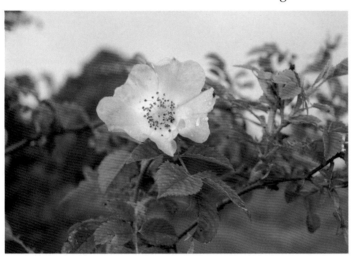

In any event, the success of the modern domesticated rose owes much to the wild form, and it is still usual for more tender species of ornamental roses to be grafted onto a wild rootstock. The petals of your garden roses can be used medicinally, if they are fragrant.

The Seals have a family story of rose grafting. Matthew's grandfather Ted Seal lived in Leicester and was a fervent gardener. For a private joke he grafted some big blowsy roses onto wild briars growing by the railway line to London.

He said he wanted to confuse the passengers and make them think the country roses near Leicester were something special. Perhaps he was one of those people who knew that thorns have roses.

Rose petal glycerite
- viral infections
- hormone balance
- menopause
- dry skin
- feeling unloved
- feeling unloving
- grief
- loneliness

Rose petal glycerite

You can use garden roses along with wild roses for this recipe, as long as they haven't been sprayed.

Pick fragrant **rose petals** and put them in a jar with a mixture of 60% **vegetable glycerine** and 40% **water**. Put the jar on a sunny window ledge or in a warm place. Stir occasionally to keep the petals beneath the surface of the liquid. You can add more petals over the season, removing any that have turned transparent. When the last petals have lost their colour, strain off the liquid and bottle. It should have a powerful aroma of rose, and taste heavenly.

Uses: 1 teaspoonful as needed for sore throats or viral infections.
For a "broken heart" or grief, mix half and half with hawthorn tincture, and take 1 teaspoonful several times a day. Rose glycerite is a pleasant addition to many herbal tinctures and formulae.
As a face lotion for dry or delicate skin, mix half and half with water, and apply daily.

Rose hip vinegar

Put 20 or 30 **rose hips** in a jar or flask and cover with **apple cider vinegar**. If you want to speed up the process, slit the skins of the hips with a sharp knife before putting them in the vinegar. Leave on a sunny window sill for about a month, then strain and bottle.

Uses: For sore throats, mix a tablespoonful with warm water, gargle, and then swallow. For colds, make a drink using a tablespoon of rose hip vinegar in a mug of hot water, sweetened to taste with honey; or use in salad dressings.

Raw rose hip syrup

Gently score a few lines through the skin of red **rose hips**, then layer them in a wide-mouthed jar with enough **sugar** to fill up all the gaps between the hips. Leave on a sunny window sill for a couple of months or until the sugar has drawn the juice from the hips and liquified. Strain off the liquid, bottle, and store in the fridge. This is a really thick and delicious syrup. Take a teaspoonful or two daily to prevent colds.

Boiled rose hip syrup

This is the more traditional way to make the syrup, and what it may lose in vitamin C content it gains in having a longer shelf life.

Measure the volume of the **rose hips** you have picked, then pour them into a saucepan with half their volume of **water** (1 pint water to 2 pints hips). Boil hips and water for 20 minutes in a covered saucepan. Allow to cool, then strain through a jelly bag. For every 2 cups of juice, add 1 cup **sugar**. Boil for 10 minutes and pour while still hot into sterilized bottles. Label bottles when cool. Take a teaspoonful or two daily to prevent colds, or more frequently as needed for sore throats and colds.

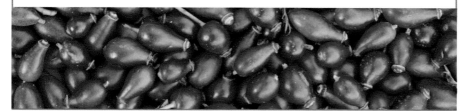

Rose hip vinegar
• colds
• sore throats
• salad dressings

Rose hip syrup
• colds
• sore throats
• source of vitamin C

In Wynter and in Somer it [Syrope of Rooses] maye be geuen competently to feble sicke melacoly and colorike people.
– Askham's Herbal (1550)

Willow *Salix alba, S. fragilis, S. nigra*

**Salicaceae
Willow family**

Description: Tall deciduous trees that frequently hybridize with each other.

Habitat: Riverbanks and other wet places.

Distribution: Widespread around the world, in a variety of damp habitats.

Species used: Crack willow (*S. x fragilis*) has higher levels of salicin than white willow (*S. alba*), which is the species mentioned in most herbals. In North America, the black willow (*S. nigra*) is the main species used.
.
Parts used: Bark, collected in spring, and leaves.

It is a fine cool tree, the boughs of which are very convenient to be placed in the chamber of one sick of a fever.
– Culpeper (1653)

The branch tips and leaves, known as willow tips… are traditionally used in many parts of South Africa to treat rheumatism and fever.
– Van Wyk et al. (1997)

Willow bark contains salicin and other aspirin-like compounds. It is used to treat pain and inflammation, but does not have the stomach-irritating or blood-thinning effects of aspirin.

Willow helps to lower fevers, and can be used as a gentle pain reliever for headaches, arthritis, gout, rheumatism, muscle aches, and lower back pain.

Willows are graceful trees often found growing by water. White willow is particularly elegant, with its silvery leaves swaying in the wind. Crack willow is so named because the fast-growing trunk often cracks and splits under its own weight. The familiar silver catkins, "pussy willow," are from the sallows, a group of willows with broader leaves.

Willows are highly adaptable trees, and will usually root readily from a stick put in the ground. Willow leaves, mashed up and soaked in water, can be used as a natural rooting hormone to help root cuttings of other plants.

Willows have many uses. The flexible shoots, mainly of osier (*Salix viminalis*), make excellent wicker baskets, and the wood of a variety of white willow is used commercially for clogs and cricket bats. Willow wood is burnt to make charcoal for drawing, and willow charcoal was once used in producing gunpowder.

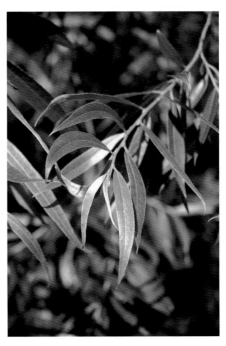

Willow contains high levels of the aspirin-like salicin, but research suggests it is actually the combination of flavonoids that is analgesic and anti-inflammatory. The modern use of aspirin began in 1763 when Rev. Edmund Stone extracted salicylic acid from willow bark for his parishioners' use. In 1853 the French chemist Charles

Gerhardt made a primitive form of aspirin. Later a German chemist discovered a better method for synthesizing the drug, and it started being marketed by Bayer in 1899. Aspirin, acetylsalicylic acid, is one of the most widely used drugs in the world today.

Interestingly, the early herbals do not focus on willow for relieving pain but more on its astringent action in stopping bleeding, diarrhea and other "fluxes." The leaves, boiled in wine and drunk over an extended period of time, were considered an effective treatment to reduce lust in both sexes.

It is possible that willow was used for pain as a folk remedy that didn't make it into herbals. Willow bark was chewed by country folk to relieve headaches and toothache, and to treat the ague, a type of malarial fever.

Today herbalists use willow mainly for pain, inflammation, and fever. Our son, who suffered from ME for several years as a young

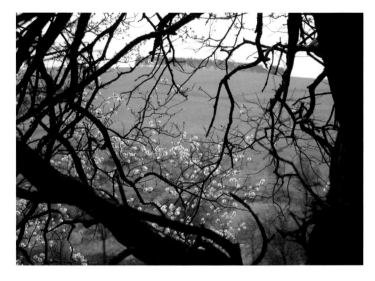

teenager, always asked for it for his headaches and muscle aches and pains. Like meadowsweet, it is effective for treating arthritis and rheumatism, and can ease the pain of polymyalgia rheumatica and fibromyalgia, for which it combines well with Guelder rose.

Note that if you are taking aspirin as a blood thinner, you cannot replace it with willow, which lacks this effect. But for long-term pain relief willow may be better for the stomach than aspirin.

Pussy willow, rural Shropshire, April

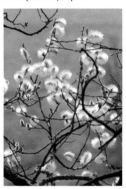

Cautions: Do not take willow if you are allergic to aspirin or while breastfeeding.

Willow bark tincture
- aches and pains
- headache
- arthritis
- rheumatism
- muscle aches
- backache
- gout
- period pain
- colds and flu
- sports injuries

Willow bark tincture

Harvest the bark in the spring, from branches where it isn't too thick. Use a sharp knife to strip thin slices of bark lengthwise off the branch on one side, taking care not to take too much from any one place.

Put the **willow bark** in a jar, and pour in enough **vodka** to cover it. Leave it in a cool dark place for a month, shaking regularly every few days. Strain off the liquid, bottle, and label it.

Dose: 1 teaspoon 3 times a day, taken in a little water when needed for relief of pain and inflammation.

Willowherb *Epilobium* spp.

Onagraceae
Willowherb family

Description: Perennials, up to about 2 ft, recognizable by small pink flowers, with four notched petals, borne on the ends of long seed-pods. These split and curl when ripe to release downy seeds.

Habitat: Gardens and other disturbed ground, woods, damp places.

Distribution: Widespread throughout the northern hemisphere.

Species: There are about ten species, used interchangeably, including American willowherb (*Epilobium ciliatum*), marsh willowherb (*E. palustre*), hoary or smallflower willowherb (*E. parviflorum*), and broad-leaved willowherb (*E. montanum*).

Related species: Rosebay willowherb has been reclassified into the genus *Chamerion* (see p163), but is closely related and has similar uses. The great willowherb (*E. hirsutum*) is not used in herbal medicine – it grows to 5 ft, has large cerise flowers and grows in ditches or by streams.

Parts used: Above-ground parts in flower.

The small-flowered willowherbs are a specific remedy for prostate problems, including benign prostate hyperplasia (BHP). Plants in this informal group help shrink the tissues, arrest cell proliferation, and normalize urinary function.

Small-flowered willowherbs are also effective for a wide range of bladder and urinary problems, for women as well as men, with the astringent and diuretic action serving to tone and detoxify the urinary tract.

The Austrian herbalist Maria Treben was the first to bring the small-flowered willowherbs to public attention in recent times. She wrote of helping hundreds of people with prostate problems by using this neglected herb.

Julie's father, living in Namibia (which still has a strong German influence from colonial days), drank willowherb tea for his prostate thirty-five years ago, but the tea is still not widely available for sale in the UK. All the more reason to grow or pick your own!

These willowherbs frequently appear as garden weeds because they like bare or disturbed soil. If you break the stem about halfway up, the plant will grow new side shoots, and you can collect from the same plant several times during the summer.

Any of the small-flowered species can be used (see panel on the left), which is handy because they

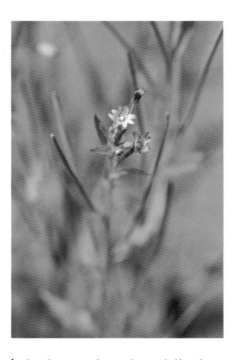

hybridize easily and are difficult to identify individually. The flowers vary in colour from deep pink to almost white, and leaf shapes range from very narrow to quite broad, and from smooth to downy.

The name willowherb comes from the willow-like leaves. The flowers of some species look like burning matches, with the bright pink buds at the end of long ovaries or unripe seed pods (or cods as the old English herbalists call them).

These writers classified willowherbs with the loosestrifes. Gerard describes the seed "wrapped in a cottony or downy wooll, which is carried away with the winde when the seed is ripe," but apparently didn't use the plant. Parkinson calls it very astringent and "effectuall both to stanch blood, restrain fluxes, heale the sores of the mouth and secret parts, close up quickly greene wounds and heale old ulcers."

While best known as a prostate remedy, these plants aren't just for men. They can help women with bladder and urinary problems too, used on their own or with pellitory of the wall, couch grass, horsetail, and bilberry leaves.

For prostate enlargement, willowherbs can be taken alongside nettle root, another effective remedy for the condition. But do consult your herbalist or doctor first.

It is well worth keeping a little patch of willowherbs in a corner of your garden. They are persistent, growing up in cracks of paving or unweeded bare soil, so once established you'll have a ready supply on hand (we know gardeners will regard these words as heretical).

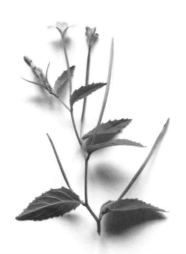

These two specimens from our garden show how variable in form small-flowered willowherbs can be in even a small area

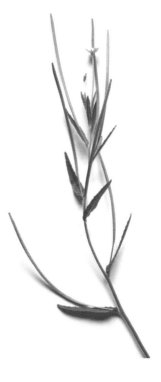

Harvesting willowherb

Havest by picking the flowering stems about halfway up. This enables the plant to produce more flowers and seeds later on. Dry in a shady place. As the plants dry, the seed pods often break open and release tiny downy seeds, so you might want to do this outdoors. You can use the whole plant, but the tea is more manageable if you discard the fluffy seeds and larger stems, then cut into small pieces with a pair of scissors and store in jars or brown paper bags in a cool dry place.

Willowherb tea

Use a heaped teaspoonful of the **dried herb** per mug of **boiling water**, and infuse for about 3 minutes. Drink two to three cups a day. Maria Treben recommends 1 cup in the morning on an empty stomach and another half an hour before the evening meal.

Willowherb tea
- prostate enlargement
- urinary problems
- bladder disorders
- diarrhea

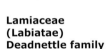

Wood betony *Stachys officinalis* syn. *Betonica officinalis*

Wood betony, often simply betony, was a significant remedy from ancient times. A Roman physician wrote a whole book extolling its virtues, and it was the herb of choice for exorcising demons and protection against all kinds of evil in the Middle Ages.

Wood betony is a nerve tonic, and through its action on the solar plexus has a wide range of benefits, especially on the digestion. It also improves circulation, and is excellent for the elderly.

Lamiaceae (Labiatae) Deadnettle family

Description: A perennial up to 18" tall, with distinctive bluntly toothed leaves in a rosette, and bright magenta flowers.

Habitat: Heaths, grassy places, and woodland clearings.

Distribution: Naturalized in Massachusetts and New York state; native to Europe.

Related species: Other *Stachys* species include lambs ear, woundworts and hedgenettles.

Identification: Wood betony can look like a purple orchid, but is easily distinguished from its relatives by its type of toothed leaves, which are unique.

Parts used: Leaves and flowers.

Wood betony is another herb that does so much that it is hard to know where to start in writing about it. It is a pretty, orchid-like but easily overlooked plant, and, appropriately, works quietly to improve health over a broad front.

As an herbal all-rounder it was known to the ancients. Culpeper (1653) relates that Antonius Musa, physician to Emperor Augustus, wrote a monograph on betony, with 47 different conditions it would treat, among them protection from both snakes and evil.

Anne Pratt, a prolific mid-nineteenth-century botanist, writes that betony was still highly valued in Italy. She quotes two Italian proverbs: "May you have more virtues than betony," as a farewell to a friend, and "Sell your coat, and buy betony," for those in pain.

John Parkinson (1640) sums up the reputation of betony in his own day, neatly indicating the link he valued of "daily experience" and ancient authority: "it is found by daily experience, as Dioscorides formerly wrote thereof, to be good for innumerable diseases."

Betony was venerated by the Celts, and its common name is thought to be a corruption of two Celtic words: "bew" for head, and "ton" for improve, making clear its power to cure head problems.

Throughout the Middle Ages this was a herb cultivated in monastic gardens and graveyards, for protection against witchcraft. Amulets of betony would be worn around the neck or placed under the pillow for personal protection.

It could be that betony's old reputation as a protector stems from its ability to help us face the fears and evils in our own minds. The *Grete Herball* (1526) made sure by combining betony with wine "for them that ben to ferfull": "gyue two dragmes of powdre hereof wt warme water and as moche wyne at the tyme that the fere cometh."

Use wood betony for...

Perhaps this echo of magic and folklore has swayed many classically trained herbalists against betony, and some modern writers are dismissive of its efficacy. We see it as an herb, like St. John's wort or vervain, that meets our ever-changing physical and spiritual needs.

Today it is best known as a nerve tonic, which strengthens the entire nervous system. Betony calms and relaxes, helping release stress and tension from both mind and body.

It is an excellent herb for insomnia stemming from nervous tension, where endless thoughts keep churning and you just can't let go and relax. Have a cup of the tea or a few drops of the tincture in the evening for deep relaxation, followed by a restorative sleep.

Betony was once used to treat madness, and can still have a useful role in some psychiatric disorders. Herbalists favor it for people coming off addictive drugs or recovering from head injuries.

Betony is beneficial for tension, migraine, and liverish varieties of headache, especially when there is a feeling of spaciness and unconnectedness, as well as in cases of frantic mental activity and scattered thoughts.

We have often seen in cottages in Kent... large bundles of the "medicinal Betony," as Clare calls it, hung up for winter use.
– Pratt (1857)

Thy wild-woad on each road we see;
And medicinal betony,
By thy woodside-railing, reeves
With antique mullein's flannel-leaves.
– Clare, "Cowper Green" (1828)

Wood betony in an English meadow, July

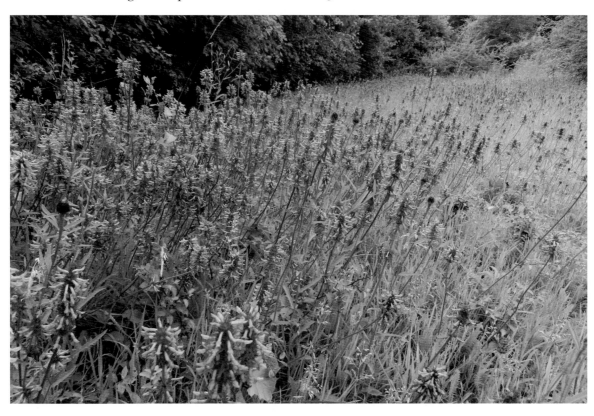

Because betony affects the solar plexus, it assists in a wide range of digestive problems, harmonizing the action of the entire digestive tract. It is helpful when anxiety, irritability or depression affect the digestion, or when digestive upsets are upsetting the mind. Betony stimulates a weak digestive tract but also soothes and calms it. It is thus helpful when there is irritable bowel syndrome, gastritis, colitis, and other conditions with gut inflammation and tension.

These actions make betony the perfect remedy for "butterflies in the stomach" and for reconnecting us to "gut instincts." When we are "too much in our heads," it can bring us down to earth, grounding our reactions and feelings.

Betony also improves concentration and memory, which, combined with its calming qualities, makes it a good choice during examinations or other stressful times in our lives when we need to be able to focus and concentrate.

With positive effects on memory, circulation, and digestion, betony is an ideal herb for older people or anyone recovering from long-term illness. It will gently warm and invigorate the whole bodily system, increasing mental and physical strength. It also improves the appetite and supports those who are too thin in regaining healthy weight.

Betony increases tone throughout the body, so can assist with prolapses of the uterus and other organs. It is useful in weak labor, excessive menstrual bleeding, poor respiration, debility, and liver and gallbladder problems.

A 2013 study on 66 women showed its effectiveness in treating polycystic ovary syndrome.

In general, like self-heal, wood betony is a good choice for when you don't quite feel well but don't really know what the problem is.

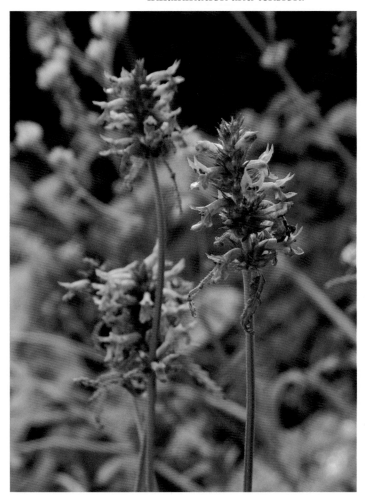

Harvesting wood betony

Pick the plant just before the flowers fully open. To dry for a tea or pillow, spread it on a screen or brown paper in the sun. When dry and crisp, put into brown paper bags or jars to store.

Wood betony tea

Use 2 teaspoonfuls of the fresh herb or 1 teaspoonful of the dried herb per cup of boiling water, and leave to infuse for 10 to 15 minutes.

Dose: 3 cups a day, or 1 cup at bedtime to relax for a good night's sleep.

Wood betony tincture

Put fresh **wood betony herb** in a blender with enough **vodka or brandy** to cover. Blend briefly, then pour into a jar and put in a cool dark place for a week. Strain off the liquid, bottle, and label.

Dose: Wood betony often works very well in drop doses. Take 5–10 drops in a little water three times a day. For insomnia, take 10 drops at bedtime. For more of a tonic effect, take 1 teaspoonful three times a day.

Wood betony ointment

Pick a handful of **wood betony leaves**. Put them in a small saucepan with half a cup of **extra virgin olive oil**. Using a low heat, warm gently, just below simmering, until the leaves have lost their green colour and are quite crisp. Strain, returning the oil to the pan.

Add half an ounce of **beeswax** and warm until it melts. Stir well and pour into jars. Leave the lids off until the ointment sets, then label and store in a cool place until needed.

Wood betony pillow

Sew a small cloth bag, leaving one end open. Fill loosely with dried wood betony leaves. Some dried lavender flowers or rose petals can be added for their fragrance. Stitch or tie up the open end, and place the bag under your pillow.

Wood betony, hawthorn and horseradish formula

Mix 5 parts **wood betony tincture**, 4 parts **hawthorn tincture or syrup** and 1 part of **horseradish vinegar**. This formula stimulates and warms, improving digestion, circulation, and memory.

Dose: 1 teaspoon morning and afternoon as a tonic for older people or anyone recovering from a long illness. Also great for exam time!

Wood betony tea
- insomnia
- digestive problems
- headache
- poor circulation
- low appetite
- muscular tension
- nightmares
- sinus congestion
- watery, irritated eyes
- head colds
- chills and fevers

Wood betony tincture
- headache
- feeling of spaciness
- digestive problems
- vertigo
- memory loss
- nervous exhaustion
- anxiety
- irritability
- poor concentration

Wood betony ointment
- bruises
- sprains
- strains
- varicose veins
- hemorrhoids

Wood betony pillow
- insomnia
- nightmares

Wood betony, hawthorn and horseradish formula
- tonic for older people
- convalescence
- exams

Caution: Do not take during pregnancy.

Yarrow *Achillea millefolium*

Yarrow or milfoil is a leading backyard medicine plant. A ready first-aid treatment for wounds and nosebleeds, it has larger uses as a circulatory system remedy that both stops bleeding and moves stagnant blood, preventing and clearing blood clots. It tones the blood vessels and lowers high blood pressure.

Yarrow is beneficial for a wide range of menstrual problems, and is a first-rate fever herb, used as a hot tea to induce sweating.

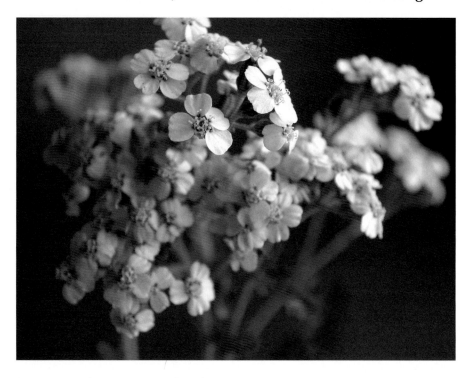

Yarrow is a famous wound and fever herb, yet today it can pass unnoticed except as a lawn weed. The legendary Achilles used it as a field dressing for his soldiers' wounds in the Trojan war, and the plant is named for him. A pity, then, he had none handy for his own fatal heel wound!

Use yarrow for...
Yarrow is our favourite remedy for nosebleeds, and we advise keeping a patch by the back door if anyone in your family suffers from them. Simply pick a few fresh leaves – available year round, though at their best in spring and fall – and rub them between your

hands to bruise them, releasing the aromatic oil. Roll the leaves into a nasal plug, insert into the affected nostril and leave until the bleeding completely stops before gently removing the plug.

Julie's father was staying with us once and suffered a really bad nosebleed in the middle of the night, but luckily we had a patch of yarrow close by and the bleeding was soon stopped.

Yarrow has a reputation of being able to start a nosebleed as well as stop one, from a time when bleeding was a traditional cure for headache and migraine. Indeed, one of the plant's old names was "nosebleed."

It is certainly as effective at breaking up congealed blood as it is at stopping hemorrhages, making it a valuable first-aid remedy for thrombosis, for blood blisters and bruises with bleeding beneath the skin, as well as hemorrhoids. If treating for hemorrhoids, take yarrow tea or tincture internally, and place a yarrow poultice or compress over the affected area.

This special ability to both stop bleeding and break up stagnant blood makes yarrow a valuable menstrual remedy. It will correct both heavy and suppressed periods, and will normalize blood flow if there is clotting.

It is also a remedy for vaginal discharge and helps prevent painful periods. Austrian herbalist Maria Treben considered yarrow "first and foremost a herb for women."

This has truth, but the plant's old names of soldier's woundwort and knight's milfoil bring us back once more to yarrow's affinity for battlefields and for being a wound-packing material, probably long before the Achilles myth was recorded. Its use paralleled the development of weapons, and it was the *herba militaris*, the herb dressing carried by battle surgeons around the world until at least the American Civil War.

Yarrow has long had a particular repute for closing bleeding wounds caused by weapons or tools made of iron. In France it is called the *herbe au charpentier* (English version: carpenter's grass) for the same reason. It is useful to know in case of domestic or outdoor accidents that yarrow's emergency help can be at hand. Find a plant, strip the leaves, crush them and pack into the wound: it is antibacterial and antimicrobial so you will not introduce infection.

The reason why yarrow is so versatile – it was known as a "cure-all" herb – is that it works to tone the blood vessels, especially the smaller veins, and lower blood pressure by dilating the capillaries. This means it has a beneficial whole-body effect through the blood system, especially on conditions related to hypertension and including coronary thrombosis.

Yarrow has proved beneficial in the treatment of so many illnesses and afflictions that no garden should be without it.
– Roberts (1983)

Achillea is an important diaphoretic herb, and is a standard remedy for helping the body deal with fever. It stimulates digestion and tones blood vessels.
– Hoffmann (2003)

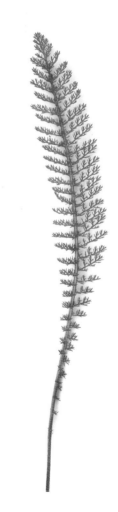

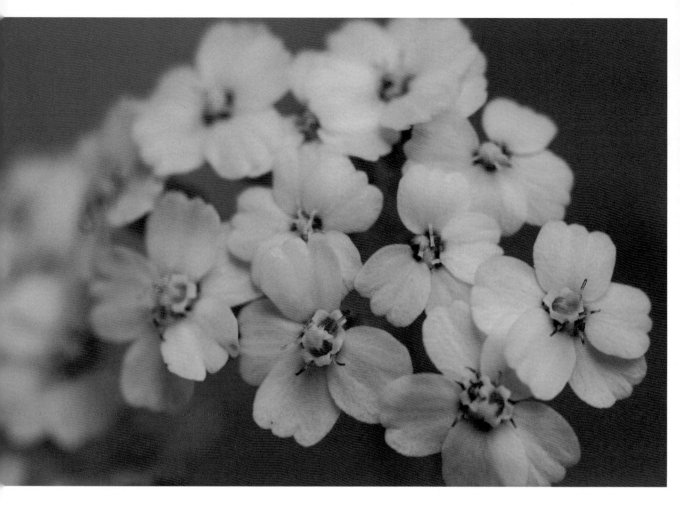

... *Any treatment for external and internal haemorrhage calls for the inclusion of Yarrow.... I cannot imagine dealing effectively with painful periods or with high blood pressure if the prescription did not include a small but positive amount of Yarrow.*
– Barker (2001)

But there is another range of bodily ills for which yarrow is well recommended, and this is in reducing fevers. By relaxing the skin, yarrow will open the pores to allow copious sweating and the release of toxins. Yarrow taken as tea or as a bath at the beginning of a fever or flu is an excellent way to reduce the body temperature. It is an herb for measles and chicken pox, and it is safe for children. It was once called "Englishman's quinine" for a claimed benefit for treating ague (a form of malaria).

The sweating / purifying / relaxing effects are enhanced, herbalists have found, by combining equal quantities of yarrow, peppermint, and elderflower in a tea, drunk as hot and as often as the patient can stand. The same mix works well as a skin lotion or in a bath. The equivalent mixture for high blood pressure is yarrow plus nettle and lime blossom, again taken as a tea.

Yarrow has various other health benefits, as befits its all-rounder status. Its effect on bodily fluids helps in cases of diarrhea and dysentery. It is effective for colic and blockages of the urogenital area, as also for stomach cramps, cystitis, arthritis, and rheumatism.

A yarrow lotion makes a good eyebath and stimulates the scalp, with traditional benefit to the hair; plugs of crushed leaves help to relieve toothache or earache.

Yarrow has a further dimension to its long human history: it is a herb of divination, used by the Druids for predicting the weather, by the Chinese for auguries (in the *Book of Changes* or *I Ching*), and by love-lorn English maidens for indicating who their true love would be. One chant from East Anglia links the yarrow of blood and the yarrow of foretelling:

Yarroway, yarroway, bear a white blow/ If my love love me, my nose will bleed now.

These were benign uses, but the past is not one-sided and yarrow also had a shadow side, being the "devil's nettle" and "bad man's plaything." For the most part it was involved in sympathetic magic, as in its part in St. John's day celebrations (see page 179).

All this virtue, and a little vice, comes with a tally of yarrow's profit and loss account. No question about it, it is one of the great presences in western herbalism. At the same time, some cautions should be noted.

Yarrow has a stimulating effect on uterine contractions, so is best avoided in pregnancy; prolonged use externally can, in some people, cause allergic rashes and make the skin ultra-sensitive to sunlight; large doses can cause headaches.

You should also be aware that the active constituents of yarrow vary from plant to plant and by locality. If you try yarrow for any of the uses we have outlined and it seems to be ineffective, go to another plant and use that.

Milfoil is always the greatest boon, wherever it grows wild in the country.... It should on no account be weeded out. Like sympathetic people in human society, who have a favourable influence by their mere presence ... so milfoil, in a district where it is plentiful, works beneficially by its mere presence.
– Steiner (early 20th century)

Yarrow by Maria Merian (1717)

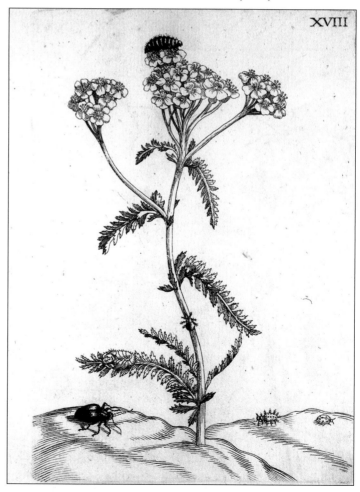

XVIII

Yarrow tea
- colds and fevers
- scanty menstruation
- heavy periods
- menstrual clotting
- high blood pressure
- to tone varicose veins
- to prevent blood clots
- tension
- weak digestion

Yarrow tincture
- scanty menstruation
- heavy periods
- menstrual clotting
- high blood pressure
- to tone varicose veins
- to prevent blood clots
- tension
- weak digestion

Fresh leaf
- nosebleeds
- cuts and wounds

Harvesting yarrow

Yarrow leaves are evergreen so can be harvested fresh almost whenever they are needed. To make a tincture or when drying it for tea, yarrow is best gathered while flowering. Note also that yarrow accumulates particulates from vehicle exhausts because of the large surface area of its flowerhead and leaves, so it is best to pick it away from busy roads.

To dry your yarrow, hang whole stems in bunches or place them on brown paper in an airing cupboard. Allow a month, and once they are dry, strip the leaves and flowers off the stems and crumble for use as a tea. Smaller stems can be chopped up with scissors, but the larger stems are usually discarded. Keep the leaves dry and you can use them for months, or find fresh leaves for a green tea.

Yarrow tea

Use 1 heaped teaspoonful of **dried yarrow** per cup or mug of **boiling water**, and let it infuse for 10 minutes. Strain and drink hot.

Dose: For colds and feverish conditions, drink a cupful hot every two hours until there is an improvement, and continue drinking three cups a day until you are well. For chronic conditions, drink three cups a day. For fevers, yarrow combines well with mint and elderflower. Use externally as a wash for cuts, and as a hair rinse for a healthy scalp and shiny hair.

Yarrow tincture

Chop up **fresh yarrow leaves and flowers**, and put in a jar. Pour in enough **vodka** to cover, put the lid on and place the jar in a dark cupboard for two weeks. Shake it every few days. Strain and bottle.

Dose: 20 drops in water, three times a day.

Ointment for hemorrhoids

Gently heat 1 oz **dried yarrow** and 1 oz **dried raspberry leaf** or 1 oz **horse chestnut leaf** with 1 cup **extra virgin olive oil** in a small saucepan for 15 minutes, stirring frequently. Strain out the herbs and return the oil to the pan. Add about 1 oz **beeswax** and stir until melted. Use enough beeswax to set the ointment – test a few drops on a cold saucer as you do when making jelly. If you live in a hot climate or it is summer, you will want to use more beeswax than if the weather is cold. If your ointment is too runny, melt it again and add more beeswax.

Apply the ointment externally a couple of times a day as needed. It can also be used on bruises, varicose veins, and thread veins.

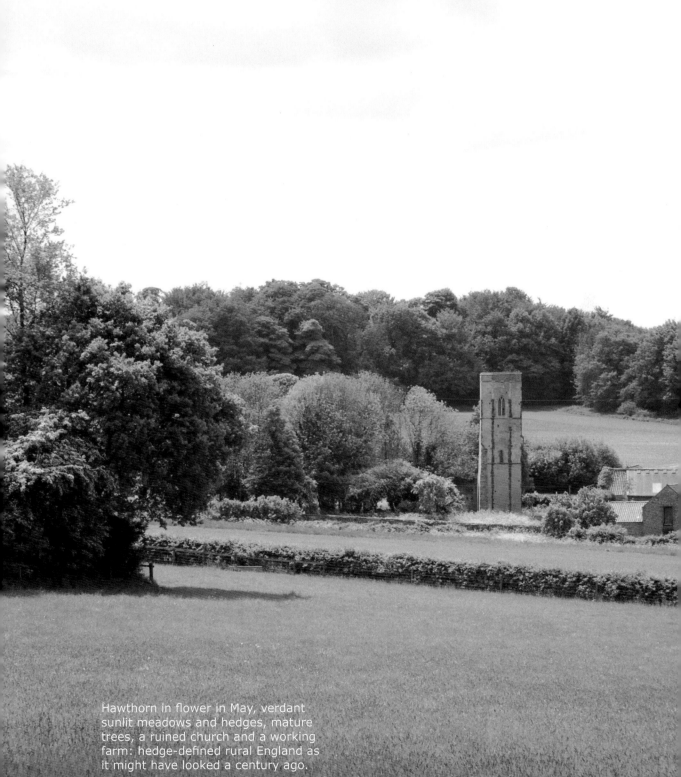

Hawthorn in flower in May, verdant sunlit meadows and hedges, mature trees, a ruined church and a working farm: hedge-defined rural England as it might have looked a century ago.

Notes to the text

Full citation given in first reference only, thereafter author and page number. Original year of publication is in square brackets; place of publication London unless otherwise noted; PubMed references are to (date) and online reference number

Introduction [9]: For an accessible summary of British hedgerow history, see Oliver Rackham, *The Illustrated History of the Countryside* (2003), 75–89; Hew DV Prendergast & Helen Sanderson, *Britain's Wild Harvest: The Commercial Uses of Wild Plants and Fungi* (2004), 64.

Harvesting from the wild [10]: James Green, *The Herbal Medicine-Maker's Handbook: A Home Manual* (Berkeley, CA, 2000), 10; Steven Foster & James Duke, *A Field Guide to Medicinal Plants and Herbs of Eastern and Central North America* (Boston, MA, 1999); nettle and elderflower from William Woodville, *Medical Botany*, 4 vols (1790–3), courtesy of John Innes Foundation Historical Collections, Norwich.

Relevant North American legislation on harvesting wild plants is found in the US Plant Protection Act (PPA), June 2000, which consolidates previous law. The US Department of Agriculture (USDA) is the federl agency responsible through the PPA, for regulating the growing, sale, and import of commercial plants and for keeping a noxious weeds register. The USDA website, www.usda.gov, gives the links to state legislation.

The Endangered Species Listing Program, 1999, controls the federal schedule of endangered species. No such plant is inluded in this book.

There is no general law against harvesting wild plants unless they are endangered, threatened, or illegal. Ownership dictates whether you can legally harvest in a particular place, and usually the permission of the owner is required or advised. Picking in declared wilderness, state, and national parks and by many freeways is usaally forbidden. For an overview of protocols and common sense on harvesting, see the UK code of conduct on www.bsbi.org.uk.

AGRIMONY [20–23]: Woodville, *Medical Botany*, IV, 254, courtesy of John Innes Foundation Historical Collections, Norwich; Matthew Wood, *The Book of Herbal Wisdom* (Berkeley, CA, 1997), 85–92 passim; Anne Pratt, *The Flowering Plants and Ferns of Great Britain*, 5 vols (1857), II, 218; John Parkinson, *Theatrum Botanicum* (1640), 597.

BILBERRY [24–27]: "hunter-gatherer": Richard Mabey, *Food for Free* (2000 [1972]), 100–1; Fraughan Sunday: Geoffrey Grigson, *The Englishman's Flora* (1975 [1958]), 282; "mucky-mouth pies": Mabey, *Flora Britannica* (1997), 163; Mrs. M Grieve, *A Modern Herbal*, ed. Mrs. CF Leyel (1998 [1931]), 99–100; James Duke, *The Green Pharmacy* (Emmaus, PA, 1997), 318; Nicholas Culpeper, *Complete Herbal* (1995 [1653]), 33; Abbé Kneipp, qtd Jean Palaiseul, *Grandmother's Secrets*, trans. Pamela Swinglehurst (1976 [1972]), 48.

BIRCH [28–31]: Baron Percy, quoted in Palaiseul, 50–1.

BLACKBERRY, BRAMBLE [32–35]: Walt Whitman, "Song of Myself" 2, stanza 31, *Leaves of Grass* (New York, 1855); Jonathan Roberts, *Cabbages & Kings* (2001), 17; Dennis Furnell, *Health from the Hedgerow* (1985), 44–5; Carol Belanger Grafton, *Medieval Herb, Plant and Flower Illustrations* [CD-Rom and book] (New York, 2004), image 165; Julian Barker, *The Medicinal Flora of Britain and Northwestern Europe* (West Wickham, Kent, 2001), 171.

BURDOCK [36–39]: "official": British Herbal Medical Association, *British Herbal Pharmacopoeia* (1996), 49; Green, *Herbal Medicine-Maker's Handbook*, 35.

CHERRY [40–41]: "Wildman" Steve Brill & Evelyn Dean, *Identifying and Harvesting Edible and Medicinal Plants* (New York, 2002 [1994]), 119; Grigson, 177; (2012) 3510330.

CHICKWEED [42–45]: Brill & Dean, 138; (2012) 17078633; Susun Weed, *Wise Woman Herbal: Healing Wise* (Woodstock, NY, 1989), 122.

CLEAVERS [46–49]: Culpeper, 73; Parkinson, 568; Maria Treben, *Health through God's Pharmacy* (Steyr, Austria, 1983 [1980]), 10–11; (2016) 27085941; John Pughe, trans., *The Physicians of Myddfai* (Felinfach, Wales, 1993 [1861]), 444; John Evelyn, *Acetaria: A Discourse on Sallets* (1699 [Brooklyn, 1937]), 12.

COMFREY [50–53]: names: Deni Bown, *The RHS Encyclopedia of Herbs & Their Uses* (1995), 206; Bocking 14: Henry Doubleday Research Association, www.gardenorganic.org.uk; Norfolk recipe: Book of Culinary Recipes, 1739–79 (Norfolk Record Office, RMN 4/5), fo. 4; Dr. John R Christopher, *School of Natural Healing* (Springville, UT, 1996 [1976]), 337; Staiger (2012) 3491633; Norman Grainger Bisset & Max Wichtl, eds, *Herbal Drugs and Phytopharmaceuticals* (Stuttgart/Boca Raton, 2001 [1989]), 485.

COUCH GRASS [54–57]: Culpeper, 93; *civice*: Audrey Wynne Hatfield, *How to Enjoy Your Weeds* (Worcestershire, 1999 [1969]), 47; *King's American Dispensatory*, by Harvey Wickes Felter & John Uri Lloyd (1898), www.henriettesherbal.com; Parkinson, 1175; Bisset & Wichtl, 242.

CURLED DOCK [58–61]: Weeds Act 1959, www.defra.gov.uk; seeds: Maida Silverman, *A City Herbal*, 3rd edn (Woodstock, NY, 1997 [1977]), 57; chants: Roy Vickery, comp., *A Dictionary of Plant-Lore* (Oxford, 1997 [1995]), 107; Tswana women: Margaret Roberts, *Margaret Roberts' Book of Herbs* (Johannesburg, 1983), 61; David E Allen & Gabrielle Hatfield, *Medicinal Plants in Folk Tradition* (Portland, OR/Cambridge, 2004), 98; Shiwani et al. (2012) 3506869; Maria Sibylla Merian, *Erucarum ortus alimentum et paradoxa* *metamorphosis* (Amsterdam, c1717), courtesy of John Innes Foundation Historical Collections, Norwich; Culpeper, 91; old herbalists: Thomas Bartram, *Bartram's Encyclopedia of Herbal Medicine* (1998 [1995]), 459; "superlative remedy": Matthew Wood, *The Practice of Traditional Western Herbalism* (Berkeley, CA, 2004), 152; jaundice recipe: Mary Norwalk, *East Anglian Recipes*, 2nd edn (Dereham, 1996 [1976]), 40.

DANDELION [62–67]: English / Chinese names: Silverman, 50–1, 53; William Coles, qtd Silverman, 51; US salad industry: Brigitte Mars, *Dandelion Medicine* (Pownal, VT, 1999), 18; quotation, Mars, 1; (2010) 3018636.

ELDER [68–73]: Chambers: qtd Chris Howkins, *The Elder* (Alderstone, Surrey, 1996), 20; John Evelyn, *Sylva* (1664), ch. XX, 17, www.gutenberg.org; Ria Loohuizen, *The Elder in History, Myth and Cookery* (Totnes, 2005); cordials: Prendergast & Sanderson, 24–7; Norfolk recipe: Book of Culinary Recipes, 1739–79 (NRO, RMN 4 / 5), fo. 14.

FIGWORT [74–77]: names: Grigson, 325; Ningpo figwort: Dan Bensky & Andrew Gamble, *Chinese Herbal Medicine Materia Medica*, rev. edn (Seattle, WA, 1993 [1986]), 69; Michael Moore, *Medicinal Plants of the Mountain West* (Santa Fe, NM, 1979), 78; "organizing construct": Wood, *Book*, 21; Tooker: qtd Carole Levin, "Elizabeth I and the Politics of Touch", digitalcommons.unl.edu (1989), 199; John Pechey, *The Compleat Herbal of Physical Plants*, 2nd edn (1707 [1694]), 92; La Rochelle: Lesley Gordon, *A Country Herbal* (Exeter, 1980), 80; Peter Holmes, *The Energetics of Western Herbs*, 2 vols, 2nd edn (Boulder, CO, 1994 [1989]), II, 656; Malcolm Stuart, *Encyclopedia of Herbs and Herbalism* (New York, 1979), 261; Elizabeth Blackwell, *A Curious Herbal* (1739), pl. 87; "bite": Graeme Tobyn et al., *The Western Herbal Tradition* (Edinburgh, 2011), 303; (2010) 3870064; (2017) 5651059; (2015) 4365673; (2003) 12673026; (2002) 11807962.

GUELDER ROSE, CRAMPBARK [78–79]: Gerard: Grigson, 380;

Rosemary Gladstar, *Herbal Healing for Women* (New York, 1993), 175, 239; Dr. Christopher, 431.

HAWTHORN [80–85]: Pratt, II, 269; Dr. Green: Bertram, 215; Jennings: HP Whitford et al., *A Treatise on Crataegus* (Cincinnati, 1917), www.soilandhealth.org; Peter Conway, *Tree Medicine* (2001), 170; "Fair Maid": Blanche Fisher Wright, illus., *The Real Mother Goose* (New York, 1916), www.gutenberg.org; (2010a) 20148500; (2010b) 3249900; (2013) 3891531); hawthorn berry leather: Ray Mears, "Wild Food", BBC2, 31.1.2007, and *Wild Food* (2007), 216–17.

HONEYSUCKLE, WOODBINE [86–87]: English woodland: Furnell, 98; twizzly canes: Katherine Kear, *Flower Wisdom* (2000), 89; yellow-flowered: Christopher Hobbs (herbal workshop, 2007); *shuan huang lian*: Duke, 93–4; Anne McIntyre, *The Complete Floral Healer* (1996), 147; Parkinson, 1461.

HOPS [88–89]: John Gerard, *The Herball*, ed. Marcus Woodward (1994 [1597]), 213; Laurel Dewey, *The Humorous Herbalist* (East Canaan, CT, 1996), 92; Evelyn, *Acetaria*, 19; George III: Mabey, *Flora Britannica*, 64; "official": *Br. Herb. Pharm.*, 106.

HORSE CHESTNUT [90–93]: "park": figure cited *Independent*, 24.8.2006; Turkey: McIntyre, 52; Chris Howkins, *Horse Chestnut* (Addlestone, 2005), 20–1; World War I: Howkins, 29–32; David Hoffmann, *Medical Herbalism* (Rochester, VT, 2003), 524.

HORSERADISH [94–95]: Parkinson, 861; Philippa Back, *The Illustrated Herbal* (1987), 75; (2016) 4924378; Pechey, 197.

HORSETAIL [96–99]: Furnell, 102–4; "drumsticks": Palaiseul, 154; "moth-eaten asparagus": Hatfield, *Weeds*, 75; (2015) 4441770; Galen, qtd Mrs. Grieve, 421; Treben, 26–9.

LIME, LINDEN [100–02]: Barker, 237; Conway, 271.

LYCIUM [103–07]: David Winston & Steven Maimes, *Adaptogens* (Rochester, VT, 2007), 178–81; Lu Ji and Chinese

saying, Winston & Maimes, 179; protecting UK hedgerows: Department for Environment, Food and Rural Affairs, www.defra.gov.uk 15.1.03; goji as food: Food Standards Agency, www.food.gov.uk 18.6.07; Duke of Argyll: Mabey, *Flora Britannica*, 300; aphrodisiac: Duke, 192.

MALLOW [108–11]: *Br. Herb. Pharm.*, 127–30 (leaf & root); Treben, 31–2; Cobbett, qtd A. Lawson, *The Modern Farrier* [1842], 282–4; Gabrielle Hatfield, *Memory, Wisdom and Healing* (Stroud, 1999), 40–2; *Hortus Floridus* (1614–16), courtesy of John Innes Foundation Historical Collections, Norwich; Culpeper, 156, 159; mallow tea: Richo Cech, *Making Plant Medicine* (Williams, OR, 2000), 182; "far from roads": Furnell, 122; Cicero: Clinton C. Gilroy, *The History of Silk, Cotton, Linen, Wool, …*(New York, 1843), 191–202, www.biodiversitylibrary.org.

MEADOWSWEET [112–15]: Turner: Grigson, 154; Chaucer: Mrs. Grieve, 524; Parkinson, 593; Cuchulainn: Tess Darwin, *The Scots Herbal* (Edinburgh, 1996), 149; Palaiseul, 208; Cech, 183.

MINT [116–20]: "fishes": Palaiseul, 211; Gerard, 155; William Thomas Fernie, *Herbal Simples Approved for Modern Uses of Cure* (Philadelphia, 1897), 342, www.gutenberg.org; Parkinson, 35; "official": *Br. Herb. Pharm.*, 149; sekanjabin: from Persian recipes; Rumi: qtd www.superluminal.com.

MUGWORT [121–25]: "female remedy": McIntyre, 57; northern saying: Susan Lavender & Anna Franklin, *Herb Craft* (Chieveley, 1996), 371; Sir John Hill, *The British Herbal* (1756), qtd Keith Vincent Smith, *The Illustrated Earth Garden Herbal* (1979), 100; insecticide: Pughe, *Myddfai*, 53; Silverman: quote and *Leech-Book*, 92, 94; moxa: Thornton, 695; tobacco, Manx festival: Mabey, *Flora Britannica*, 370.

MULLEIN [126–29]: Odysseus: Homer, *The Odyssey*, trans. EV Rieu (Harmondsworth, 1979 [1946]), 163; quaker girls: Wood, *Herbal Wisdom*, 493; Hildegard: Wighard Strehlow & Gottfried Hertzka, *Hildegard of Bingen's*

Medicine, trans. Karin Anderson Strehlow (Santa Fe, NM, 1988), 21; Dr. Quinlan: Allen & Hatfield, 250; Moore, *Medicinal*, 113; Dr. Christopher, 345.

NETTLE [130–35]: "springtime herbalism": James Green, *The Male Herbal* (Freedom, CA, 1991), 92; Milarepa: *The Oxford Companion to Food*, ed. Alan Davidson (Oxford, 1999), 532; Dr. HCA Vogel, *The Nature Doctor* (Edinburgh, 1990 [1952]), 369; Hatfield, *Weeds*, 93; Merian, *Erucarum ortus*; nettle-eating: Piers Warren, *101 Uses for Stinging Nettles* (2006), 71; Sir John Harington, *Regimen Sanitatis Salernitanum* (1607), qtd Keith GR Wheeler, *A Natural History of Nettles* (Victoria, BC, 2005), 48; Weed, 171; Duke, 371.

OAK [136–39]: "necessary": Grigson, 269; bark "official": *Br. Herb. Pharm.*, 145; Moore, 116; "half-pay": Grigson, 273; Hoffmann, *Medical*, 497; German: Bisset & Wichtl, 403; Culpeper, 182.

PELLITORY OF THE WALL [140–41]: Parkinson, 437; Culpeper, 192; Norfolk recipe: Anon., *Archdale Palmer's Recipes 1659–1672* (Wymondham, Leics, n.d.), unpaginated; asthma weed: www.weeds.org.au; Mrs. Grieve, 624.

PLANTAIN [142–47]: sacred herb: Grigson, 356; lawns: Ken Fern, *Plants for a Future*, 2nd edn (East Meon, Hants, 2000 [1997]), 144; footprint: Gordon, 135–6; *Archdale Palmer's Recipes*; "Indian bandaid": JT Garrett & Michael Garrett, *Medicine of the Cherokee* (Rochester, VT, 1996), 57; Abbé Kneipp, qtd Palaiseul, 250; Bessie Smith: Darwin, 138; Dr. Christopher, 57; Merian, *Erucarum ortus*.

RAMSONS [148–51]: Hippocrates: www.bmj.com; Mrs. Grieve, 344; Abbé Kuenzle, qtd Treben, 37; Plants for a Future database: www.pfaf.org.

RASPBERRY [152–54]: Ida: *Oxford Companion to Food*, 653; Juliette de Baïracli Levy, *The Complete Herbal Book for the Dog* (1971 [1955]), 59; John Parkinson, *Paradisi in Sole: Paradisus Terrestris* (1629 [New York, 1976]), 558.

RED CLOVER [155–57]: Scott: *Guy Mannering* (1815), ch. 3; Hatfield, *Weeds,*

38–9; Dr. Christopher, 61; Matthew Wood, pers. comm., 9 Jan 2008; "official": *Br. Herb. Pharm.*, 161; phyto-estrogens: Ruth Trickey, *Women, Hormones & the Menstrual Cycle* (Crows Nest, NSW, 2003 [1998]), 402–4.

RED POPPY [158–61]: and war: e.g. Grigson, 57; Myddfai: Pughe, 414; Pechey, 192.

ROSEBAY WILLOWHERB, FIREWEED [162–65]: Singerweed: Roy Vickery, *Plant Lore Notes and News* (Dec. 1998); Roger Phillips, *Wild Food* (1983), 77; Felter & Lloyd, *King's American Dispensatory*, www.henriettesherbal. com; Carol Rudd, *Flower Essences* (Shaftesbury, Dorset, 1998), 52; (2013) 23796429.

SELF-HEAL [166–70]: Chinese background: Henry C Lu, *Chinese Natural Cures* (New York, 1994), 204–5; Parkinson, 528; *Brunella*: Stuart, 247; Gerard, 145; Duke, 256–7, 273.

SHEPHERD'S PURSE [171–73]: Barker, 146; Ryokan poem: trans. John Stevens, *Dewdrops on a Lotus Leaf: Zen Poems of Ryokan* (Boston, MA, 1996).

SORREL [174–75]: Channel Islands: Hatfield, *Memory*, 55; Evelyn, *Acetaria*, 42–3; sour milk: Silverman, 146; Parkinson, *Theatrum*, 745; Essiac: (2006) 17212569; Sinupret®: (2011) 22112724; Mességué: *Health Secrets*, 265.

ST. JOHN'S WORT [176–81]: "hyperikon": Wood, *Book*, 307; Parkinson, 574; Mrs. Grieve, 708; MAO: Dewey, 137; Germany: Larry Katzenstein, *Secrets of St. John's Wort* (1998); Alfred Lear Huxford: qtd Anne Pratt, *Wild Flowers* (1852), 109; herbs of St. John: Grigson, 85–6; Klamath weed: Grigson, 88–9; Australasia: Sir Edward Salisbury, *Weeds & Aliens* (1961), 208.

SWEET CICELY [182–84]: Gerard, 244; Culpeper, 66; Furnell, 165.

TEASEL [185–87]: bath of Venus, eg, Allen & Hatfield, 275; fulling: Mrs. Grieve, 754; TCM: Bensky & Gamble, 349; Wood, *Book*, 234–7; lyme: Stephen Harrod Buhner, *Healing Lyme* (Randolph, VT, 2005).

VERVAIN [188–90]: prayer: TF Thiselton Dyer, *The Folklore of Plants* (Llanerch, Wales, 1994 [1889]), 285; Myddfai: Pughe, 448–9; Parkinson, 676; marriage and *verbenarius*, McIntyre, 233; Pechey, 241; Pratt, IV, 210.

WHITE DEADNETTLE, ARCHANGEL [191–93]: names: Mrs. Grieve, 580; Gerard, 158; "too common" and quote: Barker, 370.

WILD LETTUCE [194–95]: wild vs commercial: Brill & Dean, 246; lactucarium and 1771: Stuart, 210; "official": *Br. Herb. Pharm.*, 185; Galen and "eunuch's plant": Palaiseul, 184; Min: Penelope Ody, *Essential Guide to Natural Home Remedies* (2002), 128; "o'er much": www.easyhomeremedy.com.

WILD ROSE [196–201]: Vitamin C, wartime use: Mabey, 192; Anacreon: qtd Maggie Tisserand, *Essential Oils for Lovers* (1999 [1993]), 97; Bartholomew: qtd Eleanour Sinclair Rohde, *The Old English Herbals* (New York, 1971 [1922]), 49; Pechey, 202; Milto: Tisserand, 96; Pliny: Stuart, 253; dagger, other names: Back, 55; love-charm, Germany: Pamela Allardice, *Aphrodisiacs & Love Magic* (Bridport, Dorset, 1989), 21; gall: Grigson, 174; Askham's Herbal: Rohde, 60.

WILLOW [202–03]: Culpeper, 272; Ben-Erik van Wyk et al., *Medicinal Plants of South Africa* (Pretoria, 1997), 222; (2007) 17704985; (2011) 21226125; www. aspirin-foundation.com, www.pfaf.org.

WILLOWHERB [204–05]: Treben, 49; Gerard, 114; Parkinson, 549.

WOOD BETONY [206–09]: Culpeper, 30, 31–2; Pratt, IV, 189; Parkinson, 616; *Grete Herball*: Rohde, 72; John Clare: qtd Pratt, *Wild Flowers*, www.books.google. com; (2013) 23307315.

YARROW [210–14]: "herb for women": Treben, 50; "cure-all": Barker, 460; Margaret Roberts, 31; Hoffmann, *Medical*, 523; Barker, 460; East Anglian saying: qtd Keith Vincent Smith, 136; Rudolf Steiner [n.d.]: qtd Smith, 136; Merian, *Erucarum ortus*.

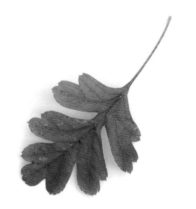

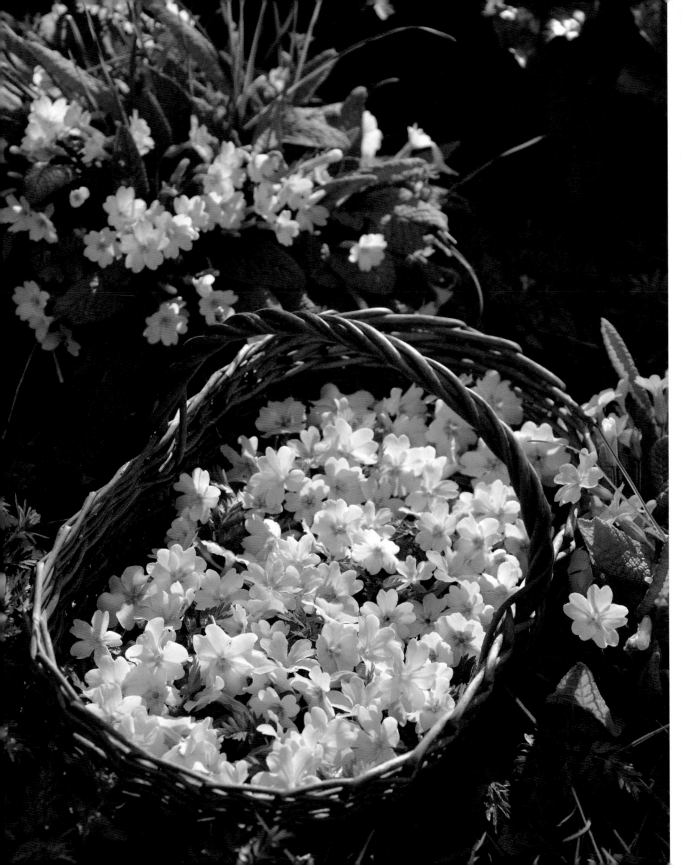

PART II: BACKYARD MEDICINE FOR ALL
A GUIDE TO HOME-GROWN HERBAL REMEDIES

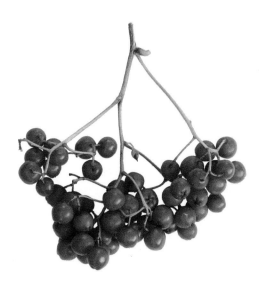

Illustration: rowan berries

Contents

Preface 7
Introduction 9
Harvesting from the wayside 10
Using your wayside harvest 13

* For all references and sources, see Notes to the Text, starting on page 430

Preface

We wrote this book because we saw around us a wealth of plants growing abundantly, which have medicinal uses that people have largely forgotten. These plants were once valued and widely used, but over time fell out of fashion and were bypassed because of a focus on the herbs of commerce.

Many readers of our earlier book *Hedgerow Medicine* have noted our hint there that we had another 50 or more plants in mind for similar treatment. In *Backyard Medicine for All* we have made room for these and a few more, including cognate species in a single chapter – such as primrose and cowslip; silverweed, tormentil and cinquefoil – or family groups, eg cranesbills, speedwells and thistles.

This is in effect a sequel to *Hedgerow Medicine*, with a similar locale and rationale. It has the same layout, with its strong visual emphasis, and the same sequence of information. As the subtitle suggests, we focus on largely forgotten medicinal plants that grow by roads or paths in the countryside or in the city.

Wayside plant medicine may start for you with reading a book like this, but the aim is for you to go out and practise it. Even Mr Squeers, the almost-illiterate headmaster in Dickens' *Nicholas Nickleby*, would agree. On Nicholas' first day at school, Squeers says:

"When the boys knows this out of book, he goes and does it. Where's the second boy?"
"Please, sir, he's weeding the garden."
"To be sure. So he is. B-O-T, bot, T-I-N, bottin, N-E-Y, bottiney, noun substantive, a knowledge of plants. When he has learned that bottiney means a knowledge of plants, he goes and knows 'em. That's our method, Nickleby.
"Third boy, what's a horse?"

And where do we 'go and know' for our practical lessons? To what the late Roger Deakin called *the undiscovered country of the nearby*. Waysides of old have become the road verges of today, and these everyday, nearby but overlooked ecosystems are significant wild plant communities.

Each chapter has an introductory section that puts the plant(s) into historical and botanical context, and its forgotten or traditional medicinal uses; the Use For section describes current medicinal applications; and a new final section, Modern Research, selects from published clinical work about the plant (mainly from the PubMed database). We dislike animal studies for several reasons but have included some as they can inspire further exploration.

The medicinal recipes have an important role. We subscribe to the advice of noted herbalist Christopher Hedley: *Don't buy a herbal book if it doesn't have recipes!* Making a medicine from it is the ultimate relationship with a plant, and we hope you will move from the armchair to the roadside, with due cautions noted, and try these recipes for yourself.

But, why 'forgotten' plants? Mostly these are plants that were once in the herbal pharmacopoeia but have been dropped as chemical medicines replaced them, and as the pharmacopoeias themselves shrank. Once out of the 'official' lists, plants are no longer commercially attractive and disappear from everyday use and familiarity.

Herbal knowledge has been declining since a peak in the mid-17th century, when John Parkinson included some 3,800 herbs in his great herbal. But we can do something about it. Contemporary American herbalist David

Winston, writing in 2005, made a plea that we heartily endorse: *One way of correcting this problem is the expansion of our pharmacopoeias by the inclusion of unused but effective indigenous and introduced species. There are hundreds of such herbs available that have long histories of usage by peoples who depended on these plants for their health and well being.*

Winston offers about a hundred plants for an 'American extra pharmacopoeia'. Indeed, several of them overlap with our choices (eg chicory, cow parsnip/hogweed, ground ivy, ox-eye daisy and purple loosestrife).

What are our rules for a plant's inclusion in this book? We cover plants we have had experience of; local abundance on waysides (eg navelwort is common in the west but not otherwise in the UK); we wanted to include juniper and centaury but they are endangered in the wild, so we didn't; ease of identification; being non-poisonous (eg we explain at length how other Apiaceae species differ from hemlock); and above-ground parts rather than roots.

Harvest with respect is our belief, so don't pick more than you need even where a row of hogweed stretches to the horizon along your roadside. It will be there tomorrow, unless the council mower happens to pass by.

❀ ❀

Writing a book like this is a collaborative process, not only between ourselves as co-authors but also within a wider herbal community. Our heartfelt thanks go to: Julian Barker, Charlotte du Cann, Danny O'Rawe and Mark Watson for acting as expert sounding boards in our contents-selection process; to Julia Behrens, Alice Bettany, Andrew Chevallier, Nikki Darrell, Chris Gambatese, Barbara Griggs, Karin Haile, Simon Harrap, Glennie Kindred, 7Song, Cathy Skipper and Davina Wynne-Jones for herbal wisdom, freely shared; and to Christine Herbert for (as usual) reading every word and offering us acute comments – and letting us photograph or pick plants in her smallholding. We also thank the Forgotten Herbs Facebook group, and forager friends Mina Said-Allsopp, Robin Harford and Monica Wilde.

To Merlin Unwin, Karen McCall and Jo Potter of Merlin Unwin Books our renewed thanks for getting the carrot/stick ratio just right.

We are grateful to a number of institutions, including the Wellcome Library, the British Library and the Norfolk County Council library service. We especially thank our local bibliographic treasure-house, the John Innes Historical Collections and outreach curator Dr Sarah Wilmot.

We have acknowledged sources in the Notes to the Text, and thank copyright holders for permission to include extracts from their work. If we have overlooked or been unable to locate copyright owners we will gladly add details in a later edition. Needless to say, the opinions expressed here are our own, and we take responsibility for them.

Thanks also to Julie's many patients who, wittingly or not, have contributed to this book. Don't worry, you remain anonymous.

Finally, our respect to the plants themselves. We owe them everything, for, as John Ruskin wrote over 150 years ago:

All the wide world of vegetation blooms and buds for you; the thorn and the thistle which the earth casts forth as evil are to you the kindliest servants; no dying petal nor drooping tendril is so feeble as to have no help for you.

Julie Bruton-Seal & Matthew Seal
Ashwellthorpe, Norfolk
November 2016

Introduction

Jesus' Parable of the Sower starts with the seeds that fall by the wayside – *and the fowls came and devoured them up* (Matthew 13.4). This wayside is hard and impenetrable, unsuitable ground for hand-spread seeds to germinate. In effect they were bird food.

The parable next has seeds falling on stony ground, which grew but scorched in the sun because they had no root. Seed scattered on thorny ground germinated but was choked by weeds. The seed on fertile ground flourished, and gave varying levels of fruit.

The parable explains different levels of faith. But what concerns us here is an undertone: in the battle of agriculture and nature, cultivated crops must win against weeds, or we all die. 'Falling by the wayside' is a metaphor for losing out, giving up and being forgotten, as morally inferior. Waysides are marginal land, between public road and private farmland, lacking the status and value of either.

Yet European and other pre-industrial waysides were once vibrant spaces, tracks where multitudes of people and livestock moved between fields and villages, while ancient droveways saw cattle led hundreds of miles to distant urban markets. Carts and carriages used animal power, and as draught horses or cows grazed the wayside vegetation they also fertilised it. It was a wayside golden age for wild flowers where meadows met mud tracks, and grass was kept short.

Fast forward to today, and livestock is moved by truck, people drive rather than walk, fields are over-fertilised, roads are metalled over, mass levels of traffic emit nitrous oxide pollutants, and hedges and roadsides are cut by mowers owned by councils or landowners. The wayside wild plants are often mown in early summer, when all but spring plants have yet to complete their life cycle, and the sward is left uncollected, leading to excess nitrogenous content in the soil. This favours nitrogen-loving summer species like hogweed (cow parsnip), nettle and bramble, which choke other plants – thorny ground indeed.

The plant conservation charity Plantlife estimates that 97% of British meadows have gone since the 1930s. No wonder that the few remaining animal-based rural economies in places like parts of Romania, Sardinia, Poland or Amish lands in Pennsylvania are celebrated, a reminder of the lost wealth of ancient meadowlands and waysides.

Yet all is not a forgotten memory. Plantlife estimates that about 700 species of wild plants still grow on Britain's road verges, some 45% of the nation's flora. And there are nearly 320,000 miles (500,000 km) of these verges. They are effectively the residual habitat of lost meadows, and they are already managed. And sometimes protected: we live near Wood Lane Road-verge Meadow, Long Stratton, home of the endangered sulphur clover.

Taking 'road-verge' as the modern equivalent of 'way-side' opens everything up. Why not locate and use some of these abundant, free, easily identified (in most cases) and wiry wild wayside plants for our own medicine? This book invites you to step off the 'beaten track' and offers you the means to do so, including the legalities and practicalities of collecting wayside plants for medicinal use.

Harvesting from the wayside

Harvesting wild plants for food or medicine is a great pleasure, and healing in its own right. We all need the company of plants and wild places, whether a wayside, an old wood, a remote moor or seashore or even our own garden. Gathering herbs for free is the beginning of a valuable and therapeutic relationship with the wild. Here are a few basic guidelines to get started.

Why pay others to frolic in the luscious gardens of Earth, picking flowers and enjoying themselves making herbal products? You can do all that frolicking, immersing yourself in wondrous herbal beauty, and uplifting your mind and spirit. Making your own herbal medicine both enhances your happiness and boosts your immune system.
– Green (2000)

Herbs are to be gathered when they are fullest of juice which is before they run up to seed; and if you gather them in a hot sunshine, they will not be so subject to putrifie: the best way to dry them is in the Sun ... Let Flowers be gathered when they are in their prime, in a sunshine day, and dried in the Sun. Let the Seeds be perfectly ripe before they be gathered. Let them be kept in a dry place; for any moisture, though it be but a moist air, corrupts them.
– Culpeper (1653)

The process of gathering wild herbs for medicine – our own term for this is medicinal foraging – is straightforward. You identify the right plant and pick it at the right time, then make a simple home medicine. The benefits are aptly expressed by James Green (quote alongside), and the desiderata have not changed in the 350-plus years since Nicholas Culpeper gave his advice (below left).

Identification
Perhaps the most important thing is to ensure you have the right plant. A good field guide is essential – we like *Harrap's Wild Flowers* by Simon Harrap – and there are numerous phone apps for wild plants. A herb mentor is invaluable: many herbalists offer herb walks. Check our Resources page (437) to contact practitioners in your area.

For distribution maps and plant identification, the Botanical Society of the British Isles has a regularly updated site: see www.bsbi.org. In America the USDA maps both wild plants and crops (www.usda.gov).

Where to collect
Choose a place where the plant you are harvesting is abundant and vibrant. Woods, fields and minor roads are best, though some of our plants are also found in the city. Avoiding heavy traffic is safer for you and your lungs, and plants growing in quiet places are less polluted. Park carefully and be aware of traffic at all times.

Remember that hedgerows next to fields may receive crop sprays and waysides may be sprayed, as well as being mown (often just when you are ready to collect).

When to collect
Harvest herbs when they are at their lushest. Pick on a dry day, after any morning dew has burned off. For aromatic plants the sun's energy is vital, so wait for a hot day and pick while the sun is high, ideally just before noon.

Harvest only what you need and will use; leave some of the plant so it will grow back. When picking above-ground parts of a plant, only take the top half to two-thirds. Never harvest if a plant is the only one in a particular area.

Collecting equipment
Very basic: think carrier bags or a basket, and perhaps gloves, hat, scissors or secateurs. Be sensible: blackthorn and sea buckthorn call for more protection than veronica. Be aware that carrying a knife with

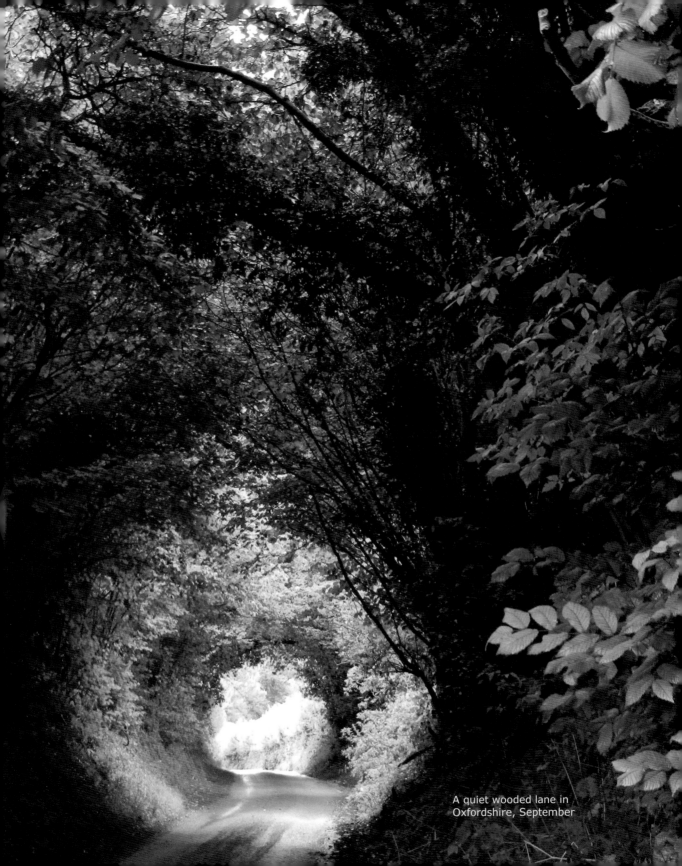

A quiet wooded lane in
Oxfordshire, September

a blade of more than 75mm long may be a legal offence. If you are harvesting roots take a small shovel or digging fork.

We have included a few roots in our recipes. It is important not to over-harvest these, as you are usually killing the plant (exceptions include ground elder). The roots we have selected are widespread and often classed as weeds.

Collecting for sale

This book describes medicinal foraging for personal use rather than collecting for sale, either directly as in fungi to a restaurant or for making medicines or cosmetics to sell. Other laws and regulations apply when selling is involved, including health and safety approval of your equipment.

We do however like the story of Dr Christopher (1909–83), the American naturopath and herbalist, who in the lean post-war years worked as a gardener in the mornings. He kept the 'weeds' he had unearthed, notably plantain, took them home and made medicine from them. Then he sold this back to his clients!

Legal guidance

Custom in the form of common law still protects the right to wild-gather the 'four Fs' of fruit, foliage, fungi and flowers, for personal use and not resale. Roots are somewhat different, as the law recognises: it's one thing to smell a neighbour's rose, another to pick its petals and yet another to dig it up without permission.

In practical terms you should seek an owner's permission

before unearthing roots anywhere outside your own garden, but picking above-ground parts of plants anywhere will generally be condoned if done discreetly and moderately. There are seldom prosecutions for medicinal harvesting.

Note that private land should be marked with a notice board, and you can theoretically be charged with trespass if you ignore such a notice. Waysides may be owned privately or be public land. Many nature reserves prohibit any picking.

Rare plants are protected by the Wildlife and Countryside Act 1981, and a list of these plants is regularly updated. No such plants are included in this book, and we would not expect to make medicine from an endangered species.

Note that legislation differs in Scotland and Scandinavian countries, with more 'right to roam' embedded in law than in England and Wales. For the text of relevant legislation, see www.legislation.gov.uk.

Storing your plants

It's a good idea to make your medicines on the same day as you pick them, if you can. And the best way to store your plants is in the medicinal form you have made, whether preserving in alcohol or glycerine, honey, vinegar, ghee, as tea or ice cubes, and so on, as outlined in the next section.

Don't forget to label any container with the plant's name, date and place collected.

Using your wayside harvest

Herbs can be used in many different ways. Simplest and most ancient is nibbling the fresh plant, crushing the leaves to apply them as a poultice or perhaps boiling up some water to make a tea. Many of the plants discussed in this book are foods as well as medicines, and incorporating them seasonally in your diet is a tasty and enjoyable way to improve your health.

But because fresh herbs aren't available year round or may not grow right on your doorstep, you may want to preserve them for later use. Follow these guidelines.

Equipment needed
You don't need any special equipment for making your own foraged medicines. You probably already have most of what you need.

Kitchen basics like a teapot, measuring jugs, saucepans and a blender are all useful, as are jam-making supplies such as a jelly bag and jam jars. A mortar and pestle are handy but not essential. You'll also need jars, bottles and labels for these.

There is a list of suppliers at the end of the book to help you source any supplies or ingredients you may need (see p220).

It is a good idea to have a notebook to write down your experiences, so you'll have a record for yourself and can repeat successes. Who knows, it could become a family heirloom like the stillroom books of old!

Drying herbs
The simplest way to preserve a plant is to dry it, and then use the dried part as a tea (infusion or decoction: see overleaf). Dried plant material can also go into tinctures, infused oils and other preparations, though these are often made directly from fresh plants.

To dry herbs, tie them in small bundles and hang these from the rafters or a laundry airer, or spread the herbs on a sheet of brown paper or a screen. (Avoid using newspaper as the inks contain toxic chemicals.)

Generally, plants are best dried out of the sun. An airing or warming cupboard works well, particularly in damp weather.

You can easily make your own drying screen by stapling some mosquito netting or other open-weave fabric to a wooden frame. This is ideal, as the air can circulate around the plant, and yet you won't lose any small flowers or leaves through the mesh.

A dehydrator set on a low temperature setting is perfect for drying herbs as well as summer fruit.

Storing dried herbs
Once the plant is crisply dry, you can discard any larger stalks. Whole leaves and flowers will keep best, but if they are large you may want

The 'Virtues' of a herb are its strengths and qualities; its inner potency, expressions of its vital spirit and of the way it is in the world. The way a herb is in the world will inform it of the way to be in your body. We prefer this term to the more modern 'uses'. Herbs do not have uses. They have themselves and their own purposes. – Hedley & Shaw (2016)

to crumble them so they take up less space. They will be easier to measure for teas etc if they are crumbled before use.

Dried herbs can be stored in brown paper bags or in airtight containers such as sweet jars or plastic tubs, in a cool place. If your container is made of clear glass or other transparent material, keep it in the dark as light will fade leaves and flowers quite quickly.

Dried herbs will usually keep for a year, until you can replace them with a fresh harvest. Roots and bark keep longer than leaves and flowers.

In looking at medicine-making we start with the familiar teas and tinctures, then move on to often-forgotten but still valuable methods.

Teas: infusions and decoctions
The simplest way to make a plant extract is with hot water. Use fresh or dried herbs. An **infusion**, where hot water is poured over the herb and left to steep for several minutes, is the usual method for a tea of leaves and flowers.

A **decoction**, where the herb is simmered or boiled in water for some time, is best for roots and bark. Decoctions stored in sterile bottles will keep for a year or more if unopened.

Infusions and decoctions can also be used as mouthwashes, gargles, eyebaths, fomentations and douches.

Tinctures
While the term tincture can refer to any liquid extract of a plant, what is usually meant is an alcohol and water extract. Many plant constituents dissolve more easily in a mixture of alcohol and water than in pure water. There is the added advantage of the alcohol being a preservative, allowing the extract to be stored for several years.

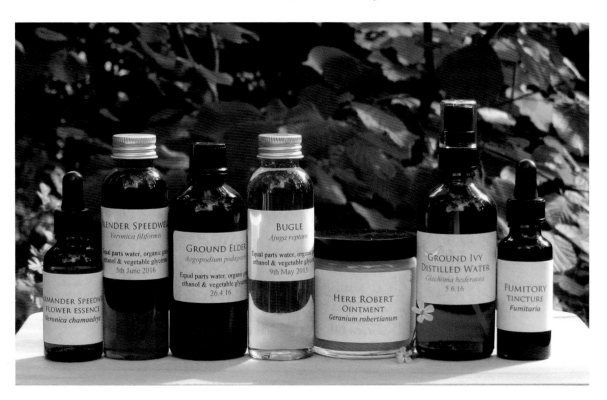

The alcohol content of the finished extract needs to be at least 20% to adequately preserve it. Most commercially produced tinctures have a minimum alcohol content of 25%. A higher concentration is needed to extract more resinous substances, such as pine resin.

For making your own tinctures, vodka is preferred as it has no flavour of its own, and allows the taste of the herbs to come through. Whisky, brandy or rum work quite well too. Wine can be used, especially for dried herbs, but will not have as long a shelf life because of its lower alcohol content.

To make a tincture, you simply fill a jar with the herb and top up with alcohol, or you can put the whole lot in the blender first. The mixture is then kept out of the light for anything from a day to a month to infuse before being strained and bottled. The extraction is ready when the plant material has lost most of its colour.

Tinctures are convenient to store and to take. We find amber or blue glass jars best for keeping, although clear bottles will let you enjoy the colours of your tinctures. Store them in a cool place. Kept properly, most tinctures have a shelf life of around five years. They are rapidly absorbed into the bloodstream, and alcohol makes the herbal preparation more heating and dispersing in its effect.

Wines and beers
Many herbs can be brewed into wines and beers, which will retain the medicinal virtues of the plants. Elderberry wine and nettle beer are traditional, but don't forget that ordinary beer is brewed with hops, a medicinal plant.

Other fermentations
There are other fermentations that use a combination of yeasts and bacteria. Sourdough bread is one example, but more relevant here are drinks such as kefir and kombucha. The starter grains are usually available on eBay.

There are two kinds of kefir, one made with milk and one made with sugar and water. We find the latter a really useful drink that can be flavoured with various herbs, such as in our sea buckthorn recipe on p160.

Glycerites
Vegetable glycerine (glycerol) is extracted from vegetable oil, and is a sweet, syrupy substance. It is particularly good in making medicines for children, and for soothing preparations intended for the throat and digestive tract, or coughs. A glycerite will keep well as long as the concentration of glycerine is at least 50% to 60% in the finished product.

Glycerine does not extract most plant constituents as well as alcohol does, but preserves flavours and colours better, and is particularly good for flowers. Glycerites are made the same way as tinctures, except the jar is kept in the sun or in a warm place to infuse.

Many herbalists like to add a small amount of alcohol to their glycerites to help preserve them, and to make them less sweet.

Glycerine is a good preservative for fresh plant juices, in which half fresh plant juice and half glycerine are mixed, as it keeps the juice green and in suspension better than alcohol. This preparation is called a succus.

Gemmotherapy extracts
Gemmotherapy is nothing to do with gem stones but rather uses the buds, shoots and sometimes root tips of trees and shrubs. The idea is that the embryonic tissue in the growing tips contains all the information of the whole plant, as well as various hormones not present elsewhere in the plant.

Buds are collected when they are plump but still firm, just before they open. Shoots are picked green, when they emerge from the dormant twigs. Because picking off the growth tip of a tree branch stops that part producing leaves, it needs to be done respectfully, not taking too many from any one plant.

For extracting the chemistry of buds and shoots, a mixture of equal parts water, alcohol and glycerine has been found most effective. If you are using vodka or another spirit that is 50% alcohol (or more usually 40% alcohol and 60% water), simply use two parts alcohol to one part glycerine.

We have found this an effective mixture for roots and leaves too, and often prefer it to making a standard tincture or glycerite.

Vinegars

Another way to extract and preserve plant material is to use vinegar. Some plant constituents will extract better in an acidic medium, making vinegar the perfect choice.

Herbal vinegars are often made from pleasant-tasting herbs, and used in salad dressings and for cooking. They are also a good addition to the bath or for rinsing hair, as the acetic acid of the vinegar helps restore the natural protective acid pH of the body's exterior. Cider vinegar is a remedy for colds and other viruses, so it is a good solvent for herbal medicines made for these conditions.

Herbal honeys

Honey has natural antibiotic and antiseptic properties, making it an excellent vehicle for medicines to fight infection. It can be applied topically to wounds, burns and leg ulcers. Local honeys can help prevent hayfever attacks.

Honey is naturally sweet, making it palatable for medicines for children. It is also particularly suited to medicines for the throat and respiratory system as it is soothing and also clears congestion. Herb-infused honeys are made the same way as glycerites.

Oxymels

An oxymel is a preparation of honey and vinegar. Oxymels were once popular as cordials, both in Middle Eastern and European herbal traditions. They are particularly good for cold and flu remedies. Honey can be added to a herb-infused vinegar, or an infused honey can be used as well.

Electuaries

These are basically herbal pastes. They are often made by stirring powdered dried herbs into honey or glycerine, but also by grinding up herbs, seeds and dried fruit together. Electuaries are good as children's remedies, soothe the digestive tract and can be made into tasty medicine balls or truffles.

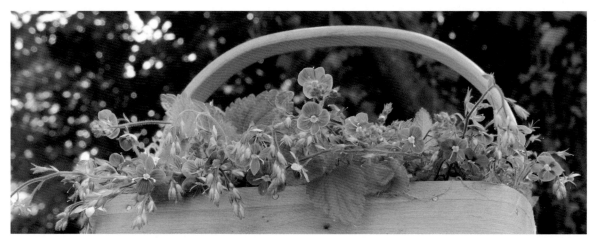

Syrups

Syrups are made by boiling the herb with sugar and water. The sugar acts as a preservative, and can help extract the plant material. Syrups generally keep well, especially the thicker ones containing more sugar, as long as they are stored in sterilised bottles.

They are particularly suitable for children because of their sweet taste, and are generally soothing.

Herbal sweets

While we are not recommending large amounts of sugar as being healthy, herbal sweets such as coltsfoot rock and peppermints are a traditional way of taking herbs in a pleasurable way.

Plant essences

Plant essences, usually flower essences, differ from other herbal preparations in that they only contain the vibrational energy of the plant, and none of the plant chemistry. They have the advantage of being potent in small doses. Julie nearly always dispenses flower essences for her patients alongside other herbal preparations as they help the herbs do their job.

To make an essence, the flowers or other plant parts are usually put in water in a glass bowl and left to infuse in the sun for a couple of hours, as in the instructions for our forget-me-not essence on page 291. This essence is then preserved with brandy, and diluted for use.

Distilling herbs

While distilling essential oils from plants requires large plant quantities, it is simple to distil your own herbal waters or hydrolats.

Simply use a stockpot or other large saucepan with a domed lid that can be put on upside-down. One with a glass lid is best, as you can see what's going on inside. Put a collecting bowl in your saucepan under the centre of the lid, raised on a brick or upturned bowl above the water around it, which contains the plants. Heat the pot so that the water starts to become steam; this collects inside the lid and drips down into your collecting bowl. Ice cubes (or frozen peas!) on the upturned lid speed up the condensation. Keep on low heat until your collecting bowl is nearly full. Pour the distilled herbal water carefully into sterile bottles. There are many videos on YouTube showing you how to do this.

If you want to make larger quantities, we recommend the traditional hand-made copper alembics still being produced in Portugal. See www.al-ambiq.com

Distilled plant waters keep quite well, but do not have any preservatives, so are often dispensed in spray bottles to keep them from contamination. They are good as face washes and eyebaths, and can be taken internally. They are gentler than tinctures, but effective.

Infused oils

Oil is mostly used to extract plants for external use on the skin, but infused oils can equally well be taken internally. Like vinegars, they are good in salad dressings and in cooking.

We prefer extra virgin olive oil as a base, as it does not go rancid as many polyunsaturated oils do. Other oils, such as coconut and sesame, may be chosen because of their individual characteristics.

Infused oils are also known as macerated oils, and should not be confused with essential oils, which are aromatic oils isolated by distilling the plant material.

Ointments or salves

Ointments or salves are rubbed onto the skin. The simplest ointments are made by adding beeswax to an infused oil and heating until the beeswax has melted. The amount of wax needed will vary, depending on the climate or temperature in which it will be used, with more wax needed in hotter climates or weather.

Ointments made this way have a very good shelf life. They absorb well, while providing a protective layer on top of the skin.

Ointments can also be made with animal fats or hard plant fats such as cocoa butter, and with plant waxes such as candelilla.

Butters and ghees
Butter can be used instead of oil to extract herbs, and, once clarified by simmering, it keeps well without refrigeration, making a simple ointment. Clarified butter is a staple in Indian cooking and medicine, where it is called ghee. It is soothing on the skin and absorbs well, plumping up the skin. Herbal butters and ghees can also be used as food.

Skin creams
Creams are a mixture of a water-based preparation with an oil-based one, to make an emulsion. Creams are absorbed into the skin more rapidly than ointments, but have the disadvantages of being more difficult to make and of not keeping as well.

Creams are best refrigerated, and essential oils can be added to help preserve them. Creams are better than ointments for use on hot skin conditions, as they are more cooling.

Poultices
The simplest poultice is mashed fresh herb put onto the skin, as when you crush a plantain leaf and apply it to a wasp sting. Poultices can be made from fresh herb juice mixed with slippery elm powder or simply flour, or from dried herb moistened with hot water or vinegar.

Change the poultice every few hours and keep it in place with a bandage or sticking plaster.

Fomentations or compresses
A fomentation or compress is an infusion or a decoction applied externally. Simply soak a flannel or bandage in the warm or cold liquid, and apply. **Hot fomentations** are used to disperse and clear, and are good for conditions as varied as backache, joint pain, boils and acne. Note that hot fomentations need to be refreshed frequently once they cool down.

Cold fomentations can be used for cases of inflammation or for headaches. Alternating hot and cold fomentations works well for sprains and other injuries.

Embrocations or liniments
Embrocations or liniments are used in massage, with the herbs preserved in an oil or alcohol base, or a mixture of the two. Absorbed quickly through the skin, they can readily relieve muscle tension, pain and inflammation, and speed the healing of injuries.

Baths
Herbs can be added conveniently to bathwater by tying a sock or cloth full of dried or fresh herb to the hot tap as you run the bath, or by adding a few cups of an infusion or decoction. Herbal vinegars, tinctures and oils can be added to bath water, as can a few drops of essential oil.

Besides full baths, hand and foot baths are very refreshing, as are sitz or hip baths where only your bottom is in the water.

Part of the therapeutic effect of any of these baths is the fact that they make you stop and be still, something most of us do not do often enough.

Douches
Once they have cooled, herbal infusions or decoctions can be used as douches for vaginal infections or inflammation.

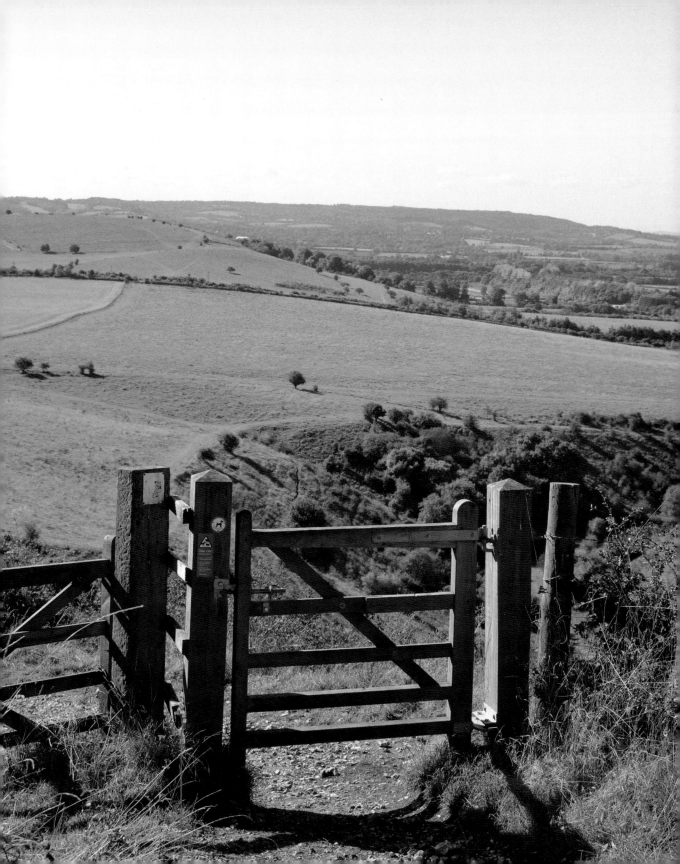

Alexanders *Smyrnium olusatrum*

Alexanders has made the switch from wild-gathered plant to cultivated and back to wild, and was both food and medicine in classical and medieval times. It lost out to celery as a commercial salad crop from the 16th century, but is now making a comeback as a winter foraged food and has intriguing possibilities in colon cancer research.

Apiaceae (Umbelliferaceae) Carrot family

Description: Tall biennial (to 1.5m or 5ft), with hairless, scented stems; leaves dark green, glossy, three-lobed; flowers yellow-white; seeds dark black ovals. Dies back in summer.

Habitat: Near the sea, by cliff and roadsides, hedgerows, forming colonies; spreading inland slowly.

Distribution: Mediterranean origin, naturalised throughout Western and Central Europe; east and southern coasts of Britain and Ireland, southern England.

Related species: Many Apiaceae are medicinal, including angelica, celery, dill, fennel and lovage. Be careful of your identification as there are several poisonous species in this family.

Parts used: All parts, including the seeds, available from autumn to spring; produces early foliage in winter.

Geoffrey Grigson (1958) says alexanders is 'happiest and most frequent by the sea'. He's right, and sturdy stands of this vigorous and stately naturalised umbellifer abound by eastern and southern coasts of Britain and Ireland.

It also seems to be pressing inland in our part of East Anglia, thriving by roadsides at least 55km (35 miles) from the Norfolk coast, perhaps responding favourably to regular winter salting of the roads.

We welcome its advance, and Julie has fond memories of picking winter alexander shoots for salad on the school run to Wroxham.

The plant's origin and names are clearly Mediterranean. Archaeological finds suggest it was being cultivated in the eastern Mediterranean in the Iron Age (c.1300–700 BC). Its roots and shoots had become a popular, if pungent, potherb and vegetable by the time of the reign of Alexander the Great in the fourth century BC.

The English name alexanders could be for the emperor, or indeed for the port in Egypt that he founded and which bore his name. The plant's Greek name *hipposelinon* means 'horse parsley or celery', which was still being used by John Parkinson in the early 17th century. In this context horse means large, according to William Salmon's herbal of 1710.

Columella, the Roman agricultural writer (AD 4–70), knew alexanders as 'myrrh of Achaea', the then current Latin name for Greece. The myrrh reference has followed the plant in its generic name *Smyrnium*. Some people do find the taste and scent to be myrrh-like, though others get more lovage in it; an old name is black lovage.

Alexanders had an early shift from wild-gathering to cultivation, and from Roman times to the 16th century or so it was more known as a food than a medicine. Its species name *olusatrum* derives from *olus* for potherb and *atrum* for black, the colour of the large seeds, which were ground as a condiment.

As both a food and medicine alexanders became a widely used monastic plant in medieval times. Many scattered inland sightings of it in Britain can be related to sites of former monastic houses. By the dissolution in the 1530s and 1540s, wild celery was being cultivated and superseded alexanders and lovage in popularity.

Currently alexanders is becoming popular again with foragers, for its fresh greens in winter and spicy seeds. We like it as a condiment to use as pepper. We actually don't find it 'peppery' but more pungent, sour, oily and nutty.

Use alexanders for …
Alexanders was classified in classic Galenic terms as 'hot and dry in the third degree', and its actions were accordingly forceful. It was found to work strongly on the urinary and digestive systems, especially the seeds.

Parkinson (1629) states that *The seede is more used physically than the roote, or any other parte.* Salmon (1710) writes that alexanders *effectually provokes Urine, helps the Strangury, and prevails against Gravel and Tartarous Matter in Reins and Bladder.*

In modern terms, Salmon was saying that alexanders was a diuretic, clearing obstructions in the urinary system, including stones in the kidneys and bladder.

Dioscorides, in the 1st century AD, knew alexanders as an emmenagogue, a herb that promoted menstruation. Salmon noted that the plant 'powerfully provokes the Terms'; it also 'expels the Birth', ie afterbirth. That is, it is a powerful uterine tonic, to be treated with caution in pregnancy.

The Monks were good Chemists, & invented many good Receipts: which they imparted to their Penitents: & so are handed downe to their great-grandchildren, a great many varieties.
– Aubrey, c.1660s

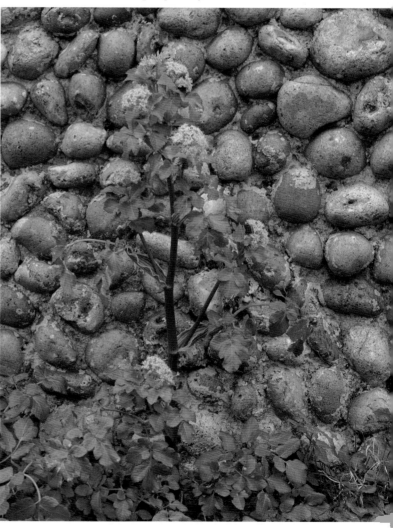

Salmon adds that a cataplasm of the bruised leaves, applied hot to the afflicted part, will dry up old sores and foetid ulcers, *and either discusses* [breaks up] *or maturates Scrophulous* [tubercular] *Tumors.*

Alexanders was included in the first London *Pharmacopoeia* (1618), meaning it was an 'official' herb of the apothecaries. But by the time Salmon prepared his herbal nearly a century later it had been dropped. It was sliding out of use in both medicine and cookery,

though there are records of alexanders root being sold to the public in Covent Garden market later in the 18th century.

Of course it does not follow that because alexanders has gone out of fashion it is no longer useful as food and a wayside medicine. The virtues the old herbalists championed remain valid, even if less used these days, and furthermore clinical experimentation is opening up some new possibilities.

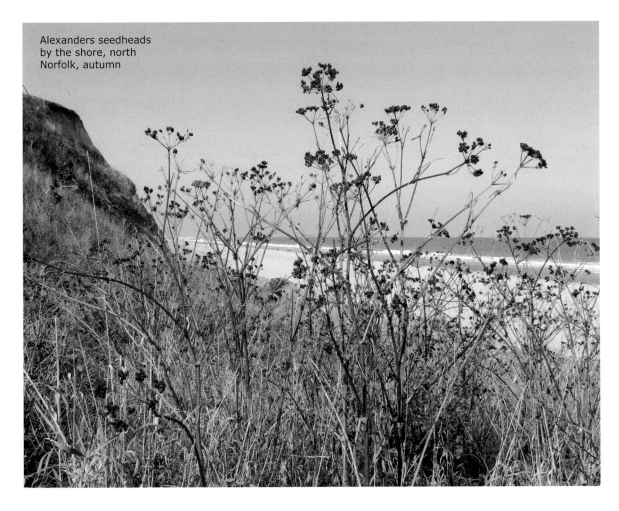

Alexanders seedheads by the shore, north Norfolk, autumn

Modern research

One area of recent interest is alexanders essential oil. Italian researchers found (2014) that the oil from the flowers induces apoptosis, or cell death, in human colon carcinoma cells. The oil has high quantities of isofuranodiene, a known anti-cancer agent.

Another intriguing finding (2012) is that this oil is strongly effective against candida, a fungal infection.

There is also a suggestion (2008) that alexanders has a comparable biomedical action to zedoary (*Curcuma wenyujin*), a type of Chinese ginger and source of a traditional remedy called Ezhu.

Ezhu is prescribed in China as an essential oil for liver, gastric, lung and cervical cancer, and its active principle, furanodiene, is the same. Perhaps alexanders could be a Western Ezhu in waiting?

Its certain aromatic or pungent flavour … would be too strong for modern tastes.
– Pratt (1866)

… although it be a little bitter, yet it is both wholsome, and pleasing to a great many, by reason of the aromaticall or spicie taste, warming and comforting the stomack, and helping it digest the many waterish and flegmaticke meates [that] *are in those times* [winter and spring] *much eaten.*
– Parkinson (1629)

Harvesting alexanders

The green herb is best harvested in winter or very early spring, before the stalks become stringy. The seeds can be harvested once they turn black, and the stems are no longer green.

A tisane for the stomak

The tisane (tea) recipe, taken from the *Syon Abbey Herbal* of 1517, may be the first English reference to alexanders as a medicinal plant (preceding the usually referenced one in William Turner's *Herball* of 1562). This quartet of four Apiaceae roots as a hot tea makes for a powerful stimulant to a sluggish stomach.

Take rotis [roots] *of Fenell, Alisaundre* [alexanders], *Parsyly and Smalach* [celery], *a godehandfull, well and clen, washen and wel stanpid* [crushed] *in a morter & seth* [boil] *hem in a pottel* [pot] *of water to the half and do therto a littil hony and clens it and drink it at even and at moroun* [morning], *ix sponfull at oones* [at one go].

Alexanders black butter sauce

Collect the seeds in the autumn when they are ripe. Grind them in an electric spice mill or coffee grinder. They are best freshly ground in small quantities as needed, sieving to remove any larger chunks as these can be quite chewy.

Melt 2 tablespoons **butter** with 1 tablespoon **olive oil**. Add 2 cloves **garlic**, crushed. Cook gently for a few minutes, then add 2 to 3 teaspoons **ground alexanders seeds**, and heat through.

Serve stirred into pasta, or as a dipping sauce for bread. Quite heady!

Root tisane
- sluggish digestion
- gas and griping pains
- urinary gravel
- urinary infections

Alexanders black butter sauce
- stimulates digestion
- urinary gravel

Caution
Avoid alexanders seed during pregnancy.

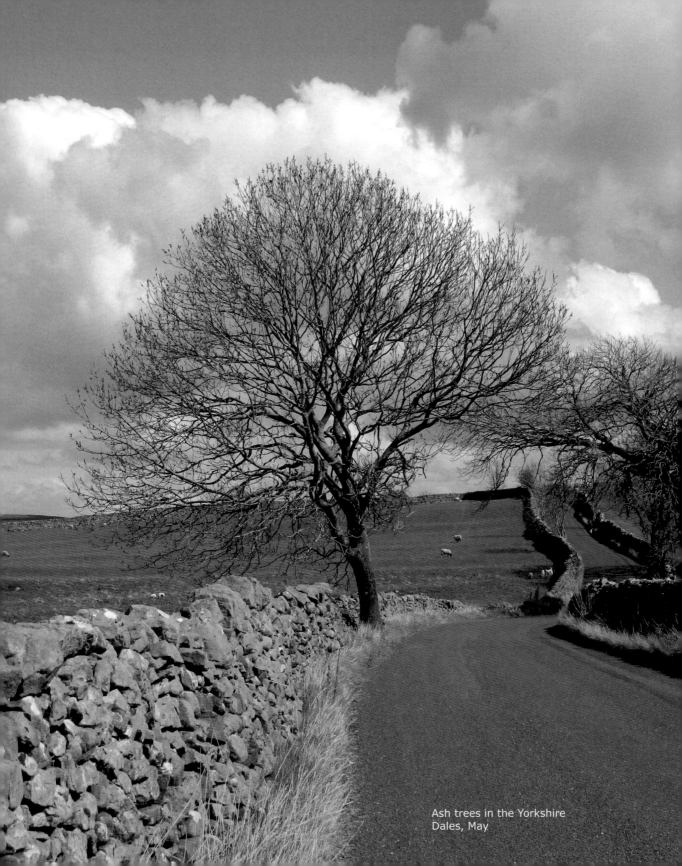

Ash trees in the Yorkshire
Dales, May

Ash *Fraxinus excelsior*

Ash has been a common British tree since Neolithic times, known as both a highly adaptable wood with a huge range of uses and as a folk medicine. It is currently in the news because it is endangered by ash dieback, a fungal disease.

Britain recognised officially in 2012 that its 126 million or so *Fraxinus excelsior* (European ash) trees were under attack by ash dieback, an almost incurable fungal condition arriving in ash trees imported from mainland Europe. The dieback manifests in the tree crowns and leaf mass, and affects saplings more readily than mature trees. Estimates in late 2015 put up to 90% of British ash trees at serious risk.

Identified first as *Chalara fraxinea*, ash dieback has been subject to intensive research, which has moved its name on twice – it is now known as *Hymenoscyphus fraxineus*. The early genome research into the fungus was carried out in the wood at the back of our house in Norfolk – and our village has the unintentionally ironic name of Ashwellthorpe.

Another threat to ash trees is the emerald ash borer, a small destructive beetle endemic to North America and now rampaging through Russia, though not found yet in the UK. It destroys a full-grown ash in three years, while *Hymenoscyphus* might take five or ten.

In cash terms, estimates say ash wood adds £100 million

Oleaceae
Olive family

Description: Grows to 30m (100ft) tall, erect, deciduous; grey bark, knobbly brown and yellow flowers, large black conical buds, bright green pinnate leaves with 7–13 oval leaflets.

Habitat: Widespread, though prefers lowland and limestone; most abundant in eastern/southern Britain.

Distribution: Native to Northern Europe, Central and East Asia; sometimes forms woods, but also prominent in mixed woods, copses and hedgerows. Found in eastern Canada and north-eastern US.

Related species: *F. americana* (white ash); *F. angustifolia* (narrow-leaved ash); *F. chinensis* ssp. *rhynchophylla* (Chinese ash); *F. ornus* (manna ash).

Parts used: Bark, leaves, buds, fruit and seeds [keys], sap.

Here comes Betty and biochar!

The research community is not giving up on ash just yet.

In April 2016 a report by a joint British and Scandinavian team said a 200-year-old Ashwellthorpe ash tree nicknamed 'Betty' gave cause for hope.

'Betty' had three genetic markers for resisting dieback, even while living next to infected trees. The team think other British ashes share Betty's tolerance, and selective breeding may lead to resistant ash woodlands one day.

Another hopeful sign is biochar. Biochar is fine-grained charcoal made from burnt biomass, and is well known to gardeners and growers.

What is new is that enriched biochar (with added seaweed and worm casts) has lent resistance to ash dieback in an experiment in Essex, reported in 2015.

The tantalising promise is that adding biochar to ash tree roots will prevent fresh infections by fungal spores, notably those of dieback.

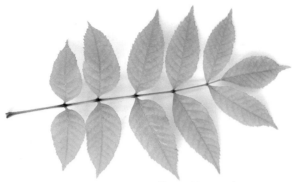

annually to Britain's economy; while ecologists remind us that ash provides a home for some 45 living species.

Even ash's glorious past has been questioned. It has long been identified as the Norse Tree of Life, Yggdrasil, with its roots in the lower world and its leaves in the heavens. But some scholars believe there has been a mistranslation, because Saga sources insist the tree is evergreen – it may be yew.

Use ash for …
But herbal accounts offer some much-needed narrative relief. Old herbals called ash **bark** a dry bitter tonic and astringent, with anti-inflammatory and febrifuge properties. In practice this meant an ash bark decoction or tincture was drunk to clear the liver and spleen, bring down malarial fevers or ague, and also externally treat arthritis and gout.

Ash bark was often used for fevers before South American tree barks like cinchona and quinine were imported. A French herbalist calls ash *a classic family remedy for intermittent fevers as a decoction or a powder with honey.*

In Traditional Chinese Medicine (TCM) ash bark is called *Qin Pin*, with properties of clearing heat, eliminating toxins and drying internal dampness. It is used for treating diarrhoea and dysentery, and leucorrhoea.

Ash **leaves** are known as diuretic and laxative, in addition to having the properties of the bark. They were used in teas for treating gravel and small stones in the kidney, as a purgative (often combined with senna pods), and for reducing the pain of gout and water retention (dropsy). An old name for ash was gout tree.

The leaves have an old reputation as a slimming aid. William Langham wrote in 1583: *To become leane, drinke the iuice of Ash leaues now and then with wine.* Ash leaves are still included in some modern slimming formulas.

Ash **buds** have also been used for their analgesic (pain-killing) properties in arthritis and as an anti-inflammatory for relieving synovial and joint pain. The practitioners of gemmotherapy (who use spring-time buds and fresh shoots) support these uses.

Ash **fruit and seeds** (known as keys) are sometimes pickled for eating, with a caper-like taste when preserved in salt and vinegar. The keys have an ancient reputation for relieving flatulence, and as an aphrodisiac, at least in Morocco (using *F. oxyphylla*).

In French herbal tradition ash keys are *a remarkable diuretic in cases of dropsy* (Palaiseul), used in tea or powder form with honey.

The bark and leaf **sap** of some ash varieties is sweet, and known as manna. The foremost of these is *F. ornus*, the manna ash. Manna was once used as a children's laxative.

Ash is a highly versatile wood: it made arrows, wheels, tools, handles, frames and sporting accessories such as baseball bats, snooker cues and hurley sticks ('the clash of the ash' in Ireland is two hurley sticks colliding).

The writer Robert Penn (2015) tested this versatility in a novel way. He felled a large ash and commissioned craftsmen to make useful objects out of it. A year's work yielded 126 of these, with even the sawdust useful as a fuel. Ash makes excellent firewood, even when freshly cut.

Modern research

Spanish research using ash keys showed diabetes-tackling potential by lowering blood sugar levels; a wound-healing effect was demonstrated in *F. angustifolia* extracts (2015); liver fibrosis from carbon tetrachloride was reduced by *F. rhynchophylla* ethanol extracts (2010); *F. excelsior* seed had a hypoglycaemic effect in reducing blood sugars (2004).

A European Medicines Authority monograph on *F. excelsior* (2011) confined itself to confirming use of ash as a diuretic and in pain relief.

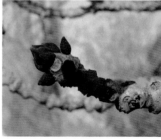

Ash buds in spring

Ash bud extract
- pain
- arthritis
- joint pain

Ash leaf tea
- constipation
- urinary gravel
- gout
- dropsy
- to lose weight
- fevers
- soothes a dry throat

Harvesting ash

Harvest ash leaves in summer. They can be used fresh or dried for winter use. Ash buds are gathered in spring, as they start to swell but just before they start to open.

Ash bud extract

Put your **ash buds** in a small jar. Mix enough **vodka** and **vegetable glycerine** to cover them, in the proportion of 2 parts vodka to 1 part glycerine. Leave for a month, shaking occasionally, then strain and bottle.

Dose: 10 drops three times daily

Ash leaf tea

Use one or two fresh **ash leaves**, or a rounded teaspoon of crumbled dried leaves, per mug of **boiling water**. Leave to brew for 10 to 15 minutes, then remove the leaves and drink. This tea can be drunk several times a day, as needed.

Avens *Geum urbanum, G. rivale*

Avens, also called wood avens or herb bennet, had a stellar medieval reputation, then retreated to more mundane uses as a potherb and moth repellant, but seems to be valued again as a rose family astringent and fever-reducing herb. Its virtues include safety, abundance and a surprising scent of cloves.

**Roseaceae
Rose family**

Description: Wood avens *(Geum urbanum)* is a hairy perennial, to 70cm (3ft), with bright yellow flowers of 5 petals, 5 long sepals; three-part greyish leaves; a bur of brownish hooked fruits. Water avens *(G. rivale)* has beautiful, nodding purply-brown flowers.

Habitat: Wood avens is found in woodland, but is also common in gardens and hedgesides; water avens needs more moisture and shade.

Distribution: Widespread and native in British Isles, Eurasia generally. Water avens is native to US; wood avens, an introduced species to US.

Related species: Mountain avens *(Dryas octopetala)* is a rare alpine; hybrid geum *(G. x intermedium)* is a fertile cross of wood avens and water avens.

Parts used: Roots.

Where [avens] root is in the house, the devil can do nothing, and flies from it; wherefore it is blessed above all herbs. – Ortus Sanitatis *(Garden of Health)* (1491)

It is what lies under the earth that elevates wood avens into herb bennet, the 'blessed *(benedictus)* herb'. The name is thought to precede the lifetime of St Benedict, the monastic innovator (c.480–c.547), and refer to an older reputation that avens root would ward off evil spirits and dangerous beasts.

Avens itself is a name of uncertain origin; one supposition is that it is from the Spanish term for antidote. The genus name Geum has a more precise meaning from the Greek *geno*, to smell pleasant,

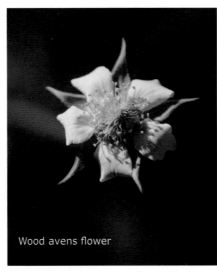
Wood avens flower

in reference to the clove-like smell of the root in spring and autumn.

It is the essential oil eugenol that gives the fragrance to avens root, as it does to cloves, nutmeg, cinnamon, basil, lemon balm and other aromatic spices and herbs. In avens itself, Polish research (2011) indicates that the time of harvest and age of the plant do not affect the amount of eugenol present.

This finding suggests that old harvesting rules of digging avens on 25 March were only partly true, and autumn roots are as potent. We have dug up the reddish-brown root of avens on several occasions, and find its smell varies in intensity according to time and place. If it doesn't smell, it could be because it is a non-fragrant hybrid geum or that the eugenol is not available; either way, it's best to return such roots to the ground.

The root is dried slowly to preserve the essential oil, and is ready when it becomes brittle. It is crushed for medicinal use, or in older times as a flavouring for a medicinal beer and wine.

Parkinson in 1640 noted: *Some use in the Spring time to put the roote to steepe for a time in wine, which giveth unto it a delicate savour and taste, which they drinke fasting every morning, to comfort the heart, and to preserve it from noisome and infectious vapours of the plague, or any poison that may annoy it.*

Avens is an antiseptic, but was not a success as a plague herb – what could be? It gradually became known as little more than a foraged potherb and broth ingredient, and a workmanlike deterrent to moths, but may be due for a herbal comeback.

Rose family astringents

We owe this category to Finnish herbalist Henriette Kress (2011). She draws attention to both the number of mild astringent herbs in the Rosaceae and the fact that they are largely interchangeable in medicinal action.

So, she writes, 'if you read that strawberry leaf works for diarrhoea, you may substitute any other astringent herb'. And, 'if you can't find anything at all, use black tea [*Camellia sinensis*, in the Theaceae], instead'. This could be a valuable guideline in your own wayside medicine-making.

Rose family astringents included in *Hedgerow Medicine* were agrimony, blackberry, hawthorn, meadowsweet, raspberry and wild rose; in this book, you will find avens, blackthorn, cinquefoil, rowan, silverweed, tormentil and wild strawberry.

Use avens for …
The description 'rose family astringent' applies to avens (see box below left). The herbalist David Hoffmann explains it well: astringents contain tannins, and in effect produce a temporary leather coat on the surface of bodily tissue. This inner surface creates a barrier to infection, and reduces irritation and inflammation.

It means that astringents as a group are good wound healers, work in the gut, relieve diarrhoea and dysentery ('bloody flux'), soothe piles and fight infection.

Avens falls into this scheme, with a specialism of combating malarial or intermittent fevers; Sir John Hill in 1812 wrote: *I have known it alone cure intermittent fevers, where the bark* [= cinchona] *has been unsuccessful.*

A common wild plant neglected, but worthy of our notice. … The root is longish and large, of a firm substance, reddish colour, and very fragrant spicy smell; it is better than many drugs kept in the shops.
– Hill (1812)

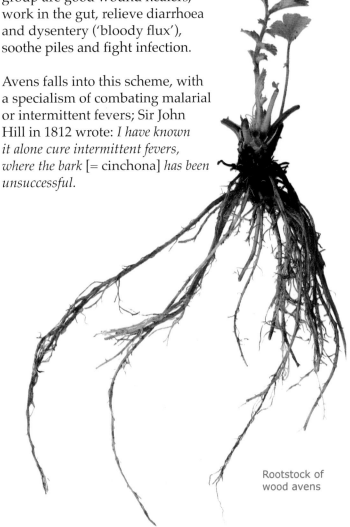

Rootstock of wood avens

Geum gee-up
• weak digestion
• poor appetite
• intermittent fevers
• convalescence
• diarrhoea

Avens mouthwash
• gum problems
• mouth ulcers

Herbalists also find avens beneficial in treatment of mouth problems, as a gargle for sore throats or an application on sore gums and mouth ulcers. The root's clove-like properties as an analgesic and antiviral help in such work, even if some 'mouth puckering' can be offputting.

The graceful water avens has similar uses, being more bitter and less aromatic (it has less eugenol in the root), and it lacks the fever-reducing benefits.

Both species are considered safe, useful remedies for everyday use.

Modern research

Polish research (2013) confirms by mass spectrometry that avens root has an essential oil and that eugenol constitutes 65–75% of it.

Romanian research (2015) gives statistical support to a posited neuroprotective activity in avens, noting a 'remarkable scavenging effect'.

More recent research (2016) proposes *G. urbanum* root as a treatment that delays α-Synuclein fibrillation in Parkinson's disease. There is no current treatment that does this.

Geum gee-up

This avens root chai uses a mixture of native aromatics and hard-to-replace spices. Into a pan of boiling water add fresh (or dried) **avens roots** chopped into small pieces (your tea and cloves); add a teaspoon-size knob of **ginger**, chopped small; a teaspoon each of **alexander** seeds (for your pepper) and ripe **hogweed** seeds (for citrus/cinnamon). Add **honey** and **milk** to taste (milk optional as it's already a lovely taste) after 10 minutes. Strain. Cooled, it will keep in the fridge for up to a week.

Avens mouthwash

An avens root tea, with or without the chai ingredients, when cooled makes for an excellent mouthwash and gum rub.

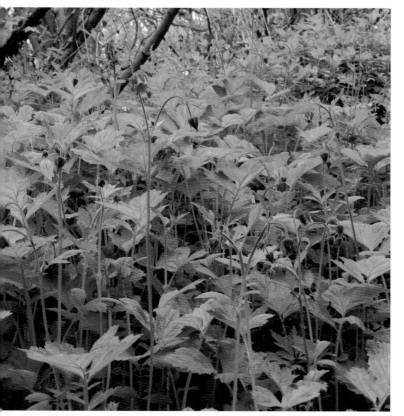

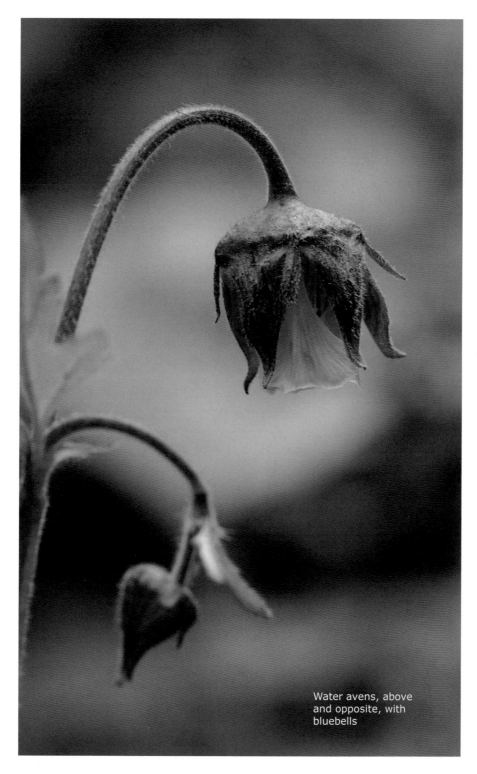

It has been said that avens is a plant that is often undervalued. There is some truth in this, for it is a sure ally against intermittent fevers, colic, diarrhoea, dysentery, circulation and liver disorders, gastric disability following acute illness, states of weakness and exhaustion, and moreover has the advantage of being easily available because it grows wild everywhere in Great Britain and Europe.
– Palaiseul (1973)

Now Geum *is fully restored in clinical practice as a safe and useful remedy.*
– Barker (2001)

Water avens, above and opposite, with bluebells

Bistort *Persicaria bistorta*

**Polygonaceae
Knotweed & dock
family**

Description: Large-leaved perennial native plant with prominent pink flower spikes in summer, like the fluffy boom microphones used in TV and films.

Habitat: Riverbanks, ponds, damp meadows.

Distribution: Locally abundant, mainly west and north of Britain. Also across northern Eurasia, introduced in north-eastern US.

Related species: Other common British Persicarias include redshank (*P. maculosa*), pale persicaria (*P. lapathifolia*), amphibious bistort (*P. amphibia*) and arsesmart or water-pepper (*P. hydropiper*).

Parts used: Leaves, roots.

Bistort root is one of the strongest astringent medicines in the vegetable kingdom and highly styptic and may be used to advantage for all bleedings, whether external or internal and wherever astringency is required.
– Grieve (1931)

Docks and sorrels are both in the Rumex genus within the dock family (the Polygonaceae) and embrace qualities ranging from medicinal docks to culinary sorrels. An emblematic member of the related Persicaria genus is bistort, which has an interesting history as both a spring food and as a medicine.

Bistort is named for its contorted black root, which looks 'twice twisted' (bis-tort). The S-shape also suggested a snake, leading to such other old country names as serpentary, snakeweed, adderwort and dragonwort.

Because appearance indicated purpose in a 17th-century mindset, bistort roots were presumed to be good to heal snake-bite, but there are few indications of this being effective, either in learned or folk herbal traditions.

The plant itself is communal, growing in great colonies in damp upland grassland, and its attractive pink spikes make it a popular bedding plant. Grigson (1958) found the bistort meadows *An uncommonly beautiful sight in the mountain meadows of the north,*

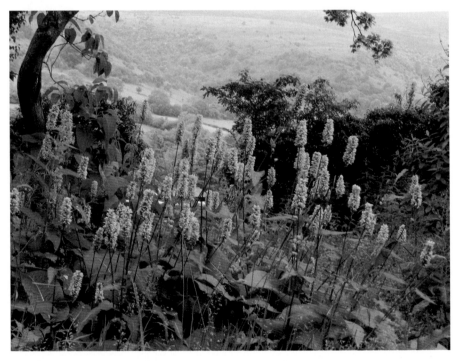

flushing the grass with pink, with spiked knaps or ears.

Bistort leaves also made for good eating as a tonic spring green. Bistort pudding was and remains food cooked in the last two weeks of Lent, hence the descriptive names of Easter mangient in Yorkshire, Easter giant in Cumberland, and passion dock in central and northern England.

Grigson proposes an interesting explanation for another name for Bistort pudding, Easter ledger or ledges. He goes back to the herbalist William Turner, who in 1548 said 'Easter ledger' was an English form of Astrologia; and Astrologia was the French name for Aristochlia or birthwort. Birthwort was an important herb in childbirth from ancient times – incidentally its other names were snakeroot or serpentary. There is

certainly an old link, weaker or stronger, with bistort as a plant of Easter and hence of new birth.

Competitive bistort pudding-making still happens each spring in the Calder valley, Yorkshire, an on-off tradition for centuries. During the Second World War, the German-supporting broadcaster 'Lord Haw Haw' (William Joyce) trumpeted that the poor Yorkshire folk had to eat grass, because they had no food. In truth they were enjoying bistort as a delicacy.

Bistort is a survival food as far afield as northern polar areas and Bangladesh. The Arctic explorer Amundsen bought bags of 'Eskimo potatoes' in the Yukon in 1905–6, probably bistort tubers, to get his team through the winter. Bistort roots are highly astringent, more so than the leaves, and could be used in tanning leather.

I found that Bistort warms and soothes the liver … helping to dispel pressure and discomfort in that region and calming that associated feeling that one's head is going to burst with stress or frustration. … I had mostly ignored this plant, thinking it was only good for gum problems and only had it because the supplier made a mistake!
– Blackwell (2014)

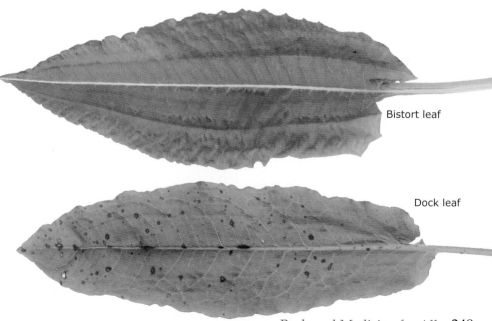

Bistort leaf

Dock leaf

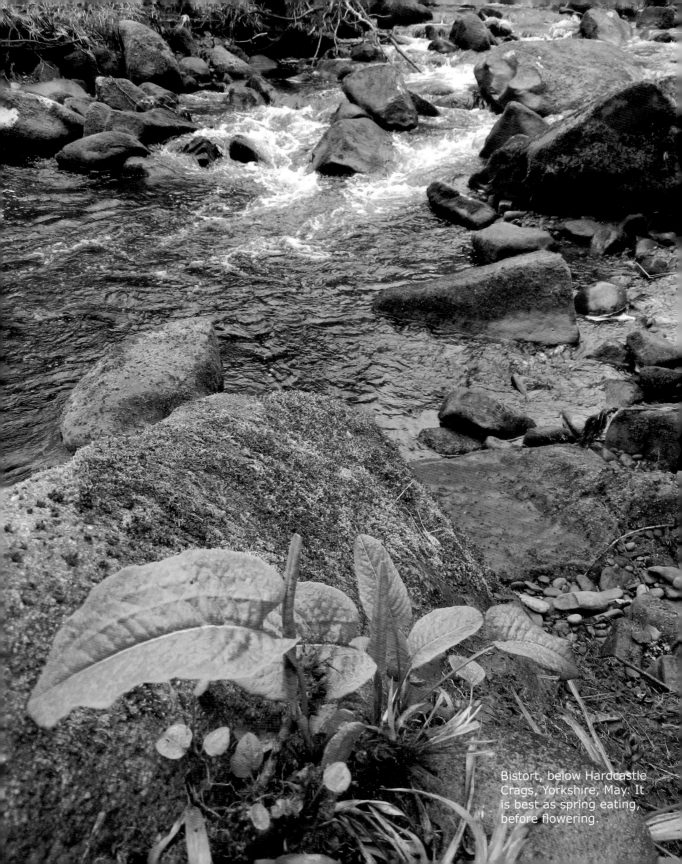

Bistort, below Hardcastle Crags, Yorkshire, May. It is best as spring eating, before flowering.

Use bistort for …

The evident astringency of bistort is combined with its 'soothing demulcent' properties to make it good eating, yet also 'a gentle yet really effective plant' (Barker).

Its actions include treatments for diarrhoea, piles, ulcers, irritable bowel, mouth, gum problems and toothache (it is partly anodyne) and many types of bleeding, as visible wounds but also internally.

Modern research

Persicaria bistorta has been under-researched, but a 2014 study of the state pharmacopoeia of the Soviet Union (last edition 1990) noted that the closely related *P. maculosa* (redshanks) was 'official'. It was available in Russian pharmacies without prescription, and used as a tea for piles, as a laxative and diuretic; a tincture was taken for blood flow as an anti-coagulant.

Other Persicaria relatives of bistort have been shown by researchers to be wound-healing (2016), antioxidant (2008), anti-cancer (leukaemia) (2015) and 'potentially therapeutic' (2011) in metabolic syndrome.

This is a gentle yet really effective plant. … I find that it co-operates remarkably well with other astringents in the treatment of peptic ulcers, diverticulosis and other irritable or inflammatory conditions of the bowel providing always that chronic constipation is not present. It is the combination of soothing demulcent with tonic astringent that makes it so valuable.
– Barker (2001)

Calderdale dock (bistort) pudding

Chop two **onions** and fry gently in **butter** or oil. Coarsely chop a few handfuls of young **bistort leaves** and some young **nettle** tops, and add to the pan with a handful of **oatmeal**. Stir and cook until the leaves are tender and the oatmeal has become moistened from their juices. Season to taste with salt and pepper, and serve hot.

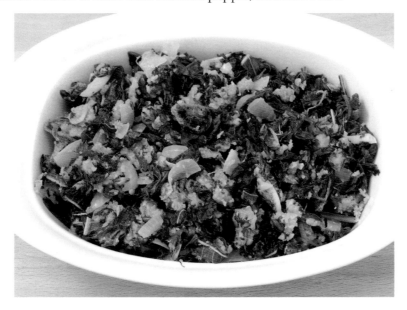

Thanks to Brenda Taylor for sharing the recipe with us: delicious!

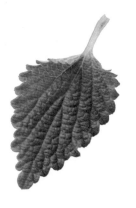

Black horehound *Ballota nigra*

A scruffy-looking wild plant, black horehound is actually an exciting 'forgotten' herb and deserves to be widely used, despite its musty smell. It is antibacterial – and notably effective against MRSA – antifungal and antiparasitic. Like its better-known cousin white horehound, it is used for coughs. It also has antispasmodic qualities and helps deal with anxiety and insomnia.

**Lamiaceae
Deadnettle family**

Description: A perennial to 1m (3ft) tall or more. Has a square stem, with dark and roughly hairy leaves; pinkish-purple flowers in whorls, late summer.

Habitat: Verges, waysides, walls and hedge bottoms, often on nitrogen-rich soils.

Distribution: Common in England and Wales, less frequent in Scotland and Ireland. Found across Europe to Asia and in North Africa; introduced to North and South America and New Zealand.

Related species: *B. africana*, kattekruid or kattekruie, is used in southern Africa for fevers, insomnia, piles and liver problems. *B. glandulosissima* is used similarly in Turkey.

Parts used: Flowering tops.

Eclipsed by its white horehound cousin, this plant offers valuable potential – even though its name *Ballota* comes from a Greek word meaning 'rejected', apparently because cattle refused to eat it.

White horehound (*Marrubium vulgare*) is the species more likely to be found in herb gardens, with its fuzzy white leaves, white flowers and tidier habit. A well-known cough remedy, its bitterness was sweetened by making horehound candy.

The name horehound has been given many derivations, but the most likely is from Old English *harhune*, meaning hoary or hairy plant. 'Father of English botany' William Turner (1548) had his own name for black horehound – 'stynking horehound'.

Some writers say white horehound tastes better. We disagree. Though black horehound is musty, we find it less disagreeable than the related red deadnettle or hedge woundwort, and the tincture and tea are really quite pleasant.

Black horehound tends to follow human settlement as it likes the rich nitrogenous soils found there and in places where livestock have been kept (as do elder and nettle).

One area it is appreciated is the Western Cape of South Africa and north to Namibia. The leaves are used to treat fevers and measles, and children would dance around *Ballota africana* singing 'dis 'n lekker kruie' (O what a lovely herb).

Domestically, the dried square stems of black horehound were used as wicks for butterlamps or night lights, and the leaves burnt to drive off biting insects.

Most writers suggest that black horehound is no longer used, and that the white is better, but we find black horehound actually has a wider medicinal range.

Its champion is the early 20th-century English herbalist Richard Hool; contemporary American herbalist Matthew Wood deserves credit for highlighting Hool's well-argued passion for the plant.

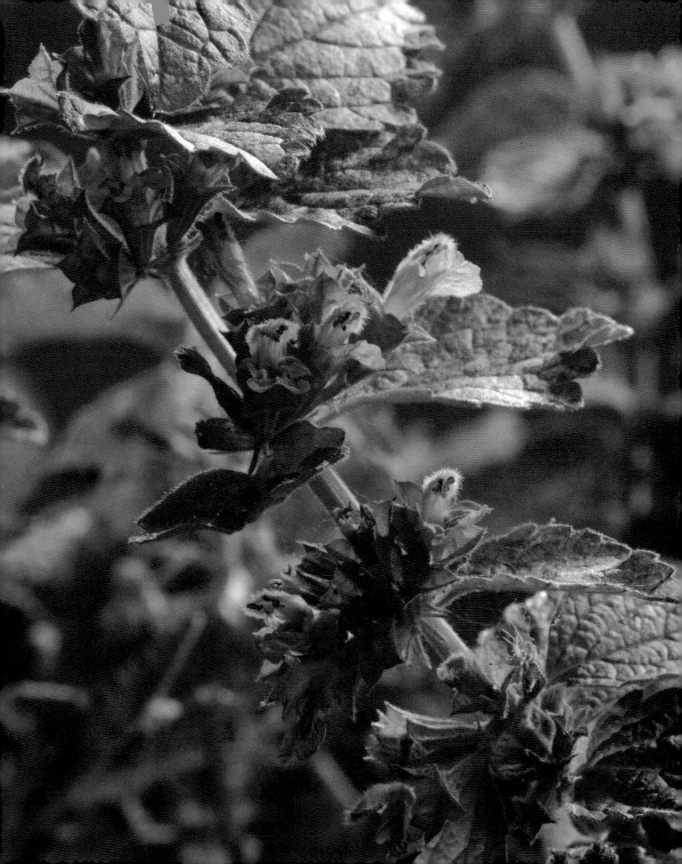

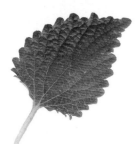

Black Horehound is one of the most efficacious remedies we have for the cure of biliousness, bilious colic, and sour belchings. In the above complaints it is as near a specific as any remedy well can be. The relief it affords is both prompt and certain, for if only a leaf or a piece of the stem be chewed, and the juice swallowed, it will be found to act as if a current of electricity had passed into the stomach, allaying all the symptoms momentarily.
– Hool (1924)

… an excellent remedy for calming nausea and vomiting when the cause lies within the nervous system rather than in the stomach.
– Hoffmann (2003)

Hool gives a remarkable case where some postal workers requested his help for one of their co-workers who was down with the cholera – loss of control of the bowels, shivering, trembling, sweating, and weakness. … He sent them off with ballota, telling them not to worry. By afternoon one of the men returned to say their co-worker was back at work, joking and laughing, as usual.
– Wood (2008)

Use black horehound for …

One of the most useful actions of black horehound is in treating nausea, particularly arising from motion or travel sickness and from inner ear problems, where ginger might be considered. It is also a good match with ginger or mint.

The pungency and bitter flavour of black horehound indicate its benefits for digestion. It appears to increase the flow of bile and has a protective action on the liver. In southern Italy it was traditionally used in cases of malaria to treat the swollen spleen and liver that accompany the disease.

Black horehound's antispasmodic effect works well for menstrual cramps, and for normalising menstruation generally. It is helpful for treating irregular periods, and lack of menstruation as well as heavy periods [see box].

Like white horehound, black horehound is excellent for coughs. It is an expectorant, helping clear mucus out of the lungs, and as an antispasmodic is useful for dry, tickly coughs and asthma. In the past it was used to treat bronchitis as well as consumption (tuberculosis of the lungs).

We have found that it calms nervous over-activity, releasing muscle tension and anxiety. It can be helpful in cases of insomnia if the leaf tea is taken before bed.

Black horehound also has tonic properties, and makes a reputable remedy for tiredness and debility, low energy and general weakness, especially if accompanied by a loss of appetite. Hool also used it as a diuretic in treating oedema, and for internal gravel.

An ancient use, going back two thousand years to Dioscorides, was to bruise the leaves with salt to dress and heal dog bites (but this is not where 'hound' came from!). He also advocated mixing the leaves with honey for cleansing infected wounds and ulcers.

Black horehound as normaliser

In suppressed, and also in excessive, menstruation it is simply wonderful. It may seem contradictory to the ordinary reader to say that it may be prescribed in what are generally considered to be opposite conditions of the system; but when it is understood that in either case the disturbance of the physiological condition is simply due to a loss of equilibrium, and that the Black Horehound exerts such an influence as will restore the necessary equilibrium, it will be seen that it may be intelligently applicable to either case.

It should always be remembered that disease arises from obstruction, and that until this obstruction is removed and any injury to the part is repaired, there is always a disturbance of the equilibrium of the blood circulation and the nerve force.

– Richard Lawrence Hool, *Health from British Wild Herbs,* 1924 [1918]

Modern research

An Italian study (2010) found that extracts from three medicinal plants (*Ballota nigra, Castanea sativa* and *Sambucus ebulus*) were effective against MRSA. These anti-pathogenic plant extracts inhibited quorum sensing (QS) pathways, and may be a useful alternative to antibiotics in an age when increased bacterial resistance to antibiotics is a growing problem.

Animal and *in vitro* studies on species of *Ballota* have indicated its use to protect the liver, eg in a rat study (2008) *Ballota undulata* was found to lower blood glucose, increase insulin and reduce blood cholesterol levels.

A 2003 *in vitro* study compared the antimicrobial and antifungal effects of ethanol tinctures of 16 Turkish species of *Ballota*, finding they were 'good' antimicrobials and 'excellent' antifungals.

A 2014 study found *Ballota nigra* to be effective against the trypanosomatid protozoan parasite that causes Leishmaniasis.

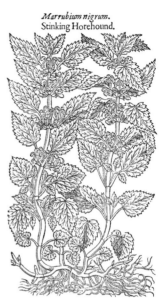

Marrubium nigrum.
Stinking Horehound.

Black horehound, woodcut in Gerard's *Herball* (1597)

Harvesting black horehound

The above-ground parts are used, especially the flowering tops, and can be gathered when flowering in summer and autumn. Use fresh to make tincture or dry for later use as tea.

Black horehound tincture

A simplified tincture method for fresh herbs can be followed: fill your chosen jar with **black horehound**, pressing it down to eliminate air pockets. Then add your **alcohol**, at a dilution of 20% of alcohol. We use diluted pure grain alcohol but commercial vodka is equally good. Half vodka and half water will give roughly the required dilution. Fill to the brim and push down any plant left sitting above the fluid level.

Leave your tincture bottle in a dark location for a month or so, at least until the plant content has been extracted. Pour the contents through a sieve into a clean bottle, stopper this and label. The flavour is slightly salty and sweet.

Dosage: a teaspoon three times a day. The taste is palatable, though still 'medicinal'.

Black horehound tea

Steep fresh or dried tops of flowering **black horehound** in **boiling water**, for 5 to 10 minutes, according to taste. It is pleasantly bitter.

Black horehound tincture
- muscle tension
- anxiety
- cramps
- low energy
- liver protective
- coughs
- bronchitis
- menstrual problems
- nausea

Black horehound tea
- stimulates digestion
- nausea
- coughs
- insomnia

Blackthorn *Prunus spinosa*

**Rosaceae
Rose family**

Description: A large shrub/small tree (to 4m, 14ft), suckering into dense thickets; simple oval leaves; black wood, bearing lateral shoots that develop into fearsome spines and from which delicate white blossoms with long golden stamens emerge in spring; these become small blue-black plums in autumn (the sloes).

Habitat: Woods, hedgerows, waysides, railway cuttings.

Distribution: Common in Britain, apart from Scottish Highlands. Widespread in Europe, western Asia, introduced to eastern North America, New Zealand.

Related species: Other European Prunus species, eg wild cherry (*Prunus avium*), cherry plum (*P. cerasifera*), bird cherry (*P. padus*). In North America, black cherry (*P. serotina*) and fire cherry (*P. pensylvanica*) are superficially similar.

Parts used: Flowers, bark, fruit (sloes).

Blackthorn's delicate white flowers are a reviving sight in spring, deserving their name 'lady of pearls'. A rose family astringent, its flowers are 'loosening' for intestinal pain whereas the fruit, or sloes, is 'binding' – a country remedy for diarrhoea, as well as gathered for the celebrated gin. Research is adding antioxidant and anti-tumour potential to its reputation.

The blackthorn is a wild ancestor of the cultivated plums, and is a relative of apricots, cherries, peaches and almonds. These were all classified by Linnaeus within the Prunus genus of the Rosaceae family.

Sloes, the fruit of blackthorn, have been dug up in Swiss lake dwellings dating from some 6,000 years ago. The famous mummy known as Ötzi, found in an Alpine glacier in 1991, and dated to 5,300 years ago, had stones from dried sloes near the corpse.

Unlike the cultivated Prunus species, blackthorn itself remains a wild, somewhat dangerous but valuable presence in hedgerows and woods.

Why use the emotive term 'dangerous'? The obvious answer is blackthorn's vicious thorns, which can be several inches long, and carry an old reputation of puncturing leather shoes or jerkins and causing wounds that never heal. A modern explanation is that when the thorn tip breaks off deep inside the skin it carries algal or fungal contamination. Infected blackthorn spines can introduce painful sinovitis and granuloma, often linked with fever.

Blackthorn wounds were so much part of everyday awareness that the translators of the King James Bible in 1611 were probably referring to blackthorn when talking of a 'thorn in the flesh', the 'messenger of Satan'.

Blackthorn was considered sinister in the 17th century for another reason, as the black wood staff was used by witches. A notorious example was the sorcerer Major Thomas Weir (1599–1670), who was burned at the stake in Edinburgh; his blackthorn rod, the agent of his magic, was thrown into the flames too.

Less dramatically, the dense wood of blackthorn made good teeth for hay rakes or walking sticks; in Ireland it was used as a club or shillelagh. Blackthorn burns well and slowly, and makes an impenetrable hedge.

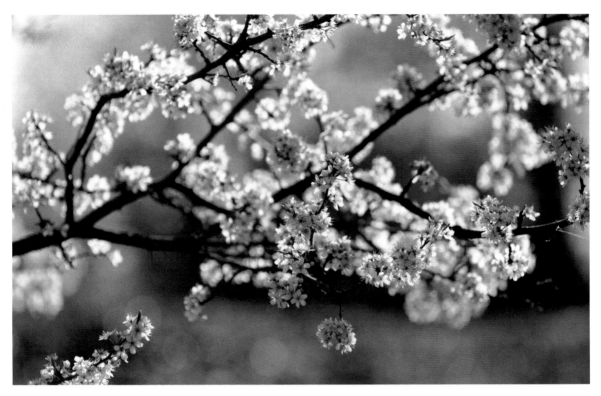

Use blackthorn for...

Blackthorn's early spring **flowers**, fresh and delicate, delight the eye with their lightness and prominent stamens; they were once called 'the lady of pearls'. They also have medicinal value for easing stomach and intestinal pain.

John Parkinson in 1640 wrote that drinking the distilled water of the flowers, preserved in white wine ('sacke') overnight, *is a most certain remedy tried and approved, to ease all manner of gnawings in the stomacke, the sides, heart or bowells*.

Other former uses for blackthorn flowers include easing the pain and reducing the severity of cystitis and gravel, gout and dropsy (oedema). The effect is diuretic, laxative and 'loosening'.

Blackthorn **bark and roots** are highly astringent (as is the whole plant), and their tannins have been used to tan leather and make a black marker ink. Medicinally, they produce a strong decoction used to treat asthma and reduce fever. Blackthorn was among the country plants, alongside tormentil and blackberry, most often used against diarrhoea.

Blackthorn **leaves** are small and oval, much like ordinary tea, and indeed were once used as a tea adulterant. They make for a bitter drink or mouthwash and gargle for mouth ulcers. Used externally,

This spiny shrub ... might well be called 'the regulator of the stomach' since, by a happy scheme of nature, its flowers loosen the bowels and its fruits bind them.
– Palaiseul (1973)

At the end of October go gather up sloes, Have thou in readiness plenty of those, And keep them in bedstraw or still on the bough To stay both the flux of thyself and thy cow.

— anon, 19th century

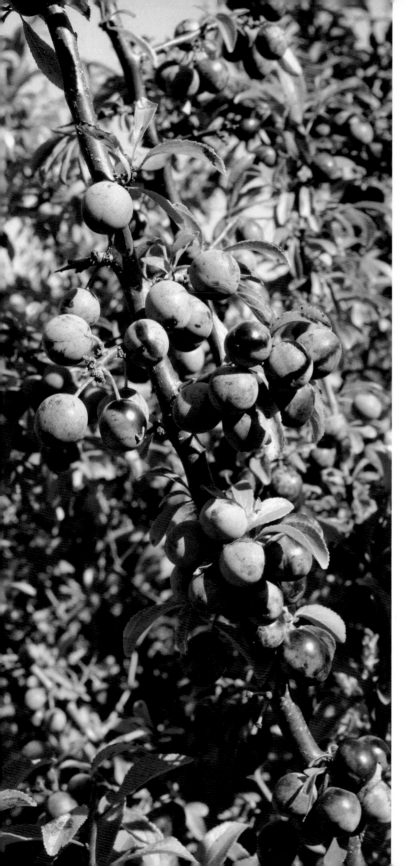

like any astringent, they will relieve skin inflammations.

Blackthorn **berries** or fruit are of course its sloes. Their taste was well described by Sir John Hill (1812): *very austere when unripe, but pleasant when mellow.* The old wives' tale of waiting for the first frost to sweeten the sloes is borne out by the chemical change induced by freezing conditions.

Freezing reduces the sloes' tannin levels and increases those of its sugars – whether you have collected your sloes and put them in the freezer or have left them on the bush. The astringency remains but the palatability improves, especially if the sloes are made into a syrup or wine.

Sloe wine was so tasty that, in the early 18th century, it was used *by fraudulent wine merchants in adulterating port wine. … It has been stated that there is more port wine (so called) drank in England alone, than is manufactured in Portugal.*

Julie's own experience bears out the tonic effects of the fruit. She was once recovering from appendicitis, and a German friend gave her a three times-decocted sloe syrup recipe. This settled her whole abdominal region.

Whereas the effect of blackthorn flowers is 'loosening' that of the sloes is 'binding', hence useful for treating cases of diarrhoea and dysentery and other bodily 'fluxes'. Sloes were also good against warts: a sloe was rubbed on the wart and then thrown over the shoulder. Sloes preserved in vinegar are a Western equivalent of the Japanese *umeboshi*, or dried, salted plums.

Modern research

Italian work in 2009 showed high antioxidant activity in fresh sloe juice, which acted as a cytoprotective.

Portuguese research (2014) using enriched phenolic extracts of wild fruits of sloes, strawberry tree and two species of rose displayed strong antioxidant and anti-tumour properties in each.

Isotonic drinks made separately from fruit of maqui, açaí and sloes, mixed with lemon juice, demonstrated higher antioxidant and biological effects than commercial isotonic drinks (2013).

A quick sloe syrup

Gather your **sloes** carefully in autumn, then freeze for a while. Transfer to a large jar; whatever your quantity, cover them with **vegetable glycerine**. Stopper the jar and place on a sunny windowsill. After about two months the liquid becomes a rich warm red. Drain off the depleted berries, put the syrup into a clean bottle, and label. Take a teaspoonful daily as a tonic.

Sloe spiced brandy

Don't be hung up on needing your sloes to be combined with gin: any alcohol is a good preservative.

A herbal friend tried this recently, tincturing **sloes**, **cardamom** and **fennel seeds** in **brandy**. The spices worked together beautifully, softening and mellowing the sloes' astringency; the bits of fruit left in the mixture tasted sweetish, rather like morello cherries.

A quick sloe syrup
- sore throats
- winter tonic
- disturbed digestion
- weak digestion

Sloe spiced brandy
- weak digestion
- dyspepsia
- lack of appetite
- sore throats
- winter tonic

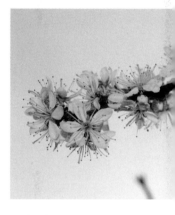

… the flowers of the blackthorn make the most harmless laxative and should be to the forefront of every family medicine chest. … So collect those blackthorn flowers, boil them for a minute, and drink a cupful of the infusion each day for three days. It acts very gently, without in any way upsetting your system; and yet it will purge you thoroughly. I recommend it also as a stomachic, depurative, and to fortify the stomach.
– Abbé Kneipp (1894)

Which thorn is it?

British people often say in late winter: Oh, the blackthorn is early this year. Usually they are wrong, because the first white-blossomed Prunus to appear in the hedgerow is cherry plum (*Prunus cerasifera*).

Cherry plum is taller than blackthorn (to 8m rather than 4m), lacks spines and is more open in habit; it has small dark red or yellow plums.

Blackthorn flowers generally appear (before the leaves) in massy drifts from early spring. Stems and branches are a dark wood, on which some side shoots form vicious spines 50cm (2in) or more long; blue-black fruits (sloes) follow.

The creamy white or pink flowers of hawthorn (*Crataegus monogyna*) appear later still when its leaves have already appeared, usually in May; hawthorn has shorter thorns than blackthorn, and red berries (haws). It is sometimes called May tree and whitethorn.

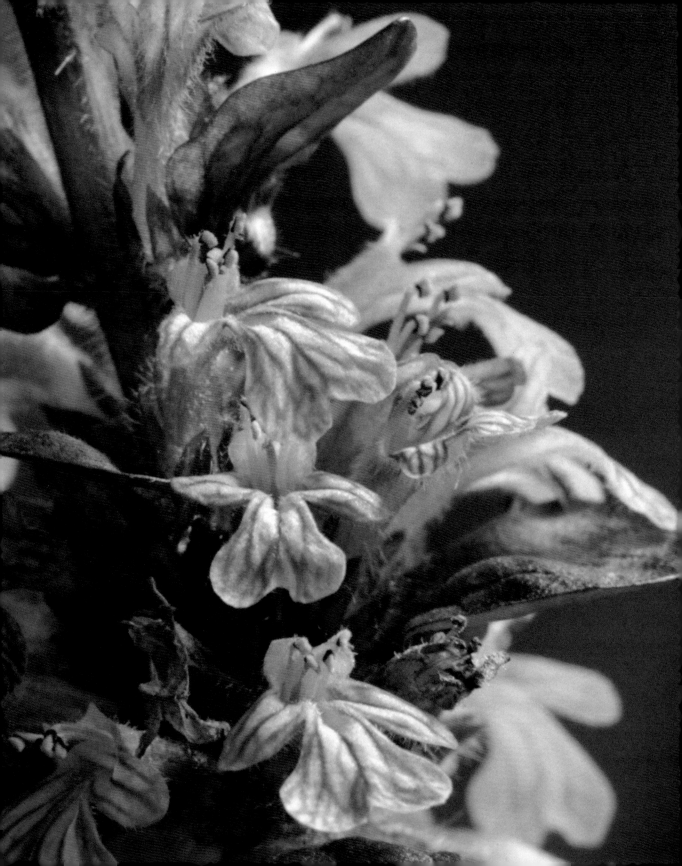

Bugle *Ajuga reptans*

Bugle was once one of the leading wound herbs, but this use is now all but forgotten. In our experience, bugle can be a useful treatment for aligning bones and dislocations, and it retains value as a mild analgesic and first aid standby.

**Lamiaceae
Deadnettle family**

Description: A creeping, colony-forming perennial with glossy dark green or purplish leaves, and blue flowers in whorls on spikes in spring and early summer.

Habitat: Found in woods and damp meadows.

Distribution: Common throughout the British Isles and across temperate Europe, north Africa and western Asia. Naturalised in the Americas and New Zealand.

Related species: There are over sixty species in the genus found around the world.

Parts used: Aerial parts.

Bugle is often grown in gardens as a ground cover for damp or shady places, and is available with purple and variegated leaves as well as the standard dark green. It spreads by extending stolons (runners) from the parent plant to form an attractive mat.

Gerard (1597) wrote that it was much planted in gardens in Elizabethan England, so it has been popular for a long time.

Bugle, sanicle and selfheal were reputed to keep the surgeon away, with many variations on the popular saying in herbal literature.

Because bugle is sometimes called bugleweed, it is often confused with the other plant of that name, *Lycopus virginicus* (see p312), but their uses are quite different.

Other common names include carpenter's weed and sicklewort, which indicate bugle's wound-healing properties in work situations, as does the old name of 'middle consound'. The consounds were wound-healing herbs, comfrey being the greater consound, and selfheal the lesser.

Use bugle for ...

In his English translation of the *Pharmacopoeia Londinensis* (1653) Nicholas Culpeper left no doubt about his admiration for bugle as a healing herb. He described it as excellent for falls and inward bruises for it dissolved congealed blood. It helped 'stoppings' (congestion) of the liver. It was of 'wonderful force' in curing

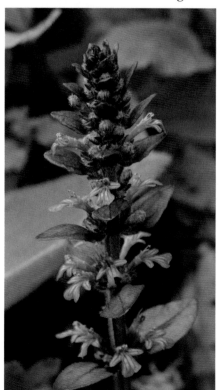

Bugle stands bravely on parade in the most cheerful and healthy colonies, in woods or in damp grass.
– Grigson (1958)

wounds and ulcers, and helping broken bones and dislocations. He added: *To conclude, let my Countrymen esteem it as a Jewel.*

Bugle had later champions, like the botanist Edward Baylis (1791), who devoted 13 pages of his herbal to its virtues, and particularly advocated it to treat the spitting of blood (as in incipient tuberculosis).

But after William Kemsey (1838) – who believed an ointment of bugle leaves and flowers was *good for all sorts of sores and old ulcers* – bugle seemed to slip out of official medical recognition. The gradual rise of antibiotics was one of the factors that led to the decline of herbal treatments for tuberculosis, and indeed wounds.

We would say the time is right to re-evaluate. It's good knowledge to have that bugle is a quietly effective first aid treatment for cuts, burns, bruising, sores and mouth ulcers or inflamed tonsils (quinsy). Scrunched-up bugle leaves on the affected part, either direct or via a wine decoction or poultice, are easily applied.

Pharmacological research shows bugle contains plentiful iridoid glycosides, including harpagide (as does the southern African herb devil's claw, *Harpagophytum procumbens*). Harpagide has a vasoconstricting effect on smooth muscle, which means both plants have blood-staunching properties.

Bugle is sometimes condemned as being only a mild analgesic. But let's rather say it is a safe one that acts gently to take the pain out of old wounds as well as fresh ones. We find it works well with a daisy ointment for bruises; with honey for sores and ulcers; and as a bugle distilled water for mouth issues.

Green's *Universal Herbal* of 1820 makes the interesting point that bugle is unlike most astringents when taken internally in that it does not produce costiveness (constipation), *but rather operates as gentle laxatives.*

Another role for bugle, we suggest, is as an alternative to the North American herb boneset (*Eupatorium perfoliatum*) for aligning bones, ligaments and tendons. This is less an innovation than recovering a traditional use (see quotes, left).

One experience of our own was that bugle tincture applied externally rapidly relieved a pinched nerve, while feeling more unctuous and tonic than boneset for the same purpose.

Modern research
Several traditional uses of closely related species of *Ajuga* have been confirmed in animal trials, and may well apply to *A. reptans*.

For example, *A. remota*, an anti-malarial herb in common use in East Africa, was shown (2011) to be effective in curing mice given doses of malaria; use of *Ajuga* in diabetes mellitus control was confirmed in diabetic rats treated by *A. iva*, a Mediterranean bugle species (2008a), with toxicity in the animals' livers, kidneys and pancreas much reduced.

Another species, *A. decumbens*, produced positive effects in Chinese research on osteoporosis and arthritis in mice (2008b), confirming traditional uses for human joint pain treatment.

These are laboratory findings rather than human clinical trials, of course, but how interesting to muse – and insist on appropriate research – whether *Ajuga reptans* shares potential with its cousins for treating malaria, diabetes, osteoporosis and arthritis.

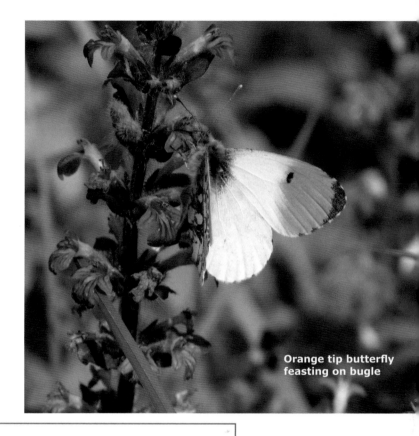
Orange tip butterfly feasting on bugle

Bugle tincture
Fill a jar with **bugle** flower spikes and leaves, then top up with 50% **vodka** or whisky and 50% **water**. Leave for a month or until the flowers have lost their colour, then strain, bottle and label.

Bugle elixir
Fill a jar with **bugle** flower spikes and leaves. Fill the jar ⅔ full with **vodka**, then top up with **vegetable glycerine**. Leave for a month or until the flowers have lost their colour, then strain, bottle and label.

Dosage: Take a teaspoonful three times daily.

Bugle ointment
Put **bugle** in a small saucepan with enough **extra virgin olive oil** to cover it. Simmer gently for about 20 minutes, then strain out the plant material. Measure the oil, and return it to the pan. Add 10g **beeswax** for every 100 ml of oil, and stir on low heat until melted. Pour into jars and allow to cool before putting the lids and labels on. Bugle combines well with daisy, yarrow and selfheal in an ointment.

Bugle tincture, externally
- back pain
- stiff necks
- joint pain
- injuries
- broken bones
- aching muscles

Bugle elixir
- hot liver
- gallbladder problems
- rapid heart beat
- anxiety
- persistent coughs

Bugle ointment
- cuts & grazes
- bruises
- blood blisters
- painful joints
- burns

Butcher's broom *Ruscus aculeatus*

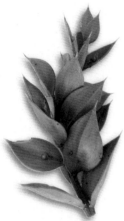

Butcher's broom offers surprises in its family (it is an asparagus), form (its 'leaves' are modified stems) and palatability (it is a thorny plant with edible shoots). It had an engaging association with butchers which gave us its common name, and has enjoyed a surge of pharmacological interest for treating varicose veins and haemorrhoids, and potentially conditions of the lungs, liver and eyes.

Asparagaceae
Asparagus family

Description: Multi-branched, hairless evergreen shrub, 1m tall (3ft); glossy, spiny, dark green 'leaves' or cladodes; tiny yellow-green flowers in centre of cladodes, then scarlet berries.

Habitat: Old woodland, hedgerows, cliffs, often at base of trees.

Distribution: Local, in lowland and southern Britain, most of Europe, western Asia.

Related species: Spineless butcher's broom (*R. hypoglossum*) is smaller, with more cladodes but fewer spines, and is a rare, introduced species.

Parts used: Root and cladodes.

A growing body of research is demonstrating that butcher's broom is a valuable medicine for venous disorders ... now a common remedy in Germany.
– Chevallier (2016)

Butcher's broom is a strange plant. Known in the past as knee holly because it is spiny and grows to about a metre tall, it superficially resembles but is not a holly. It is actually an asparagus, and an unusual one in that it is an evergreen bush.

The leaves of butcher's broom are modified stems (cladodes), its true leaves being vestigial. Its small yellow-green flower yields a cherry-like, non-edible red berry in the centre of the 'leaves'. These cladodes are leathery and tough, with a sharp terminal spine, yet the young shoots are reportedly edible, like a bitter form of asparagus.

Butcher's broom, as the name suggests, had an odd and old association with meat. It was reported by Parkinson (1640) that the Italian name for the plant was *Pongitopo*, and the German was *Muessdorn*, or mouse thorn. Italian and German butchers erected little 'hedges' of the 'leaves' around the meat to keep rodents away. The berries, which ripen in autumn and stay on the bush over winter (or until birds eat them and spread the seeds), were once collected for Christmas décor and to garnish special cuts of meat. Florists have also used the berries. And indeed a switch or besom was once made from the stems to sweep the butcher's shop. Such uses are now long gone.

Use butcher's broom for ...
Butcher's broom was known as a medicinal plant to Dioscorides, the 1st-century AD herbal systematiser, and had a modest ongoing reputation as a diuretic and 'opening' herb for treating urinary, water retention, jaundice and stone or gravel issues.

In Devon, butcher's broom 'leaves' were used to beat chilblains, anticipating current uses of the plant for varicose vein treatment.

Herbalist Christine Herbert says: *My most common use is for congested menstrual problems – dysmenorrhoea/ menorrhagia, as it is good for pelvic stagnation. It's also hormone-balancing, raising oestrogen and/or progesterone as needed. It's useful in PMS, menopause, vaginal dryness.*

Modern research

The isolation from butcher's broom of the steroidal saponin glycoside called ruscogenin has reinvigorated its medicinal status.

For example, 917 Mexicans with chronic venous disorder (CVD) were given 12 weeks of treatment with ruscogenin, with marked positive effects on their symptoms and quality of life (2009).

Ruscogenin and neoruscogenin have been shown to be effective in treating chronic venous insufficiency and chronic orthostatic hypotension (OH), the pooling of blood (2000).

The other major identified area is for relief of haemorrhoids, while more recent research suggests potential use for acute lung injury, pulmonary arterial hypertension, diabetic nephropathies and under-eye puffiness.

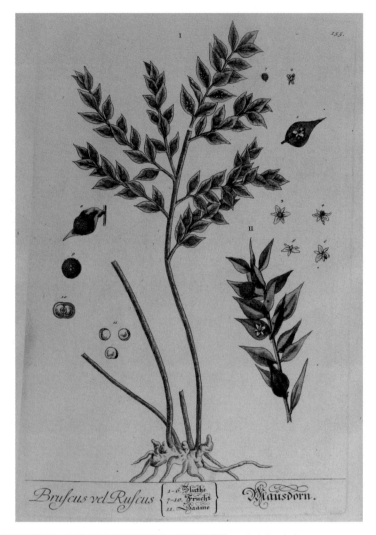

Butcher's broom, painted by Elizabeth Blackwell (1750), courtesy of the Wellcome Library

Butcher's broom infused oil & ointment
• varicose veins
• chilblains
• piles

Caution: Do not eat the berries.

Butcher's broom infused oil

A tincure or tea are often made, but an alternative for external application to varicose veins and piles is an infused oil. Pick **butcher's broom cladodes** (and root if you must) and dry them in the shade. Put into a jar and pour on **extra virgin olive oil**. Stir well. Put the lid on and place the jar on a windowsill for 3 weeks or until the colour has transferred to the oil. Strain off the oil, bottle. Label.

Butcher's broom ointment

Mix 200ml of **butcher's broom infused oil** in a small saucepan and 20g **beeswax**. Warm on low heat until the wax melts, allow to cool slightly. Pour into jars and leave to set before putting lids on. Label.

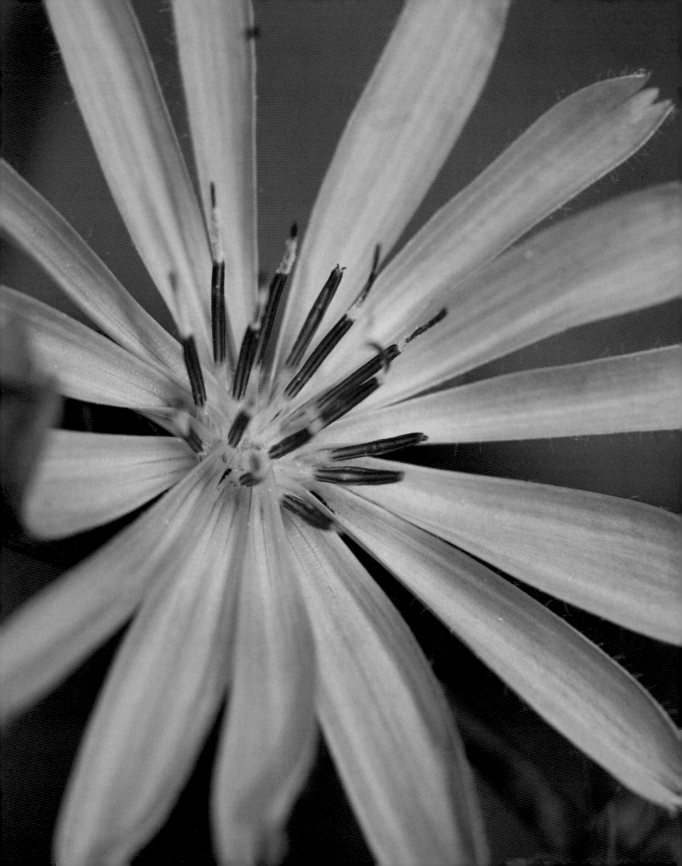

Chicory *Cichorium intybus*

Chicory is a familiar domestic presence as a coffee substitute and bitter salad ingredient, while the production of large-rooted varieties as a source of oligofructose is accelerating. These commercial emphases have overshadowed a well-established and significant herbal reputation.

Chicory is an ancient herb of India, China, Iran, Egypt and the classical Mediterranean. It was a Passover 'bitter herb' of the Israelites and can still be found in Seder ceremonies today.

Pliny records both cultivated and wild chicory growing in ancient Rome, and recommended it for headaches and as a purgative. The influential medical writer Galen (c129–c210) wrote a *Treatise on Chicory*, drawing attention to its benefits for the liver, a use that has persisted to the present day. He recommended a syrup of chicory, rhubarb and oats for the liver.

Chicory is a morning kind of plant, which closes its long blue petals in the summer afternoons. Linnaeus included chicory in his floral clock at Uppsala, where it reliably kept the time; at his latitude in Sweden it opened at 5am and closed at 10am, while in Britain its hours are 6am to noon.

The great Arabic scientist Avicenna (980–1037) also wrote on chicory, and the species name *intybus* is an anglicisation of the Arabic name,

hendibeh. Not wasting a good source-word, ancient plant-namers also transformed *hendibeh* into the related endive (*Cichorium endiva*).

The wild British and American chicory is the rough-stalked and blue-flowered species, once known as blue sailors or blue dandelion; another old English name was succory. This may have derived from the Latin *succurrere*, to run under, for chicory's depth of root.

Chicory's leaves are tender in spring, and can be foraged to be cooked or eaten fresh for their emerging bitterness; the flowers make a spectacular salad garnish. Endive hearts are blanched at an early stage to reduce their bitterness, while the related red radicchio now featuring in salads everywhere originated as a wild Italian chicory.

Chicory has become naturalised across most of North America, and is best known as a summertime highway weed. It is 'noxious' in some states, but loved by passers-by. It is *Wegwarten*, or watcher of the wayside, in Germany.

**Asteraceae
Daisy family**

Description: A stiff-stalked perennial to 1.5m (4–5ft), with striking pale blue flowers scattered up the stem; leaves light green, lance-shaped at top, larger and lobed below; deep taproot.

Habitat: Along highways, waste and rough land, field margins, often near houses; likes lime soils.

Distribution: Widespread in lowlands of southern and eastern England, occasional elsewhere; native in Middle East and Mediterranean, now naturalised in North America, Asia, Australia.

Related species: Endive (*Cichorium endiva*) is a near-relative cultivated food crop, as is radicchio. Common blue sow thistle (*Cicerbita macrophylla*) is a scattered garden escape in Britain, but has lilac flowers, oval leaves and a white sap.

Parts used: Roots, leaves, flowers.

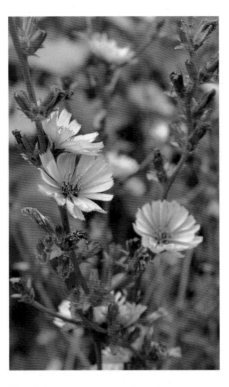

year in the Netherlands, for use in weight-control formulae and as a substrate for probiotic gut bacteria, like acidophilus.

Use chicory for...

Medicinally, chicory has been valued in traditional herbalism around the world as a bitter tonic, with diuretic and decongestant effects similar to those of the closely related dandelion.

Chicory's effect is partly dose-dependent. American herbal energetics author Peter Holmes notes that *Smaller doses are restoring, while larger ones are more draining and detoxicant.*

Chicory root as a tea, coffee or syrup stimulates digestion and appetite. It is nourishing to the taste and to the blood, and helps relieve fatigue. It reduces congestion, especially in the liver, while promoting bile production – useful in jaundice treatments.

The root and also pressed chicory juice are cooling, with a detoxing and urine-promoting effect in higher doses, and help remove oedema. Chicory has been used to relieve gout and rheumatism. For children, chicory syrup was a mild and safe laxative.

Chicory leaf tea was taken to help reduce inflammations and fever, particularly fevers arising from congestive causes in the liver; in Traditional Chinese Medicine *ju ju* (chicory) corrects liver fire.

The long taproot makes the familiar coffee substitute, often resorted to in times of blockade and coffee shortage, as in France during the Napoleonic Wars, the American South during the Civil War ('Creole' coffee) or in Britain in and after the Second World War.

'Camp' coffee, a mixture of 4% coffee, 28% chicory and sugar, first appeared in India in the 1870s as a stimulating drink for a Scottish regiment. This may have been the world's first instant coffee. It also makes excellent iced coffee.

Chicory root is cultivated commercially as a source of oligofructose, a high-fructose and low-calorie form of sugar. Some 100,000 tons is produced each

Older European traditions linked chicory with treating eye problems, including cataract. Fresh bruised leaves used to be applied on eye inflammations.

Interestingly, in TCM, the liver is strongly linked with the eye, so a 'liver herb' like chicory would be expected to be useful in both cases. In Indian tradition, juices of celery, carrot and chicory are drunk to support health of the optic nerve.

American scientist Jim Duke writes of research showing chicory reducing a rapid heartbeat but also being mildly heart-stimulating. It makes us wonder: could chicory be beneficially combined with hawthorn as a heart tonic?

Modern research

Immunotoxicity induced by ethanol was significantly restored or prevented in mice by *Cichorum intybus* treatment (2002). *C. intybus* hydroalcoholic extracts were effective (2012 research) to protect mice against experimental acute pancreatitis.

Ginger, chicory and their mixture were all found (2010) to be hepatoprotective against carbon tetrachloride intoxication in rats.

In a human study, trials with 47 people over 4 weeks showed (2015) that chicory root extract could delay or prevent the early onset of diabetes mellitus and improve bowel movement.

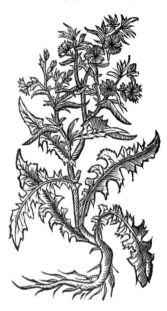

2. Cichorium sylvestre. Wilde Succory.

Wilde succory (chicory), woodcut in Parkinson, *Theatrum Botanicum* (1640)

Cardamom Camp coffee
Dig up your chicory root (this may be a tussle as it is a gnarly tap root), wash it and cut into small pieces (say 1cm or ¼ inch). It can be used fresh or roasted until it is brown, but we're going with drying it in a dehydrator (or the oven on low heat). Measure 4 tablespoons of this **dried chicory root**, 1 tablespoon **ground coffee beans**, 3 **cardamom pods** and 5 tablespoons **sugar** into 2 cups **water**. Boil and then simmer for 10 minutes. Allow to sit for 10 minutes, strain into a fresh saucepan. Simmer down to half volume – and at last you can bottle it. Keeps well in the fridge.

The result should be a thick syrup that is as good as any proprietary blend. The inulin starches have been transformed into caramelised sugars, while the cardamom tempers the bitterness.

Chicory skin toner
Pick a handful of **chicory leaves**. Mix sufficient solution of 2 parts **rosewater** and 1 part **cider vinegar** to cover the leaves. Run the mixture through a blender to make a dark green liquid. Strain into a fresh bottle. Use on the skin as a refreshing cosmetic and for minor skin blemishes.

Cardamom Camp coffee
• good for the liver
• stimulates digestion
• nourishing
• relieves fatigue

Chicory skin toner
• refreshing cosmetic
• minor skin blemishes

Cranesbill *Geranium* spp.

**Geraniaceae
Geranium family**

Description:
Cranesbills (*Geranium* spp.) and storksbills (*Erodium* spp.) are genuses within the Geranium family, with purple/pink/blue flowers and palmate (cranesbill) or pinnate leaves (storksbill); storksbills have longer 'beaks'.

Habitat: Grassland, woodland, rocks and cliffs, especially lime-rich areas.

Distribution:
Cranesbill species are common across the British Isles, mainly in lowlands, storksbills less widespread; native to Mediterranean, Middle East, also North America, South Africa.

Related species:
Herb robert (*Geranium robertianum*) is the most widespread British species [see p104], but meadow cranesbill (*G. pratense*), dovesfoot (*G. molle*), hedgerow (*G. pyrenaicum*), bloody (*G. sanguineum*) and cut-leaved cranesbill (*G. dissectum*) run it close. In eastern North America the main species is American or wild geranium (*G. maculatum*); a South African equivalent is *G. incanum* (*vrouebossie*).

Parts used: Rhizomes, leaves.

Two geranium species are most often used herbally: American cranesbill as a traditional astringent, and herb robert as a hedgerow medicine. Other wild geraniums have similar medicinal virtues and should not be forgotten.

The British native geraniums are known as cranesbills and storksbills. They are named for the comparison of the seedheads with the beaks of these once-familiar birds, and like the birds themselves may just be making a comeback.

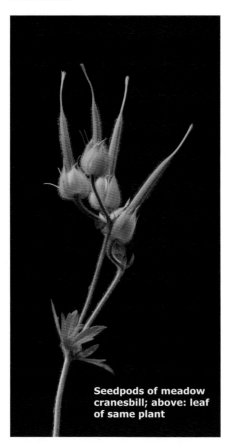

Seedpods of meadow cranesbill; above: leaf of same plant

There is an almost universal confusion between the plants in the genus *Geranium* and those tender garden plants commonly called geraniums, which are *Pelargoniums*. They are both in the family Geraniaceae, and Linnaeus had included both groups of plants under the genus *Geranium*. They were separated into two genera by Charles L'Héritier in 1789. Pelargoniums are scented, and originated in warmer climes, particularly South Africa.

Back to real geraniums. Taking two leading twentieth-century herbals as a neglect baseline, there is some way still to go: Mrs Grieve (1931) covers *Geranium maculatum*, the American geranium, but no British species, not even herb robert (*G. robertianum*); Bartram (1995) has the American species and herb robert, but no others.

Two representative older herbals feature more species. Culpeper (1653) describes 'cranebil, the divers sorts of it' among the 'official' plants of the British pharmacopoeia; he relates the uses for dovesfoot cranesbill (now *G. molle*) and adds, *I suppose*

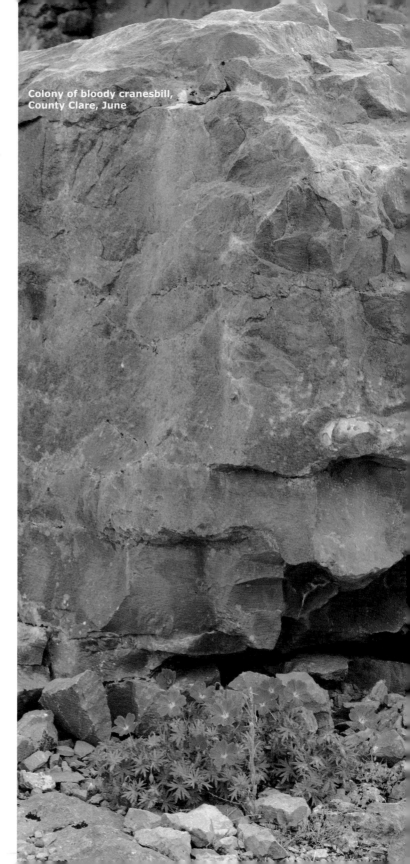

Colony of bloody cranesbill, County Clare, June

these are the general vertues of them all. Salmon (1707) itemises four garden and six wild cranesbills, saying confidently: *The Qualities, Specification, Preparations, Virtues and Uses, of all the Cranes-bills, being one and the same…*

Our forefathers evidently valued many more geranium species for their medicine, and thought their properties were broadly similar. We think that the over 400 wild geranium species worldwide (including in Britain at least 26 cranesbills and 12 storksbills) deserve some recognition.

Use cranesbills for…

As in herb robert (p104), the phytochemical signature of cranesbills is their astringency – American geranium roots have some 10–20% tannin content.

The effect of taking a cranesbill root or leaf tea, tincture or other formulation is primarily to control bodily discharges ('fluxes'), such as chronic diarrhoea, excessive menstruation and other forms of bleeding, flowing mucus and hyperacidity in the stomach (including peptic ulcers).

American herbalist Jim Mcdonald summarises his local Midwest geranium as 'a gastrointestinal astringent', which is especially good for 'tightening damp wounds in the intestines'. British botanical writer Deni Bown suggests combining American geranium with avens (*Geum*

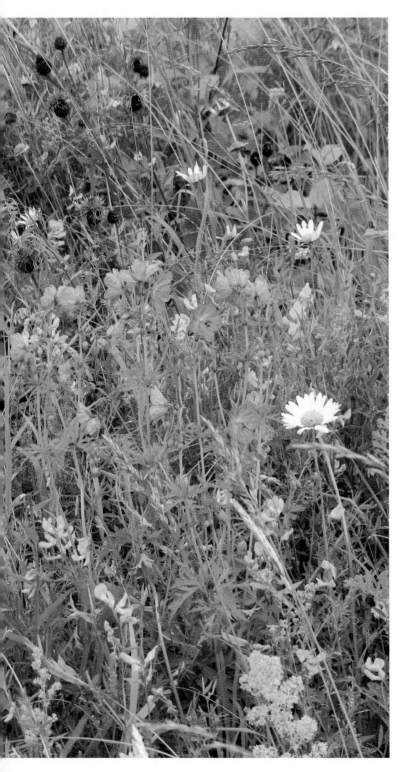

urbanum) to treat bleeding in the digestive tract and internal ulcers.

American herbalist Peter Holmes summarises American geranium (and we would suggest other species) as being 'mucostatic and hemostatic', adding piles, vaginitis and mouth ulcers as areas for its action. The late Michael Moore found crushed or powdered American geranium root as a paste helps draining of pus in wounds, gum disease or external sores.

In South Africa *Geranium incanum* is 'vrouebossie' (woman's bush), because a tea made of the leaves is a folk remedy for heavy menstruation and diarrhoea, mirroring traditional uses in Europe and among Native Americans in North America.

Another South African native relative, *Pelargonium graveolens*, or rose geranium, is a leading commercial essential oil used medicinally for similar purposes.

Mcdonald notes that American geranium roots are easily pulled up for medicine-making, and can be moderated by cooking them in milk or with cinnamon. Picking herb robert, too, can hardly be easier as it has convenient stem clusters. What are we waiting for?

Modern research
Russian work (2007) found that polyphenols in geranium and rose family species are antibacterial via antioxidant action.

Mexican research (2015) on *G. schiedeanum*, a local species of geranium, displayed hepatoprotective (liver-protecting) effects in rats by reduction of ethanol-induced toxicity.

Similarly, *Geranium macrorrhizum*, widely used in Balkan folk medicine, showed hepatoprotective potential as an antimicrobial, in addition to its astringent, wound-healing properties (2012).

It [American geranium] is perhaps the archetypal remedy for catarrhal gastritis.
– Wood (2009)

[G. maculatum] root is a reliable, average strength astringent remedy with mucostatic and hemostatic effect. … As an astringent with antisecretory action, Cranesbill root is also specifically indicated in cases of gastric hyperacidity, peptic ulcers and hemorrhoids.
– Holmes (2006)

Cranesbill ointment

Pick whichever **cranesbill** is abundant where you are. The roots will be stronger, but the above-ground parts work perfectly well.

Place in a small saucepan with enough **extra virgin olive oil** to cover the plant material. Heat gently for about half an hour or until the plant material is losing its colour and starting to become brittle. Strain the oil through a sieve into a measuring jug.

Place in a clean pan with 10g **beeswax** or 5g **candelilla wax** per 100ml of oil, and stir over low heat until the wax has all melted. Pour into jars, allowing to solidify before putting the lids on and labelling.

Herb robert and yarrow combine well with cranesbill in this ointment, as do any of the rose family astringents such as rose, agrimony, silverweed, cinquefoil and tormentil.

Use for haemorrhoids (piles), cuts and grazes.

The crushed fresh plant or root powder [of G. maculatum] made into a paste with water and applied to pus-filled ulcers or abrasions of the skin will remove the pyogenic membrane and allow draining and a reduction of pressure.
– Moore (1979)

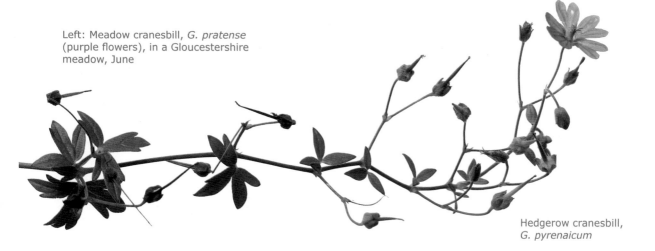

Left: Meadow cranesbill, *G. pratense* (purple flowers), in a Gloucestershire meadow, June

Hedgerow cranesbill, *G. pyrenaicum*

Creeping jenny *Lysimachia nummularia*
& Yellow loosestrife *Lysimachia vulgaris, L. punctata*

**Primulaceae
Primrose family**

Description: Creeping jenny is just a few inches high, but its creeping prostrate stems can be 50cm (18in) long; yellow cupped flowers and rounded opposite leaves; yellow loosestrife (*L. vulgaris*) is a tall, erect plant (to 150cm, 5ft), with pyramidal clusters of yellow flowers, lance-shaped narrow leaves. Dotted loosestrife (*L. punctata*) is very similar, but flowers have an orange centre and it prefers drier ground.

Habitat: Creeping jenny is found in damp, shady woods and wetter grassland; yellow loosestrife (*L. vulgaris*) in marshes, by streams and rivers; (*L. punctata*) damp places, verges, woodland margins.

Distribution: European natives, fairly common in central and southern England, and in Wales; introduced widely in US.

Related species: Yellow pimpernel (*Lysimachia nemorum*) is a widespread creeping yellow *Lysimachia*. 'Gold money herb', *jin qian cao* (*L. christinae*) is a medicinal Chinese relative.

Parts used: Above-ground parts.

Creeping jenny and yellow loosestrife are related members of the Primula family, one spreading laterally and other vertically to make imposing and attractive colonies. They share similar effectiveness in treating wounds and bleeding, 'fluxes' of various kinds and kidney and gall stones.

These two attractive yellow plants in the Lysimachia genus of the Primrose family are considered together. The first spreads out horizontally and the second forms strong vertical lines, but both have visually striking yellow and green contrasts, and share similar medicinal uses.

Neither is related to purple loosestrife, now classified in the Lythrum genus. The separate chapter on purple loosestrife (p355) looks at the reclassification and the Latin and popular names for the two loosestrifes.

As to 'loosestrife' itself, from the reputed use of the foliage to deter biting insects and hence calm restive oxen, John Parkinson (1640) comments trenchantly: *which how true I leave to them shall try, and finde it so.*

One other common name for creeping jenny deserves mention – 'moneywort'. Mrs Grieve suggests this arises from the roundish shape

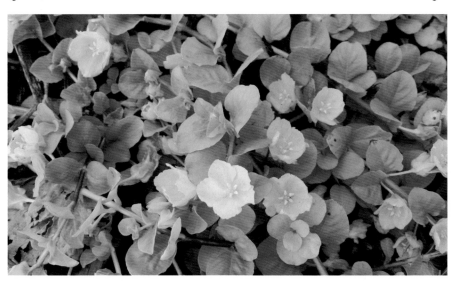

of the leaves, as they ascend the stem in pairs, resembling rows of pence. The money link is traced to William Turner (1548), the first to name the plant 'Herbe 2 Pence' and 'Two pennigrasse' (from the German *Pfennigkraut*), and confer the Latin form *nummaria* (coin).

Mrs Grieve (1931) speculates that another popular name, 'string of sovereigns', refers to the plant's golden flowers. 'Meadow runagates' and 'wandering sailor', other old vernacular names, reflect creeping jenny's spreading habit.

Use creeping jenny & yellow loosestrife for...
Those who think of creeping jenny as only a garden plant might be surprised at its medieval herbal reputation. It was known in France as a *herbe aux cent maux*, a plant for a hundred ills, in fact a panacea. It was a medicinal standby for many of the non-life-threatening but still significant things that happen. And of course it is still good for these same niggling interruptions to daily life, even if it has gone out of fashion itself.

Creeping jenny has been used since classical times, which makes its herbal history older than that of yellow loosestrife. It has generally been seen as more effective in the same healing areas. Culpeper (1653) summarises these: *Money-wort or Herb Two-pence; cold dry, binding,*

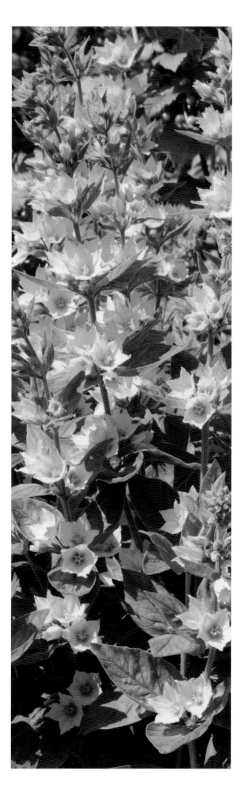

[Creeping jenny is] *singular good for to stay all fluxes of blood in man or woman, whether they be laskes* [diarrhoea], *bloody fluxes* [dysentery], *the flowing of womens monethly courses, or bleedings inwardly or outwardly, also the weaknesse of the stomacke, that is given to casting* [vomiting].
– Parkinson (1640)

[Yellow loosestrife is] *a wild plant not uncommon in our watery places, but for its beauty, very worthy a place in our gardens. If it were brought from America, it would be called one of the most elegant plants in the world.*
– Hill (1812)

Creeping jenny (far left); dotted loosestrife *L. punctata* (left), the yellow loosestrife most commonly grown in gardens

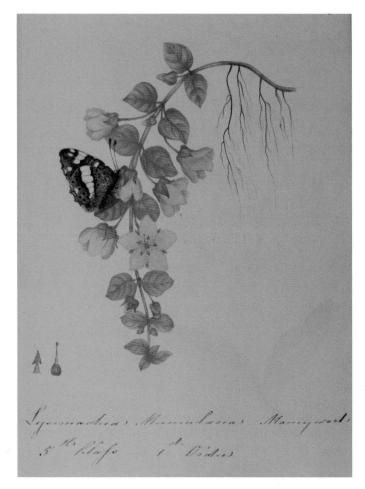

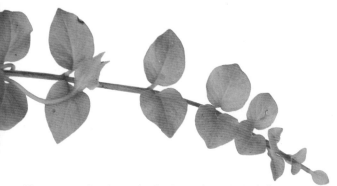

Above: creeping jenny leaf pairs and a painting of the plant; opposite: yellow loosestrife. Anna Sophia Clitherow's Watercolour Sketchbooks, c.1804–1815, John Innes Historical Collections, courtesy of the John Innes Foundation

helps Fluxes, stops the Terms, helps ulcers in the lunges; outwardly it is a special herb for wounds.

We would now say both plants are astringent, vulnerary, diuretic and antiscorbutic.

The astringency or binding property comes into play to help stop 'fluxes' of all kinds, whether upset stomach, diarrhoea or dysentery ('bloody flux').

As vulneraries, both plants healed wounds by stopping bleeding, whether old or new wounds, flowing or not, ranging from nose bleeds to piles or excess menstruation and 'whites' (leucorrhoea).

As diuretics, both plants increase urine flow, helping reduce the pain of kidney or gallstones and in some cases expel them.

Both were seen as useful against scurvy (as antiscorbutics), though their saponins, especially in yellow loosestrife, made the medicine taste soapy without added honey.

Another area of action for both plants includes the mouth, as a mouthwash for mouth ulcers, bleeding gums and quinsy (sore throat), and the lungs.

Various means have been used to take the herbs, including sipping the juice, a decoction in water or wine, the powder dissolved in water, and using the juice as a skin wash or cold compress. Fresh leaves can be applied to wounds direct or an ointment made.

L. christinae, jin qian cao, or 'gold money herb', is a related Chinese plant used to promote urination, reduce jaundice and help to expel kidney stone and gallstones. The leading Western book on Traditional Chinese Medicine describes it as *a very important herb for treating stones in both the urinary and biliary systems.*

Modern research

An aqueous extract of *Lysimachia christinae* was found to have potent hyperuricemic effects on mice (2002), ie to lower very high levels of uric acid in the blood.

At least four new saponins have been identified in Lysimachia species since 2006. In 2013 a new glycosylated triterpene 1 (named nummularoside) was isolated from the roots of *Lysimachia nummularia*. This saponin had significant activity against prostate cancer cells and glioblastoma (a form of brain cancer), while not affecting normal cells.

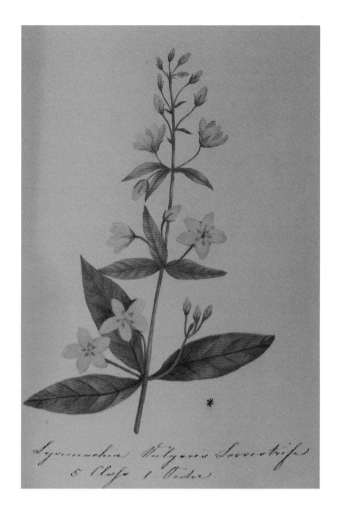

Lysimachia Vulgaris Loosestrife
5 Class 1 Order.

Twopenny tea

A healing tea is made from fresh or dried leaves and flowers of either plant. Scrunch up a handful of herb, put into a teapot, add boiling water and brew for 5 minutes. The leaves have some astringency and 'soapiness', so the taste will usually benefit from addition of honey or sugar. The effect should be soothing (demulcent) and settle upset stomachs or diarrhoea.

The cooled tea can be used as a gargle for sore throats or inflamed gums, and as a compress to place on surface wounds or skin sores. Alternatively, as with plantain, the bruised leaves themselves can be applied to the affected part.

Twopenny tea
• upset stomach
• diarrhoea
• sore throat
• minor wounds

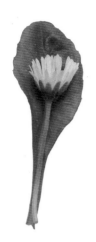

Daisy *Bellis perennis*

Daisies have long been enjoyed by poets and children, but gardeners are not so enthusiastic about the migration of these small plants from meadow to lawn. Medicinally, daisies have a somewhat neglected reputation for treating wounds, bruises and coughs, and as pain relievers. Recent clinical trials, however, offer exciting possibilities for using daisies in anti-oxidant, anti-microbial and anti-tumoural contexts.

Asteraceae
Daisy family

Description: A small perennial with rosettes of leaves hugging the ground. Flowers usually white, sometimes with red or pink on backs of petals. Petals close up at night and in cloudy weather.

Habitat: Short grass, including lawns.

Distribution: Native and common in the British Isles, Europe and western Asia. Introduced to North America.

Related species: There are 10 species in the genus *Bellis*.

Parts used: Leaves and flowers.

The daisy is universally known in temperate climes, but is sometimes specified as the English, common or lawn daisy. It is a close relative of the ox-eye daisy (see p340), and has similar medicinal uses.

Anne Pratt, the Victorian botanical writer and illustrator, explains the plant's popularity. She wrote in 1866: *How thoroughly the little wild flower is loved is told by the fact that never a poet, either of old or modern times, who has written of Nature, has forgotten to give it a line of praise.*

There's something in this. Daisy was the *dæges eage* (day's eye) to the Anglo-Saxons, and Chaucer in 1386 set the standard of affection – and confirmed daisy's status as a meadow plant: *That, of al the floures in the mede, / Thanne love I most thise floures white and rede, / Swiche as men call daysyes in our town.*

Other poets followed. Milton wrote in 1645 of *Meadows trim with daisies pied.* Shelley in 1822 called daisies *those pearled Arcturi of the earth / The constellated flower that never sets,* while in 1821 John Clare had *daisies' silver studs / Like sheets of snow on every pasture spread.*

Mrs Pratt also had a thought about why it was so easy to love the common daisy: *Perhaps there is scarcely another [flower] which has power to awaken so fully the memories of early life. … It is truly the bairnwort, the child's flower.*

The daisy is the right size for a child, and making daisy chains remains a familiar part of many children's experience. There's a story that Augustine, first archbishop of Canterbury (died AD 604), saw children outside the town busy threading daisies, and took the opportunity to preach the new religion, explaining that the golden centre of the flower was God the Father and the rays were good Christian souls.

Augustine was subtly offering a counter-ideology, a conversion narrative. The old belief was that daisies needed to be joined because evil spirits will not pass

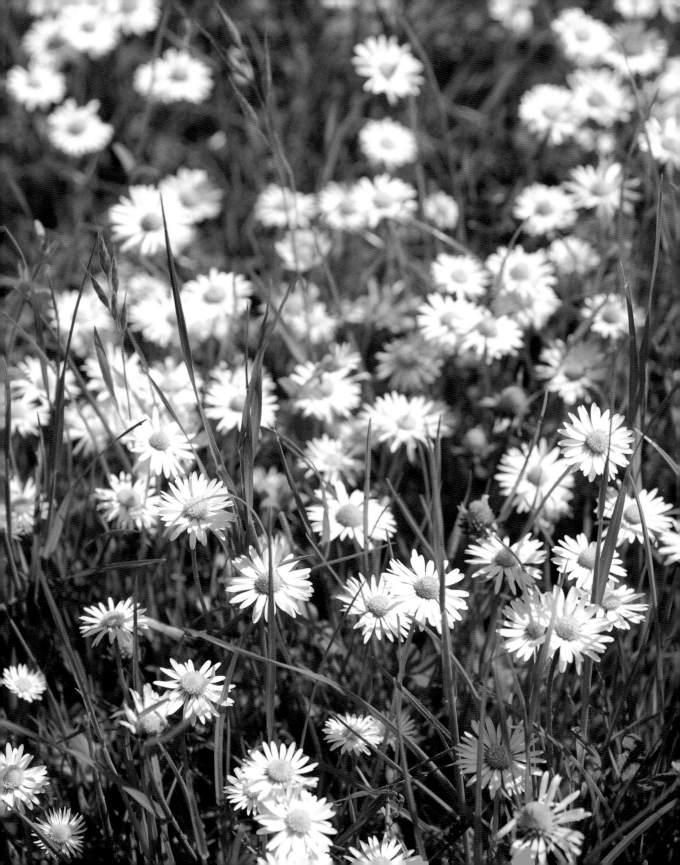

through a circle; hence daisy garlands, crowns, necklaces, bracelets and rings. This meant the daisies could be worn, and thereby prevent children of both sexes from being stolen by Little Folk, especially at May Day, when the faery kingdom is closest to us.

Some may dismiss this as 'paganism', but the passing down of daisy-chain skills from older to younger children is still with us. And so is the 'divination', if you will, of pulling off white daisy florets to the chant of 'he/she loves me, he/she loves me not'.

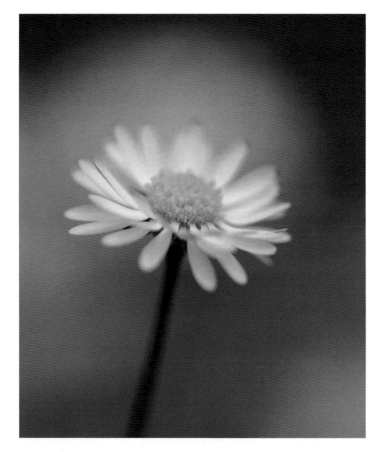

In the adult world, daisy is a plant that needs the grass around it to be short, hence its appearance in grazed meadows and of course in lawns. Despite concerted uprooting, poisoning and beheading it always returns, shining brightly, through most of the year, available to us as a forgotten but readily available healing plant.

It seems ironic that people try to kill this wild tiny aster or chrysanthemum in the lawn while working hard to keep its garden cousins flowering in the borders. But we have noticed that daisy seems to be spreading out from the garden and college lawn and back into the meadow. A decade ago we spotted wild daisies in Dartmoor and remarked how unusual that was. Nowadays we see them far more widely, and expect you do too.

Use daisy for ...
As a modern woman of a hundred and fifty years ago, Mrs Pratt says of the older medicinal uses of the plant – she mentions for oils, ointments and internal medicines – *that the men of our days have done wisely in rejecting them.* We could not disagree more.

Back in Roman times, army surgeons organised the collection of daisies by slaves to extract the juice. Bandages soaked in this juice treated sword and spear wounds. This means the plant could have links with the Latin name *bellum*, war, though most still prefer the alternative of *bellis* for beautiful.

No matter, daisy maintained a strong reputation as a wound-healing herb, often used as an ointment or salve. Parkinson wrote (1640) *that an ointment made thereof doth wonderfully helpe all wounds, that have inflammations about them, or by reason of moist humours having accesse unto them, are kept long from healing.*

Parkinson here draws our attention to daisy's cooling and drying nature, and this applies too for its renown as 'bruisewort' when used for easing the heat and pain of bruises, ulcers, skin swellings and burns. We made a daisy and mugwort ointment for an inflamed cyst on Matthew's neck, with excellent results.

Daisy is a traditional expectorant, which taken as an infusion relaxes spasms presenting as coughs and catarrh or colic. It is also a mild diuretic, which helps relieve the pain of gout and arthritis.

Daisy leaves can be used direct on the skin as a poultice for tired muscles, or added to a hot bath for generic pain relief. Gerard advocated daisies *stamped* [pressed] *with new butter unsalted*

… a wound herbe of good respect, often used and seldome left out in those drinkes or salves that are for wounds, either inward or outward.
– Parkinson (1640)

Below: Daisy therapy with Kaz

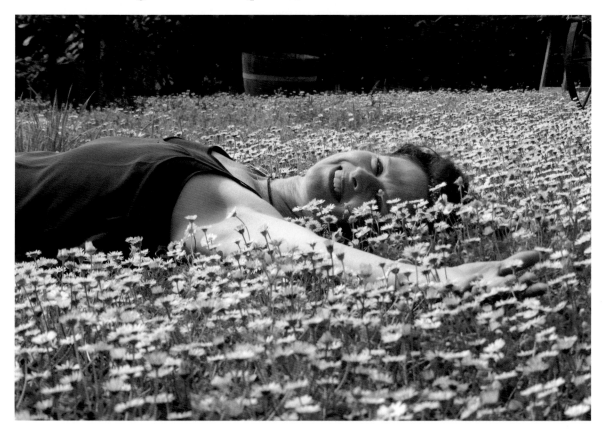

for painful joints and gout, while Parkinson preferred a tea from daisies, dwarf elder and agrimony.

A time-honoured use of daisy was to treat eye inflammations. John Wesley (1765) has a recipe (see left) that claims efficacy even *tho' the Sight were almost gone.*

Daisy is a close relative of arnica (*Arnica montana*), and is sometimes called 'poor man's arnica' as a pain reliever. Irish-based herbalists Nikki Darrell and Chris Gambatese find daisy to be the more effective, as do we. It has the added benefit of being free and local, and without toxicity.

Former internal uses for daisy in treating inflamed liver and bruising in pregnancy have dropped away, and indeed modern advice is against taking daisy internally in pregnancy.

Daisy leaves in salads add a succulent presence and a soapy or sour tang, with the white florets a bright final garnish. Herbalist Anne McIntyre likes a daisy soup, using the flowers and leaves, with added stock and ginger.

Modern research

Remarkable strides are being taken in clinical trials using daisy. Some examples:

- Daisy ointment healed wounds without scarring in 12 rats, the first scientific verification of the plant's traditional wound-healing activity (2012).
- Flavonoids isolated from daisy flowers showed strong *in vitro* antioxidant potential (2013).
- Antimicrobial activity of daisy essential oils was demonstrated (1997).
- Anti-tumour activity from saponins in daisy was shown for the first time (2014).
- Seven triterpine saponins were newly isolated from daisy flowers (2016). One of them, perennisaponin O, *exhibited anti-proliferative activities against human digestive tract carcinoma.*
- Homeopathic *Arnica montana* and *Bellis perennis* may reduce postpartum blood loss (2005).

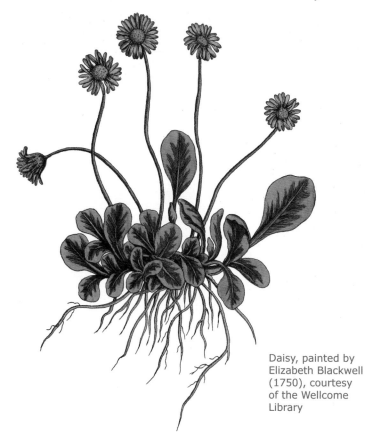

Daisy, painted by Elizabeth Blackwell (1750), courtesy of the Wellcome Library

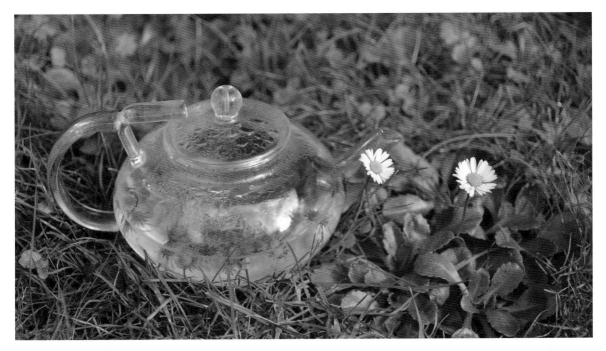

Daisy tea

While daisies can be found in flower for much of the year, we usually pick them in the spring when they are abundant, and dry them for use as a tea. Use a heaped teaspoonful of dried **daisy flowers** per mug of **boiling water**. Cover and let stand for about 10 minutes, then strain and drink. We find daisy tea has similar properties to the more familiar chamomile.

Combine with ground elder for gout and arthritis.

A daisy ointment

Make an infused oil of daisies by filling a jam jar with fresh or dried **daisies**. Pour on enough **extra virgin olive oil** to cover the flowers; press down to remove air pockets. If you have used fresh daisies, cover the jar with a cloth held on by a rubber band – this allows any moisture to escape. With dried daisies you can just use a normal jar lid.

Leave on a sunny windowsill to infuse for about a month. Then strain out the flowers, add 10g **beeswax** for every 100ml of oil, and heat gently until the beeswax has melted. Check for setting by putting a drop on a cold saucer. If too soft, add a little more beeswax. When ready, pour into clean jars and allow to cool before putting the lids on. Label.

Mugwort, plantain and yarrow also work well with daisy.

Daisy tea
- relaxing
- coughs
- painful joints
- gout

Daisy ointment
- bruising
- cuts
- grazes
- sore muscles

Caution
Avoid taking daisy internally in pregnancy

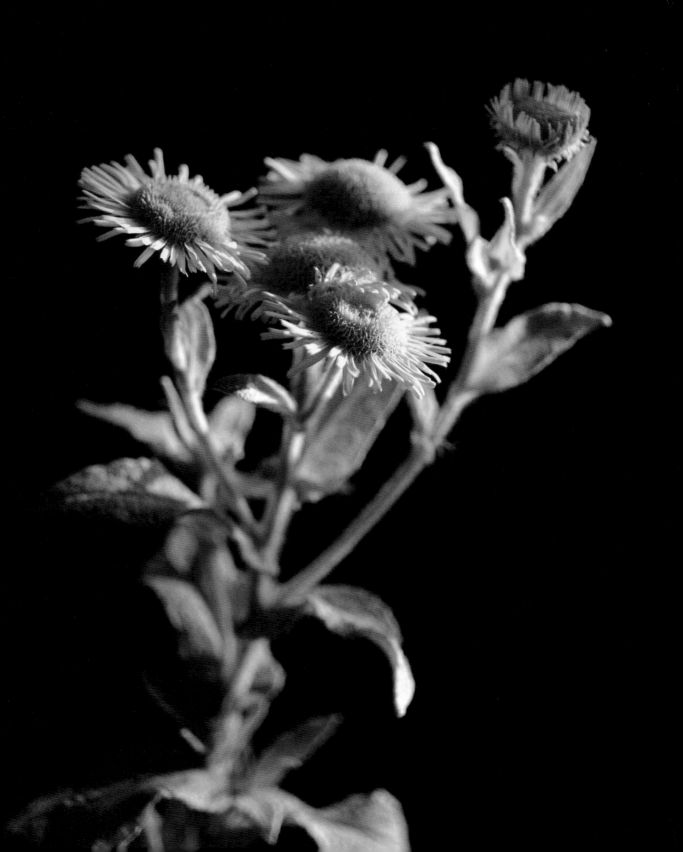

Fleabane *Pulicaria dysenterica*

Herbal names sometimes tell most of the story of a particular plant's effectiveness. Fleabane is a good example, with names reflecting traditional roles as an insecticide or repellant and for treating dysentery. It shares other medicinal actions with related members of the Aster family that should widen its use.

Fleabane is a somewhat elusive name, as it could refer to species in any of five genera within the huge family of Asters (or daisies, once called the Compositae).

These five genera are the *Inula* (notably elecampane and ploughman's spikenard); the *Dittrachia* (woody and stinking fleabane); the *Pulicaria* (common and the rare small fleabane); the *Erigeron* (blue and Mexican fleabane); and the *Conyza* (Canadian fleabane).

Our focus here is on *Pulicaria dysenterica*. The names tell it like it is: the common fleabane really does kill fleas (*Pulex* is the Latin for flea), and it has been used to tackle epidemics of dysentery.

It was Linnaeus who conferred the species name 'dysenterica', in the mid-18th century, after hearing from General Keit, a Russian army commander, that the plant had cured his soldiers of dysentery on a campaign against the Persians.

Plant names are often changed but specific medicinal qualities can persist through time and space, and remain valid today, even if the benefits are generally forgotten.

It should be no surprise that a fleabane relative (probably an *Inula*, elecampane) in Pharaonic Egypt was ground up with charcoal and the dust spread over the house to expel fleas.

Egyptian homes were plagued by rats, mice and fleas, and while cats were good against rodents, it took natron (sodium) water or fleabane to tackle fleas.

Fleas are always a corollary of civilisation, for where man goes so do they. Beds, whether of feathers for a king or straw for a peasant, attract biting creatures of various kinds, especially in the summer.

And fleas require a human response, although it was not known until relatively recent times that fleas carried bubonic plague bacteria, and nor was the link understood between mosquitoes and ague or malaria. But people were all too aware that fleas and midges were pests, and

**Asteraceae
Daisy family**

Description: Medium, untidy perennial (to about 50cm, 20in), with downy, grey-green foliage and bright yellow flowers, with flat tops and thin ray florets, above wrinkled erect leaves.

Habitat: Damp, often rough grassland, wayside ditches.

Distribution: Native to Europe and Western Asia; in Britain, southwards from Yorkshire and Lancashire (the obverse of goldenrod, which flourishes north of this area).

Related species: Many, including elecampane (*Inula helenium*), goldenrod (*Solidago virgaurea*), Canadian horseweed (*Conyza canadensis*), blue fleabane (*Erigeron acer*).

Parts used: Above-ground parts, juice, essential oil.

... though in England it [common fleabane] has never had much reputation as a curative agent it has ranked high in the estimation of herbalists abroad.
– Grieve (1931)

Fleabane, painting by Rudolf Koch and Fritz Kredel (1929), John Innes Historical Collections, courtsey of the John Innes Foundation

apothecaries like John Parkinson, writing in 1640, prescribed fleabane – for, *being burnt or laid in Chambers* [bedrooms], *it will kill Gnats, Fleas, or Serpents, as Dioscorides saith.*

The referencing of classical authority was typical of Parkinson, and he added that fleabane leaves were to be used for *bytings or hurts of all venemous creatures, as also for pushes* [pimples] *and small swellings, and for wounds.*

At that time fleabane was dried and hung in bunches in houses, or burnt in the hearth. The smell was camphorous and rather unpleasant, but as long as it killed the pests (insecticide) or deterred them (repellent) it was tolerated.

This is domestic medicine, but a close Aster relative of fleabane is the commercial-scale *Tanacetum cinerarifolium.* Once grown in the Balkans and now in Kenya, the flowerheads of this plant yield the leading non-synthetic and organic insecticide, pyrethrum.

Use fleabane for ...

Are there other uses for fleabane, apart from helping with fleas and dysentery? Parkinson hinted above at a role as a wound herb, appropriate for an astringent, and relevant for many medicinal plants among the wider Aster family.

Aster relatives, like the Canadian fleabane (*Erigeron canadensis*), are known and used for staunching blood flow topically, including for irregular menstrual bleeding and local haemorrhaging. The essential oil of this plant is often recommended in such situations, as antimicrobial and antibacterial.

The same is true for common fleabane, which ties back to its effectiveness against fleas and the pathogens they carry, no less than in treatment of dysentery.

Parkinson again: his list of virtues for fleabane included treating skin eruptions, as we have seen, and he said an extract of its leaves and flowers, boiled in wine, would help disturbed urine flow and counteract jaundice and griping pains.

In terms of method, he said the plant's juice could be swallowed and a tea or tincture made of the above-ground parts. A bath that included a quantity of the tea would be beneficial, while the distilled oil of the plant could be anointed (rubbed on the forehead) for 'fits of agues' (malarial fevers) and cold trembling.

Parkinson also cautioned that fleabane was a stimulant for the 'mother' (womb), and could cause spontaneous abortion. This warning should still be heeded.

Modern research

Ethnobotanical research seems to support Parkinson's findings. An allied species, *Pulicaria crispa*, is known in contemporary Pakistan as 'bui', and is used in syrup form to treat jaundice, ulcers, wounds and itchy skin (2012).

Research (1992) in Baluchistan found another species, *P. glaucescens* ('kulmeer'), being used in post-parturition care for women. It was boiled with other herbs, and 'gur' (raw sugarcane) added; the paste was rolled out and inserted into the vagina.

Pharmacological research has also confirmed aspects of the traditional profile. Iranian studies (2014a) on fleabane essential oil showed that it inhibited all micro-organisms tested, except for salmonella and shigella, and was partly effective against *E. coli*.

Saudi Arabian *in vivo* research (2014b) found *P. glutinosa*, another close fleabane relative, to be neuroprotective in zebra fish; the authors suggested fleabane be studied relative to human degenerative diseases, eg Parkinson's and Alzheimer's.

Caution
Avoid fleabane in pregnancy as it may stimulate the uterus.

Flea repellant bag

Fresh or dried **fleabane** can be put in a pillowcase or small **cloth bag** to deter fleas from biting in bed. Simply place the bag in the bed or under a pillow. We have found this practice very effective.

A small bag of fleabane can also be tucked into clothing or carried in a pocket to repel fleas during the day.

Fleabane tea

Pick a 3-inch sprig of fresh **fleabane** per mug of **boiling water**, and steep for 5 or 10 minutes before drinking.

This tea has surpisingly little flavour but is smooth and soothing. A larger quantity of the tea can be added to a hot bath to ease itching from a biting insect or minor irritations of the skin.

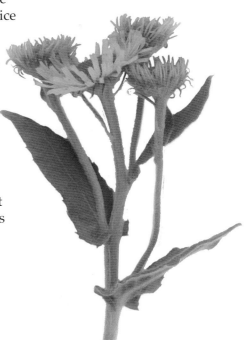

Fleabane tea
- cystitis
- infections
- dry tickly coughs
- griping pains

Forget-me-not *Myosotis arvensis*

German legends, a poet with a footnote and a steamy scene from DH Lawrence: forget-me-not is irresistible to writers! It may sound dull after all this that the plant's predominant medicinal use is a cough syrup and as a flower essence, but clinical research is now suggesting other prospects.

Boraginaceae
Borage family

Description: Annual/perennial, typically less than 50cm (20in) tall; thin hairy stems; small, terminal flowers, of striking pale blue with yellow 'eye'; daisy-like spatulate leaves; prolific in spring and summer.

Habitat: Generally fields, woods, waysides, gardens.

Distribution: Native in Eurasia and New Zealand; naturalised in US, apart from south and southwest.

Related species: Water forget-me-not (*Myosotis scorpioides*, syn. *M. palustris*) retains the old allusion to scorpions in its name, and is found at pond edges and in damp fields; wood forget-me-not (*M. sylvatica*) prefers drier rock and woodland habitats; *M. arvensis* var. *sylvestris* is the larger-flowered garden variety. Half a dozen more species are known in Britain, and about a hundred worldwide.

Parts used: Flowering tops, stems and leaves.

There is an old German legend in which God was naming all the flowers. One, a little blue flower, was overlooked. It called out, 'Forget-me-not', and God said that as all the names had gone, these very words were to be its name.

There was confusion about the plant for over 1500 years after Dioscorides (1st century AD) used the common name of 'mouse-ear' (*myosotis*), which also applied to

a type of hawkweed. John Gerard (1597) named three *Myosotis* species, but there was as yet no agreed common name.

It needed the poet Samuel Taylor Coleridge to give the plant the name we know it by today. Coleridge was travelling in Germany in the early years of the 19th century. He knew the medieval German legend of a love-struck knight, who was

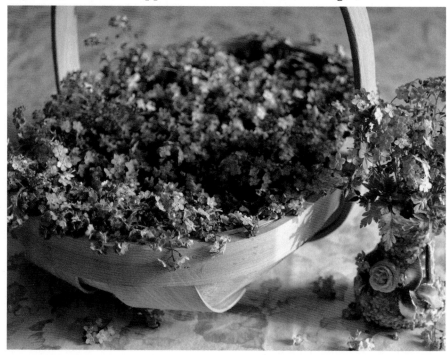

walking with his lady alongside a swollen summer river. The knight picked her a posy of forget-me-nots, but slipped and was carried away by the current. As he was drowning the knight threw the flowers to her, crying out *vergisz mein nicht*, 'forget-me-not!'

It would sound good in a German opera, but Coleridge put it in a poem, 'The Keepsake', which was published in a newspaper, and his new English name caught on (see right). We know precisely which species Coleridge was describing, because he added a footnote saying it was *M. scorpioides palustris*, water forget-me-not.

The Victorians featured forget-me-not in their language of flowers as a token of undying love.

DH Lawrence's novel *Lady Chatterley's Lover* blew such sentimentality away. The gamekeeper Mellors placed a posy of forget-me-nots on the lady's 'secret parts', as the old herbals describe them, saying *there's forget-me-nots in the right place*.

Use forget-me-not for …
Forget-me-not was known in John Parkinson's time as a source of a syrup for treating cough and 'tisicke', a consumption of the whole body as well as the lungs.

Three centuries later, Mrs Grieve (1931) confirmed the plant's affinity with the respiratory organs, notably the lower left lung.

We made a forget-me-not syrup that tasted rich, dark and densely sweet, and it did soothe the throat as it went down. Such a standard syrup was used safely for centuries to treat bronchitis, coughs, gagging and vomiting, though it is seldom used today.

Modern herbals caution that, like other members of the borage family, forget-me-not contains pyrrolizidine alkaloids, albeit in small amounts. Heat reputedly breaks them down. The flower essence is entirely safe.

Modern research
Russian clinical research (2014) has established that methyl salicylate is the principal ingredient of *M. arvensis* essential oil. This finding carries the potential for anti-inflammatory and analgesic uses of forget-me-not beyond the respiratory organs.

Clinical trials conducted on mice (2011) showed that aqueous tincture of *M. arvensis* exerts anxiolytic (anxiety-reducing) and antidepressant activity.

It was also demonstrated that essential oils of both *M. arvensis* and *M. palustris* inhibited the development of micro-organisms such as *Shigella sonnei* and *Candida albicans*. Additionally, extracts of *M. arvensis* reduced viability of *Staphylococcus aureus* and *S. faecalis*; and *M. palustris* extracts inhibited growth of *Pseudomonas aeruginosa* (2008).

Nor can I find, amid my lonely walk
By rivulet, or spring, or wet roadside
That blue and bright-eyed flowerlet of the brook,
Hope's gentle gem, the sweet Forget-me-not!
– Coleridge (1802)

8. *Myofotis Scorpioides repent. Small creeping blew Mousear.*

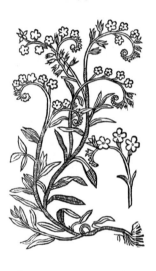

There is a Syrupe made of the juice and Sugar, by the Apothecaries of Italy and other places, which is of much account with them, to be given to those that are troubled with the cough or tisicke, which is a consumption of the whole body, as well as of the lungs.
– Parkinson (1640), with his woodcut above

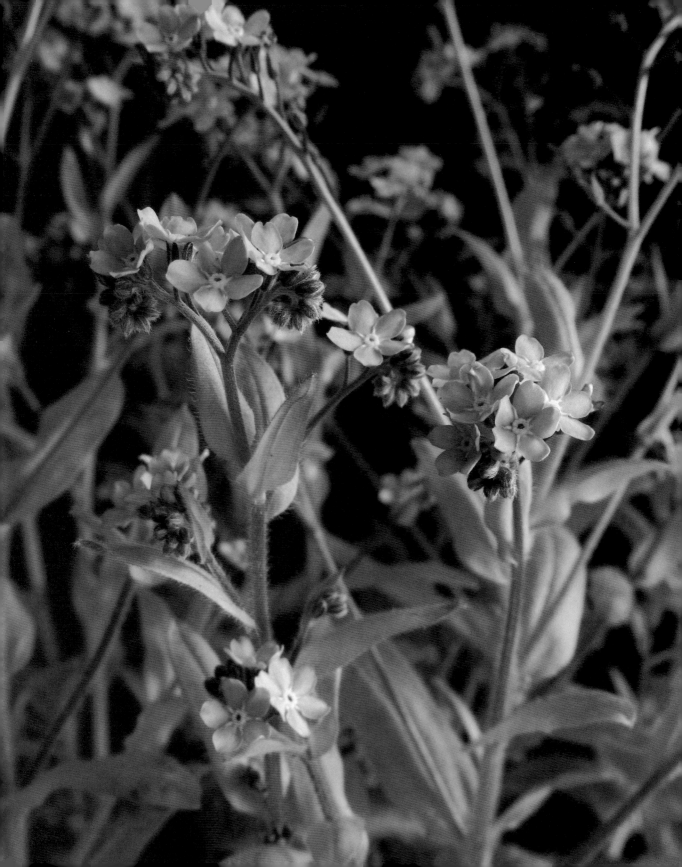

Forget-me-not flower essence

Choose a time when the flowers are at their most vibrant. Find a patch of forget-me-not growing in a peaceful sunny spot. Just sit near the plants for a while until you feel relaxed and at peace with the plants and the place. Because flower essences are based on the vibrational energy of a plant rather than its chemistry, your intention is important.

When you are ready, place a small, clear glass bowl on the ground near the plants. Fill it with about a cupful of **rain water or spring water**, then use scissors to snip off enough **flowers** to cover the surface of the water.

Leave them there for an hour or two – you can meditate on the flowers during this time, or if you prefer you can relax nearby or go for a walk while they infuse. The water will still look clear. Use a twig to lift the flowers carefully out of the water, and then use a funnel to pour the water into a bottle that is half full of **brandy.**

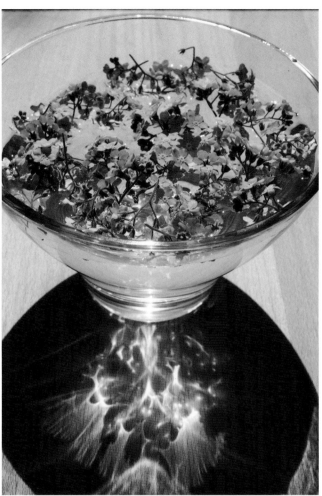

This is called your <u>mother essence</u>. Use any size of bottle you like, but a 200ml blue glass bottle works well. If any water is left over, you can drink it or water the forget-me-nots with it.

To use your mother essence, put three drops of mother essence in a 30ml dropper bottle filled with brandy. This is your <u>stock bottle</u>. With it, you can:

• put 20 drops in the bath, then soak for at least twenty minutes.
• rub directly on the skin, or mix into creams.
• put a few drops in a glass or bottle of water and sip during the day.
• make a <u>dosage bottle</u> to carry around with you, by putting three drops of stock essence into a dropper bottle containing a 50/50 brandy and water mix or pure distilled rosewater. Use several drops directly under the tongue as often as you feel you need it, or at least twice daily.

Cautions
The flower essence is completely safe, but forget-me-not contains low levels of pyrrolizidine alkaloids. Some members of this group of chemicals have caused liver damage, so the herb itself should be used with caution until more is known.

Forget-me-not essence
• grief
• clarifying
• relationships

Fumitory *Fumaria officinalis*

Papaveraceae
Poppy family

Description: Annuals, to 1m (3ft) tall, but usually shorter; many-branched stems, leaves cut fine, grey, 'smoky' from a distance; clusters of white or pink flowers with dark tips.

Habitat: Disturbed ground, fields, waysides, gardens; can grow on chalk.

Distribution: *F. officinalis* is also called common fumitory, and is widespread in the east and central British Isles, occasionally to the west; other species familiar in Europe, western Asia, widely naturalised in North America.

Related species: Three other rarer fumitories, plus six types of ramping fumitories are recorded in Britain, with much hybridisation; all share similar medicinal properties. *Dicentra formosa* (bleeding heart) and several corydalis species are also wild-growing British Fumariaceae.

Parts used: Above-ground, foliage and flowers, gathered in summer.

Common fumitory is a perky, pretty weed of field and wayside whose old name reflects its appearance as 'smoke of the earth' or *fumus terrae*. Its ancient healing reputation, especially for the liver, stomach, skin and eyes, also largely remains intact today. One modern herbalist calls it a unique gallbladder herb.

Fumitory is an important medicinal herb in both Western and Eastern traditions, and has been so since classical times. It is unusual in the sense that its principal uses – as choleretic (bile-stimulating), a tonic, a diuretic and valuable for liver, skin and eye health – have remained prominent from ancient times to today.

It was 'official', which means it was on the approved list of herbs for use by British apothecaries and doctors, in the first such list, in

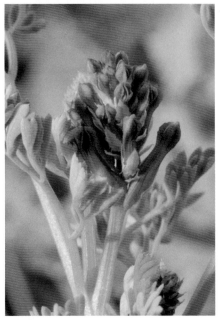

1618; and it is 'official' in the latest British list (as a choleretic) of 1996.

In 1653, the freethinking herbalist Nicholas Culpeper translated the Latin, and hence secretive, *Pharmacopoeia Londinensis* of 1618 into his own forceful English. He wrote that *Fumaria* was *cold and dry, openeth and closeth by Urine, clears the skin, opens stoppings of the Liver and Spleen, helps Rickets, Hypochondriack Melancholy, madness, frenzies, Quartan* [four-day] *Agues, loosneth the Belly*.

But what of fumitory's unusual name? Dioscorides and Pliny, some two thousand years ago, called it *kapnos*, the Greek word for smoke, because the juice of the plant made the eyes weep, as smoke does. The interesting implicit thing here is that fumitory was already in use for eye health by the Romans.

The Middle Ages had a somewhat different take. *Fumus terrae* was 'smoke of the earth', and variously meant a spontaneous growth of the plant from the ground or the 'smoky' appearance of the silvery-grey leaves from a distance. In modern terms, it is possible that its sudden appearance on wayside ground or in fields is from fumitory's ability to self-fertilise.

Fumitory smoke, 'vapours of the earth', was said to drive off evil spirits, a protection against the dark side. Shakespeare had 'rank fumiter' in Lear's 'crown': *Crowned with rank fumiter and furrow-weeds/ ... and all the idle weeds that grow/ In our sustaining corn.*

'Rank' is less a comment on the plant's scent – it's not particularly bad-smelling – than the status of fumitory, and its cousins the ramping fumitories, as a weed. Its characteristic mass of finely divided leaves in older times made manual harvesting much more onerous. Anne Pratt in 1866 thought it *among the most troublesome of weeds.*

Given the long use of 'fumitory', referencing 'smoke of the earth' both in Latin and English, it's odd that English vernacular names, as collected by Grigson (1958), have no allusions to smoke. He recorded such terms as babes in the cradle, birds on the bush, God's fingers and thumbs, jam tarts, lady's lockets and wax dolls.

We offer a new name, following up on an idea from the herb writer Gabrielle Hatfield (2007): how about 'matchsticks', for the red tip on a pinky stalk, and for referencing the old allusions to smoke?

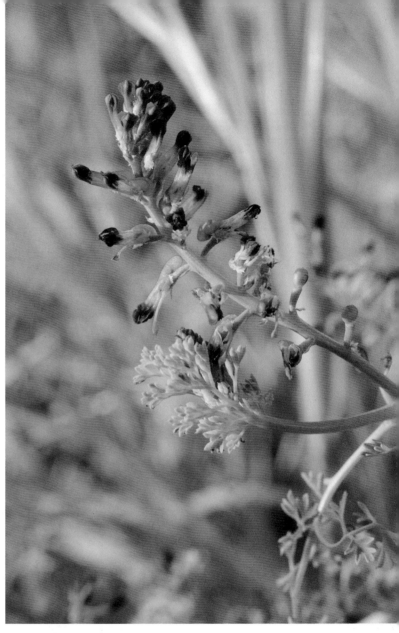

Use fumitory for ...
An important starting point is that fumitory has a reputation for safety. The European Medicines Agency monograph on fumitory (2011) collated numerous scientific studies, finding that of 710 patients tested over many years only two had experienced side effects from using the plant.

I cured a man with shocking herpes in a month with the juice and infusions of fumitory.
– Mességué (1979)

One person had suffered raised intraocular pressure and oedema, and the other a possible link to hepatitis, from using fumitory in parallel with grapevine.

The principal action of fumitory is in regulating bile flow, reducing liver stagnation and clearing liver obstructions. In particular, as Christophe Barnard points out, it keeps the sphincter of Oddi open; this muscle area affects the flow of pancreatic juices and bile into the duodenum.

Culpeper recommended boiling fumitory foliage in white wine for this 'opening' function (see quote).

The contemporary American herbalist Peter Holmes maintains that fumitory is unique among the gallbladder herbs in regulating both excess and deficiency biliary conditions (ie it is amphoteric). In the Chinese terminology Holmes uses, fumitory reduces liver qi stagnation, and as a cooling herb it modifies gallbladder damp heat.

But he adds a proviso. The array of alkaloids in fumitory has a combined dual effect, in being tonic for 8 to 10 days and then more sedative for the next 10 days.

So a patient using fumitory tea, say, for stimulating the digestion or improving bile flow would be advised to stop the treatment after 8–10 days and resume after 10 more days. Alternatively, if the more sedative, cooling range of actions is required, a three-week treatment course of fumitory can continue uninterrupted.

Fumitory is classed in the poppy family (Papaveraceae) but is not as sedative or analgesic. Nonetheless it will effectively calm the stomach as an antispasmodic, by relaxing smooth muscle and relieving constipation; it can treat migraines linked to the stomach or liver.

It is known too as a diuretic, which stimulates urinary function and can relieve gallstones and blockages in the kidney area. It is also used in weight-loss formulas in France, but these really only cause temporary moisture loss. Also in France, fumitory maintains its older reputation as a spring tonic or 'blood cleansing' herb, flowering early and reliably for mothers to force down reluctant children as a bitterish tea.

Allied with liver function and as an aspect of excretion is the role of fumitory as a skin detoxifier. The foliage of fumitory used to be gathered, put fresh into milk and boiled for use as a lotion to lighten freckles and sunburn – as one verse put it, to 'scare the tan from Summer's cheek' (see left).

Indian fumitory (*Fumaria indica*) is known as *pitpatra*, and is a plant medicine sold in bazaars for treating skin diseases like eczema and for easing swollen joints. *Pitpatra* combined with pepper is a home treatment for ague.

Modern research

In India, Gupta et al (2012), using *F. indica* in animal studies, note anti-inflammatory actions, but not antidepressant activity; these authors also add antibacterial capacity (for *Klebsiella pneumoniae*, but not for *E. coli* or salmonella), and antifungal and antioxidant properties to the fumitory register.

A more recent Indian study (2014) on the same plant suggests a use in treating fibromyalgia.

In Iran meanwhile, a study on *F. parviflora* (2011), using the full protocol of double-blind placebo controls on 44 human patients, produced conclusive evidence of the species' effectiveness in treating hand eczema.

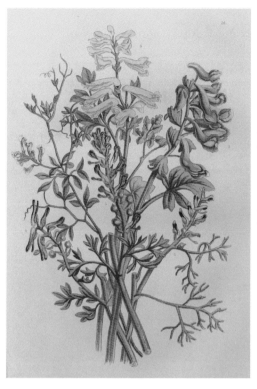

A bouquet of fumitories: common fumitory (centre) *with clockwise from lower left*: ramping fumitory, climbing corydalis, yellow fumitory, bulbous fumitory and small-flowered fumitory. Illustration from Anne Pratt, *Flowering Plants of Great Britain* Vol I (1873) pl 14, John Innes Historical Collections, courtesy of the John Innes Foundation

---

Fumitory skin lotion
As the verse (opposite) puts it, boil **fresh-gathered fumitory** in **water, milk** or **whey** to make your lotion. Put 2 handfuls of the plant into an enamel or stainless steel pan, add 1.5 cups of the chosen liquid, and boil. Simmer for 15 minutes, and leave for 15 minutes more to infuse as it cools. Pour into a jar, close and label. Store in the fridge and use freely within a week, applying morning and evening on problem skin.

Fumitory vinegar
Vinegar is a good solvent for an alkaloid-rich plant like fumitory. Choose a clean glass bottle of the appropriate size for your needs. Stuff with **dried fumitory** and fill the bottle with **white wine or apple cider vinegar**. Leave in a sunny place to macerate for a week, then strain off into another bottle. This vinegar will keep its potency for at least a year.

Dosage: 1 tablespoonful in the morning for any liver problem.

Fumitory tea
Dried fumitory is preferable for a bitter infusion: steep a heaped teaspoonful **fumitory** in **boiling water** for 5 minutes, then strain.

Fumitory skin lotion
• problem skin
• freckles
• sunburn

Fumitory vinegar
• liver stagnation
• gallbladder problems
• sphincter of Oddi dysfunction

Fumitory tea
• sluggish digestion
• lack of appetite
• spring cleanse
• liver stagnation
• gallbladder problems

Goldenrod *Solidago virgaurea*

**Asteraceae
Daisy family**

Description: Upright, untidy, with yellowish-green clusters of star-shaped, open flowers, each a small daisy; large dark green basal leaves and narrow stem leaves, variably hairy; brown seedheads.

Habitat: Invasive in wasteland and dry grassland, often on acid soils; in woodland, heathland, hedgerows and on cliffsides.

Distribution: Locally common in northern, western and southern parts of Britain and Ireland. North America. Native in Middle East.

Related species: Owing to hybridisation, the number of species is uncertain – possibly well over a hundred, most in North America. Canadian goldenrod (*Solidago canadensis*) is a common wildflower there, introduced to British Isles and an occasional alien escape.

Parts used: Flowering tops and leaves.

Goldenrod is best known as a garden flower but it has a long traditional medicinal history too, among Native Americans and Elizabethan Londoners alike. It was familiar in European medicine as a wound herb and for treating kidney stones, but now offers varied and tantalising treatment possibilities.

Goldenrod species are a familiar structural yellow presence in the wild garden, but the European goldenrod is less well known today as a powerful medicinal herb. Its genus name *Solidago* means 'to make whole or sound', a strong indication of a healing reputation; *virgaurea* is, literally, from the appearance, 'golden rod'.

The plant is also called Aaron's rod, a biblical reference to Aaron's miraculously blossoming staff, as are several other tall, wild healing perennials with spiky yellow flowers (eg agrimony and mullein).

One point of goldenrod's origin is in the Middle East, with the main European species, *S. virgaurea*, growing to 2–3 feet (0.75–1m); there are many taller native species in North America. Most abundant is Canadian goldenrod (*S. canadensis*), with feathery flower plumes up to 6 feet (2m), and a long history of Native American healing use.

Best loved of the North American varieties is sweet goldenrod (*S.*

odora) whose aniseedy aroma lends it favour as a tea herb, including in Blue Mountain Tea and formerly Liberty Tea (an ingredient of a substitute tea devised after the Boston Tea Party in 1773).

S. virgaurea had a medieval reputation as a 'woundwort' or 'Saracen's consound'. John Parkinson (1640) mentions the Arab medicine link in citing Catalan physician Arnaldus de Villanova (1235–1311), who commended its use for kidney stone and to provoke urine, as well as a sovereign wound herb to treat bruising and bleeding. Parkinson himself called it 'the best of all woundherbs'.

There was a brisk trade in imported goldenrod for such purposes in Elizabeth I's time. John Gerard (1597) notes that it once commanded a pricey half a crown an ounce in Bucklersbury, London, but after being discovered growing wild locally in Hampstead's woods its value dropped to half a crown a hundredweight.

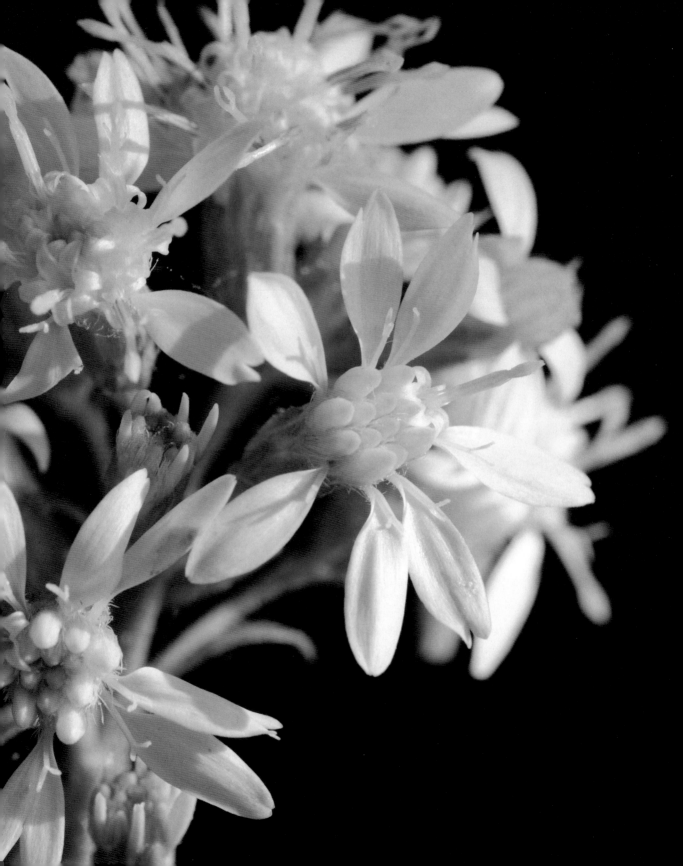

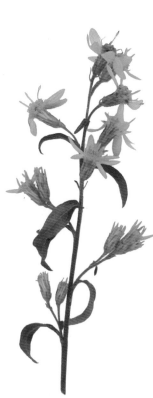

Gerard pointedly comments that this *plainly setteth foorth our inconstancie and sudden mutabilitie, esteeming no longer of any thing (how pretious soever it be) than whilest it is strange and rare.* Human psychology seems not to change much.

Use goldenrod for ...
Nicholas Culpeper's English 1653 translation of the Latin *London Dispensatory* for physicians and apothecaries captures the conventional herbal wisdom of his day for goldenrod: *hot and dry in the second degree; clenseth the Reins* [kidneys], *provokes Urin, brings away the Gravel* [calcareous deposits]; *an admirable herb for wounded people to take inwardly, stops blood &c.*

Goldenrod today is recognised among other things for its strong diuretic qualities, flushing out the system without causing loss of sodium or potassium. In Germany it is a standard kidney treatment, often preferred to pharmaceutical drugs for inflammatory diseases of the lower urinary tract. It is also used in modern irrigation therapy to prevent and break down renal and kidney calculi and gravel.

Austrian naturopath Maria Treben (1982) recommends a kidney tea made from the flowers of goldenrod mixed with species of bedstraw and deadnettle, and recounts several successful cures of otherwise intractable kidney problems. She also suggests

goldenrod as an antidepressant; the naturalist John Muir evidently agreed (see quotation).

It is regarded as a safe treatment protocol for cystitis and urethritis. It is also used as a gargle for relieving laryngitis and pharyngitis, and has been recommended as a carminative (settling the digestion).

Goldenrod has high antioxidant values – one estimate suggests seven times more than green tea. It is also antifungal, with a specific role in countering infections from *Candida albicans*, a cause of thrush of the throat or vulva.

Externally, a goldenrod ointment treated eczema, sores, ulcers and bruising; a compress made of the tea relieved muscle aches; mixed in a poultice with plantain and yarrow, it was used for burns and small wounds.

An area not highlighted in older accounts is goldenrod's value in treating upper respiratory tract disorders. This includes influenza, chronic and acute catarrh; it is 'official' for catarrh in the *British Herbal Pharmacopoeia* (1996).

The treatment would generally be a tea of the dried or fresh flowering tops and leaves. Native Americans chewed goldenrod flowers for sore throats, and also made a tea for reducing fevers. Interestingly, asthma is a condition efficiently treated by goldenrod flowers. This is despite an undeserved but persistent reputation for causing summer allergies. In North America the blame for these has been reallocated to ragweed (*Ambrosia* spp.) whose flowering season overlaps with that of goldenrod. Ragweed pollen is thought to cause over 90% of allergies in the US summer months.

Modern research

Goldenrod contains plentiful tannins, and is now recognised as an anti-inflammatory. It has been compared to diclofenac, a proprietary NSAID used for treating rheumatoid arthritis.

What is increasingly recognised (eg 2004 research) is the 'rather complex' spectrum of goldenrod's phytotherapeutic actions. It is known to be anti-inflammatory, antimicrobial, diuretic, antispasmodic and analgesic, an unusual combination of 'virtues' that offers tantalising research directions.

For example, it has been shown to be cardioprotective in rats (2014) and to treat prostatic cancer in mice (2002). Human trials are awaited.

The rhizome of a Chilean goldenrod (*S. chilensis*), sometimes called Brazilian arnica, produced (2008) a marked anti-inflammatory response in mice, by inhibiting both proinflammatory mediators and leucocyte infiltration. The same plant relieved symptoms and pain of human lumbago (2009).

Research also confirms goldenrod's anti-*Candida* credentials: a 2012 study using *S. virgaurea* showed effectiveness against two key virulence factors of *C. albicans*: the yeast-hyphal transition phase and biofilm formation.

1 Virga aurea serrata folijs.
Golden Rod with dented leaves.

Goldenrod, woodcut, Parkinson, *Theatrum Botanicum* (1640)

Caution
Goldenrod species freely hybridise, which may lead to variations in wild-gathered species' phytochemical actions. Previous herbal interpretations of goldenrod as variously 'warming' or 'cooling' may be an instance of such species variation. The general actions of goldenrod species are similar and interchangeable, but herbal users should be aware of potential variation.

Goldenrod syrup
• sore throats
• coughs
• urinary tract inflammation
• cystitis
• urethritis
• irritable bowel

Goldenrod syrup

Harvest **goldenrod** while it is in flower in the summer. Place in a pan and cover with **water**, bringing slowly to the boil. Simmer gently for a few minutes, then remove from heat. Cover the saucepan with a lid and leave overnight to infuse.

Strain off the liquid and return to a clean pan. Add 200g **sugar** to every 250ml of liquid, and bring to the boil. Stir until all the sugar has dissolved. Warm your bottles, then pour the syrup in, cap and label.

Dosage: 1 teaspoonful 3 or 4 times a day, especially for children.

If you like your syrups less sweet, try adding **fresh lemon juice** when you add the sugar. Use the juice of 1 lemon per 500 ml of liquid.

Greater celandine *Chelidonium majus*

Greater celandine might be taken for a large, leafy mustard topped by small yellow flowers, but it is in fact a poppy. Like its *Papaver* cousins, it has a stem latex and a complex array of alkaloids/enzymes, which underlie both its long-known herbal virtues and regulatory concern about its potential toxicity.

Papaveraceae
Poppy family

Description: Common perennial, 1m (3ft) tall, with relatively small lemon yellow flowers, each of four petals, on top of profuse, branched lime-green foliage, with rounded leaves; distinctive orange sap and long thin seed capsules.

Habitat: Disturbed waste land, banks, hedgerows, walls near human habitation; may often be escapes from old physic gardens.

Distribution: Native to temperate Europe, Eurasia, introduced to eastern and western North America.

Related species: No direct relative, and certainly not Lesser celandine (a buttercup). Is in a genus with but one species. Welsh poppy (*Meconopsis cambrica*) is another British yellow-flowered poppy with four petals.

Parts used: Whole plant, including orange sap (which stains but is washable) and roots.

Greater celandine has a long tradition of use in European and Chinese folk medicine (as *Bai qu cai*) as a liver and bile herb, with external applications in eye and skin health. In energetic terms, notes American herbalist Peter Holmes, its leafy green appearance with yellow flowers suggests a liver remedy, but he suggests it is better understood as *a warming cardiovascular stimulant as much as a hepatic stimulant*.

Thus, it acts to restore coronary circulation and relieve sharp chest pains (angina) brought on by over-exertion when there is inadequate blood supply to the heart. It also has an antispasmodic action, which works to relieve colic in the intestines, wheezing and coughing in the lungs, and asthma.

Greater celandine's ability to soothe bronchial spasms led to its use in treating whooping

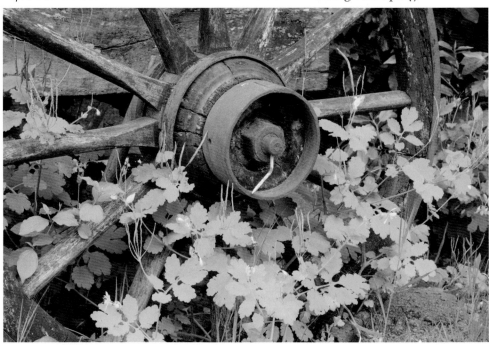

cough and bronchitis, especially in China. Holmes notes there was no equal to it in the Chinese pharmacopoeia, and it was long used in Chinese hospitals.

Use greater celandine for …
Greater celandine's stimulant effect extends to use as a bitter tea or tincture to promote sweating (as a diaphoretic), urination (as a diuretic) and irregular menstruation (as an emmenagogue). Being a uterine stimulant means it should not be taken during pregnancy.

Arising from these properties greater celandine is useful to help the body sweat out colds, flu and fatigue; relieve limb and ankle swelling (oedema or dropsy); and as a useful ingredient in gout or arthritis treatments.

Better known is the way the plant promotes bile flow (as a chloretic), alleviates the pain of gallstones, and reduces liver congestion and any related migraine headaches (as an analgesic). It has been regarded as a jaundice (hepatitis) herb, but in excess can be damaging to the liver.

British herbalist Julian Barker makes the important point that the active alkaloid and other constituents of greater celandine and their interactions vary greatly; the plant product, fresh or dried, and however extracted, is not stable, with a short shelf life; and although safe within therapeutic

limits it is potentially toxic. Dosage is key here, and any internal use of this plant should be within limits recommended by a practitioner.

It is good practice to take a break of several days in treatment after two weeks. Homeopathic use is an alternative. French herbalist Maurice Mességué recommended footbaths using greater celandine.

A still-popular use of the plant's orange sap or caustic juice is to treat corns, warts, veruccas, herpes and other skin eruptions. Old names for greater celandine, such as tetterwort (tetters are variously ringworm, herpes and eczema) and felonwort (a felon is a whitlow, an abscess of the nail), testify to folkloric usage.

We now know the sap contains protein-dissolving enzymes that destroy malignant viruses on the skin. This suggests the strength of the sap and any washes derived from it, and underlines why application should be restricted to the infected / inflamed area and not broken skin or open wounds.

One French herbalist calls external use of the plant 'irreplaceable', and claims *it will generally cause ugly cutaneous excrescences to vanish within eight days*.

A recent proponent of the use of the orange sap of greater celandine for the eyes is the Austrian herbalist Maria Treben. Her 1982 book

It wipes out herpes, deals with ringworm, literally melts away warts and corns and speeds up the healing of ulcers. … As a footbath, it regularizes women's periods, and brings them on after an abnormal stoppage.
– Mességué (1979)

… clearly, much of the story of this plant remains to be told.
– Hatfield (2007)

Caution
Greater celandine should not be taken internally during pregnancy. Its internal use is restricted in some countries.

records she applied it in drop doses on patients with cataracts, but also for her own healthy but tired eyes. At the end of a long day, when writing letters, she would wet a leaf, squeeze it, then apply the juice – *It is as if a mist is lifted from my eyes*, she wrote.

Our own view is that given the caustic strength of the raw sap it ought to be diluted if used, and under advice from your herbalist.

Modern research

Greater celandine has a mixed reputation in cancer treatment, specifically for skin and stomach cancer. This is not new: William Langham, in 1578, proposed it in an external skin cancer treatment: [For] *Kanker, wash it well with wine or vineger, and then apply the iuice of the hearbe and roots thereof.*

The European Medicines Agency has a 40-page assessment (2009) of greater celandine, and confirms its anti-tumour effects *in vitro* (on rats and mice) as 'very promising' but *in vivo* studies on mice are at an early stage. More human research, inevitably, is called for.

The same EMA report also notes a variety of dose-dependent antiviral, antioxidant, antimicrobial and anti-inflammatory effects of the plant reported in ongoing research (eg candida, herpes, RNA polio virus and *E. coli*).

This 'official' evidence is positive for such wider uses of greater celandine, a fact that should not be overlooked when considering the downside – that in some people liver toxicity results from taking it in treatments, with symptoms of fullness, gastro-enteritis, diarrhoea and other disturbances.

Because internal use of greater celandine is restricted to practitioners, we are only recommending it for external use.

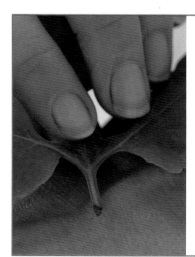

Greater celandine sap
The sap can be used any time there are green leaves of lesser celandine available, but there is generally more sap produced in warmer weather.

Break off a leaf and allow the yellowy-orange sap to emerge from the stem. Carefully apply the sap to warts or other unbroken skin blemishes. Repeat frequently, and you should see results within days.

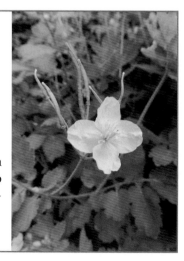

Ground elder *Aegopodium podagraria*

'Love your weeds' is an invocation that might stretch patience and credulity in the case of ground elder. Yet a positive case can be made for this garden pestilence as a traditional gout and anti-inflammatory treatment, a forage food, and most intriguingly as a potential player in the struggle against kidney and liver disease and metabolic syndrome.

Apiaceae
Carrot family

Description: Perennial, with hairless, hollow stems, rhizomes and white stolons; pinnate leaves, resembling but unrelated to elder; attractive umbels of white flowers, to 1m (3ft).

Habitat: Gardens predominantly, also waysides, disturbed ground, woodland margins.

Distribution: Native to Central Europe, Eurasia; introduced to Britain, Western Europe, North America and other temperate regions.

Related species: There are up to eight Aegopodiums worldwide but this is the common Eurasian species.

Parts used: Leaves, roots.

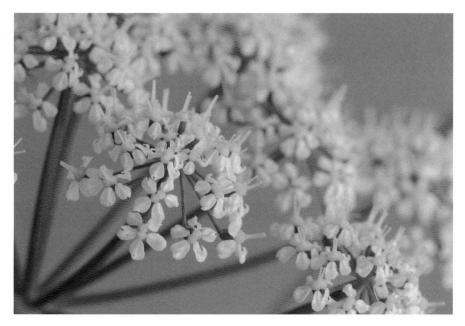

Extreme gardener Stephen Barstow describes ground elder as 'perhaps the most invasive widespread introduced plant in gardens in Europe'. So why include a terrorist of the borders in a book about wayside plants?

We had not often seen ground elder outside a garden context until summer 2015, when we visited Loughcrew, in Westmeath, Ireland. There, along a quiet road, a few hundred yards from the nearest house, was a mass of flowering ground elder. It was not just the dominant Apiaceae but the dominant plant, outmuscling nettles, herb robert, cleavers and other vigorous settlers.

So, yes, ground elder is largely a plant of gardens, but also waysides, churchyards and other disturbed habitats, sometimes as a garden discard. Its roots are said to grow up to a metre a year, and it needs only a few millimetres of root to clone itself, just as woodbine and couch grass

I have known a quantity of the roots and leaves boiled soft together, and applied to the hip in sciatica, keeping a fresh quantity hot to renew the other, as it grew cold, and I have seen great good effect from it.
– Hill (1812)

do. Incidentally, these other two invasives also have long-standing herbal uses, and we argue for ground elder in this respect. One English sufferer calls it Grelda, a 'seemingly immortal witch-weed', and Matthew's mother refused to take any rooted plants from our garden because we have ground elder. It is banned, declared toxic, in many states in the US and elsewhere.

The problem, unfortunately, is not new. In his lifetime John Gerard was as well known for his Holborn flower garden as for his *Herball* (1597). He writes with resignation: *Herbe Gerard groweth of itself in gardens without setting or sowing and is so fruitful in its increase that when it hath once taken roote, it will hardly be gotten out againe, spoiling and getting every yeare more ground, to the annoying of better herbe.*

Full of self-belief as he was, Gerard was not naming the plant after himself. St Gerard of Toul (935–994) was the patron saint of gout sufferers, and ground elder was used, even before the saint, as a home remedy for gout.

The plant had the medieval name bishopweed, perhaps because of the link between gout and the drinking habits of the higher clergy, or because ground elder was a monastic plant – useful both in the kitchen as a spring vegetable and in the infirmary for compresses and teas to relieve gout, rheumatism and sciatica.

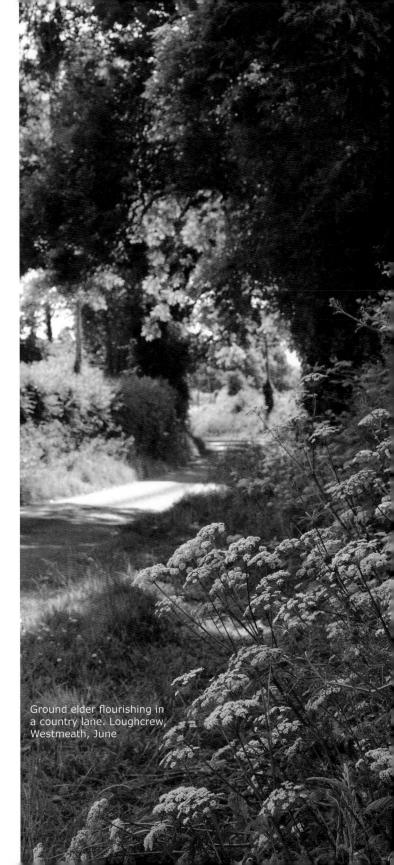

Ground elder flourishing in a country lane. Loughcrew, Westmeath, June

The species name *podagraria* is from *podagra*, or gout, so goutweed as a common name has a direct link to its observed use. The generic name *Aegopodium*, from words meaning foot and goat, is probably from the shape of the young leaves looking somewhat like the foot of a goat. American forager 'Wildman' Steve Brill believes goutweed has no effect on gout and that the common name is a corruption of the older goatweed. Few seem to agree.

The plant is thought to have had its origin in the Caucasus, Ukraine and Central Asia, spreading westwards by planting (yes, some people do this), clonal reproduction and seed dispersal (an old name is jack-jump-about).

When it arrived in Britain is moot. Some argue for a Roman introduction, others for the monastic period. Archaeological evidence from Denmark shows it was there in Iron Age times, but no similar pre-Roman discoveries have been made in Britain. Perhaps several reintroductions?

Coming up to date, Stephen Barstow is a pioneer collector and grower of unusual edible plants. What is remarkable is that he gardens near Trondheim, Norway, that is, north of the Arctic Circle. The Gulf Stream warms this area but the growing season is still very short. One of the plants he champions is ground elder, and he wants to stop its 'persecution'.

So Stephen has formed the Friends of Ground Elder as a Facebook group, with the goal of ending the chemical warfare on the plant and putting a long-overdue positive case for its use. It may be an uphill battle, but we're backing him.

Use ground elder for ...
So is goutweed good for gout? To Parkinson 'goutewort', is not named 'at randome', but *upon good experience to helpe the cold Goute and Sciatica and other cold griefs.*

This finding is widely replicated, with ground elder tea made from the leaves drunk or used externally to soak a poultice or fomentation for treating gout, sciatica, piles and diarrhoea. Julie found drinking the tea beneficial for her own sciatica one year.

The same remedy is a traditional wound herb, used for soothing burns, stings, bites and wounds externally. Tinctures are less used traditionally, though the German herbalist Tabernaemontanus (1520–90) liked to cook the plant in wine for similar purposes.

Such older medicinal uses remain available. What of cooking ground elder, as a spring green or eating raw? One forager's soup and quiche are *all the tastier from being made from the bodies of an enemy.*

We rather like its raw, anise-like taste and texture when fresh, but a little goes a long way, especially in a salad. We disguised the effect

They [ground elder patches] don't just occupy the places between the cultivated flowers. They subvert them, insinuating their white subterranean tendrils, as supple as earthworms, around and through any root system in their way.
– Mabey (2010)

I wouldn't do without it as a vegetable and I use it frequently in spring over a 6–8 week period when the fresh young growth is available. I also use it later in the summer where it regenerates after I scythe the areas where it still grows in my forest garden.
– Barstow (2014)

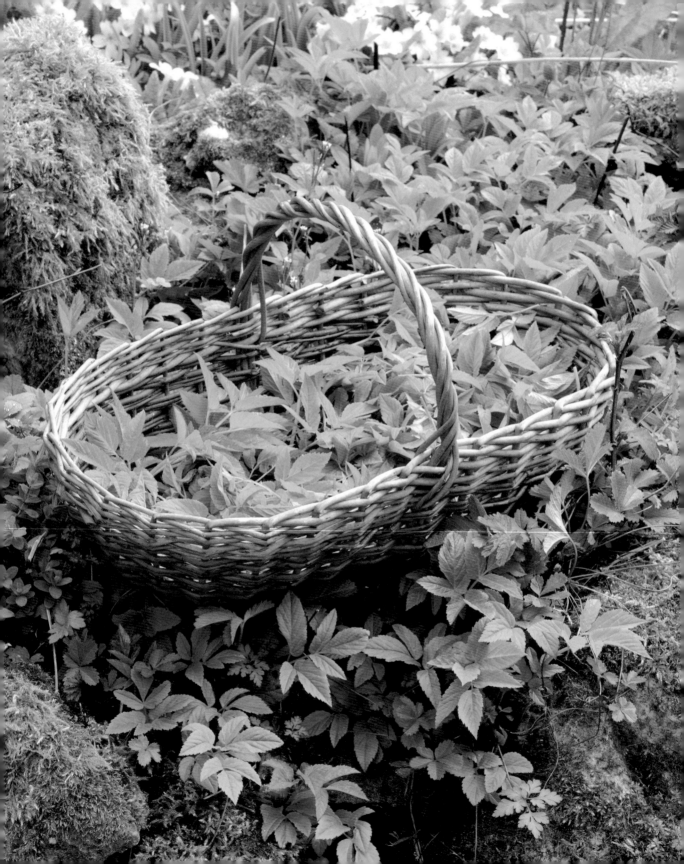

in a pleasant-tasting frittata and a sag paneer, and other cooks have used the leaves in pizza, curry and borscht. Another possibility is drying the leaves to a powder for a green smoothie, or trying the white stolons in a cooked form.

Modern research

Tovchiga et al in Ukraine trialled ground elder tincture in rat uric acid metabolism and suppression of inflammation (2014). The tincture showed protective action in kidney function, such as reducing proteinuria and hyperazotemia, and protecting the liver from carbon tetrachloride-induced hepatitis. Further, the tincture's hypoglycaemic property was found to be beneficial in metabolic syndrome treatment.

These are potentially key discoveries for application of new pharmaceuticals but also for herbal use of ground elder in these problematic areas. The next stage will be human trials.

Other research has shown that ground elder root has a type of supra-molecular protein, a lectin (1987); and that mature flowers contain falcarindiol, with proven COX-1 activity (2007).

The combination of [A. podagraria's] hypoglycemic, nephroprotective, hepatoprotective, antiinflammatory properties as well as ability to normalize uric acid metabolism can be of great value in metabolic syndrome treatment.
– Tovchiga (2014)

Ground elder frittata

This is a vegan version that we often eat, made with all sorts of wild greens, but ground elder is our favourite.

Preheat oven to 175°C (350°F). Put in a blender: 1 cup **gram flour** (chick pea flour), 2 cups **water**, ½ teaspoon **salt**, 1 or 2 peeled cloves of **garlic** and 1 teaspoon **turmeric powder.** Blend until smooth, then set aside to rest while you sauté the vegetables.

Put 1 tablespoon **olive oil** in a large skillet. Add sliced **mushrooms**, chunks of **cooked potato**, and a couple of handfuls of chopped **ground elder leaves**.

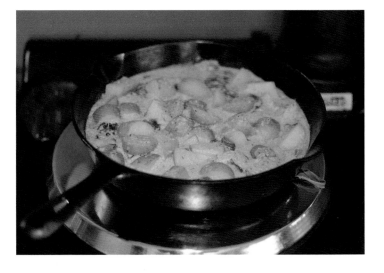

When the vegetables are cooked, pour the blended liquid over them and cook until the edges of the batter are set, then transfer into the preheated oven for 15 minutes. The frittata should be set, and gently browned on top.

Slice and serve warm.

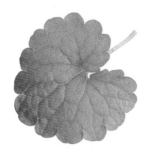

**Lamiaceae
Deadnettle family**

Ground ivy *Glechoma hederacea*

A common European and American perennial wildflower, ground ivy was once, and could be again, a home medicinal. It is best known as an expectorant catarrh-clearing herb and for head and kidney issues, but research is underlining its value as an anti-inflammatory, antioxidant and antibacterial.

Description: Low-growing creeping perennial, 20–30cm (8–12in) high. Crinkly, heart-shaped, opposite leaves; gently hairy square stems, each with 2–4 rich purple flowers in whorls, with 'Lamiaceae lip' and musty smell; underground stolons (creeping runners) can be a metre/yard long.

Habitat: Damp semi-shade in woods, scrub, hedgerows, grassland.

Distribution: Very common throughout British Isles, except west of Ireland and Scottish Highlands; widespread in northern and central Europe, east to Siberia and temperate Asia. Introduced by early settlers to North America, now common in most states.

Related species: Ground ivy is the only western species in the Glechoma genus; *G. longituba* is used as a medicinal in China. Unrelated to common ivy (*Hedera helix*).

Parts used: Above-ground parts.

Ground ivy, like many old country herbs, acquired a cluster of affectionate names. Some refer to its appearance, like cats foot (for the circular leaves); robin run in the hedge or creeping charlie in the US (for the spreading stolons); and blue runner (for the flowers).

Other names reflect its long period of use, from the Anglo-Saxons to the Tudors, as the main bitter herb for brewing and clarifying ale. It was alehoof ('hoof' meaning herb) or tunhoof ('tun', meaning the verb to brew or the cask itself), while from the French *guiller* (to brew) it became gill.

Gill was also a measure of liquid, still taught in primary school in Matthew's time – four gills make one (British) pint. The word, as Mrs Grieve mentions, also meant 'girl', so ground ivy sometimes was hedgemaid or hay maiden.

Interestingly, for a plant that was also a popular medicinal, it attracted few overtly healing names, field balm being one. And, as Geoffrey Grigson pointed out in 1958, the English 'ground ivy' itself was a 'poor name'. A version of *Hedera terrestris*, or Old English 'eorthifig', ground ivy has no relationship with ivy other than being a vine.

Use ground ivy for...
Thomas Bartram's well-regarded herbal reference book gives 'catarrh' as a keynote descriptor for ground ivy; we prefer 'clarity'. Combining the two ideas, wherever there is congestion trust ground ivy to clear it!

Ground ivy is expectorant – indeed, this is the sole function attributed to it in the latest *British Herbal Pharmacopoeia* (1996) – hence anti-catarrhal, or phlegm-clarifying, if you prefer. Bartram notes that the catarrh can be bronchial or nasal.

Ground ivy was widely used in tea form for 'inveterate coughs' and consumption (pulmonary tuberculosis), and remains highly effective in lung conditions.

Hildegard von Bingen (1098–1179) believed that ground ivy removed bad humours from the head. We

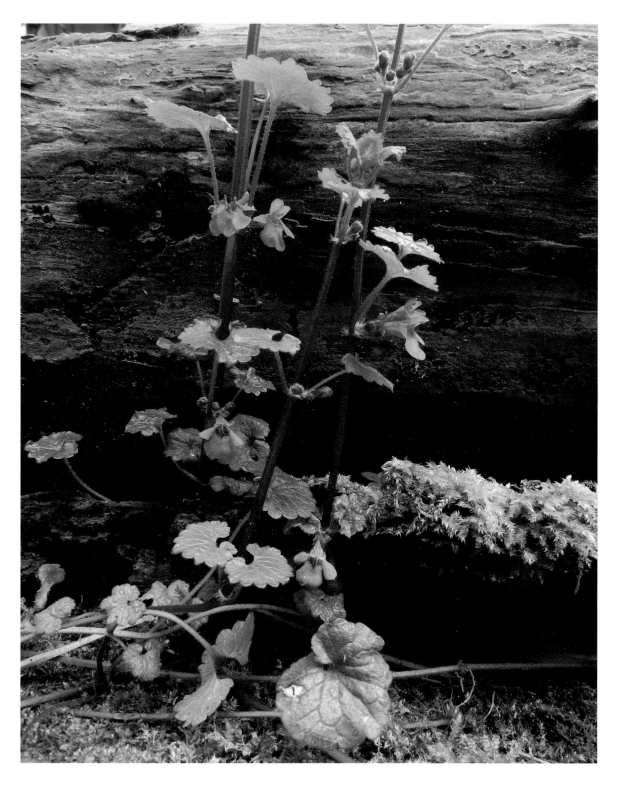

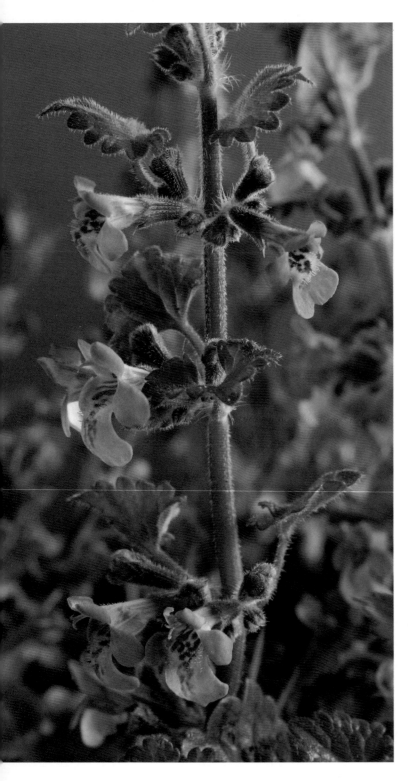

agree, and view ground ivy as the equal of rosemary as a 'head herb'.

Ground ivy is an ancient, safe herbal treatment for tinnitus, sinusitis and 'glue ear'. It makes a soothing wash for the eyes, or can be powdered and snuffed to clear the nose. As a compress it can be applied to the forehead for migraines or on 'black eyes'.

It has been useful for pain relief in toothache: William Langham in 1577 suggested: *Boile it with ginger in wine and hold thereof in thy mouth.*

It is also an 'important astringent', says Bartram, for the stomach, intestines and colon. It has a special affinity for the kidneys and bladder, as befits a diuretic herb. Poor kidney function can lead to chest congestion and breathing issues, areas ground ivy supports.

Bringing the astringent and anti-inflammatory qualities together, a recent survey recommends ground ivy for dyspepsia, gastritis, diarrhoea, irritable bowel syndrome, piles, cystitis and abdominal colic.

Another former use was as a tea to counteract 'painter's colic' or the lead poisoning from paint.

Modern research
The antimicrobial power of ground ivy was shown in 2011, when it tested as the most toxic to bacteria of the Lamiaceae species in bactericidal studies.

It was shown (2006) to inhibit nitrous oxide in conditions of macrophage-mediated inflammation, suggesting use in metabolic disease.

A traditional Japanese tea, *kakidoushi-cha*, made from *Glechoma hederacea* var. *grandis*, was found (2013) to inhibit the enzyme xanthine oxidase, making the tea protective in liver and gout issues.

Korean research (2014), testing *G. hederacea* for osteoclastogenesis, found potential for the plant's use in treating bone disorders such as osteoporosis and rheumatoid arthritis; turmeric (curcumin) and *Angelica sinensis* have shown similar potential.

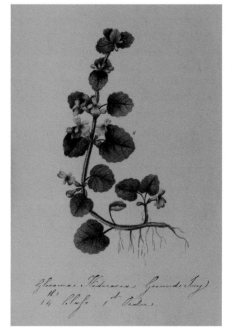

Ground ivy, from Anna Sophia Clitherow's Watercolour Sketchbooks, c.1804–1815, John Innes Historical Collections, courtesy of the John Innes Foundation

... the juice dropped into the eares doth wonderfully helpe the noyse and singing of them, and helpeth their hearing that is decayed.
– Parkinson (1640)

Meigrim [migraine], anoint the forehead and nostrels with the iuice, vinegar and oyle, or stampe [crush] the leaues with the white of an egge, & apply it.
– Langham (1577)

As a medicine useful in pulmonary complaints, where a tonic for the kidneys is required, it would appear to possess peculiar suitability, and is well adapted to all kidney complaints.
– Grieve (1931)

Harvesting ground ivy
Ground ivy is most aromatic in spring and summer (the smell varies by location), but the leaves stay green and are available most of the year.

Ground ivy clari-tea
Heat **water** (or wine or beer if you prefer) in a small saucepan, and add a few sprigs of fresh **ground ivy** for each cup of liquid when the liquid comes to the boil. Remove from heat, cover and allow to steep for 5 or 10 minutes. Strain and use the liquid.

Drink hot with honey or other sweetener, to taste. This drink once had the country name of gill tea. Most people find it has a satisfying taste and feels comforting to the throat. We mostly make ground ivy tea in the spring when it is in flower, but the leaves can be used anytime.

It can be reheated or drunk cold, as many cups a day as can be tolerated. The cold liquid can also be the basis of a compress: soak a cloth in the juice and apply to bruises, abscesses, headaches and sore eyes to take out the heat.

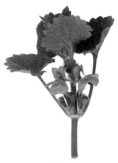

Ground ivy tea
- clears the head
- clears the mind
- congestion
- catarrh & phlegm
- stuffy nose
- tinnitus
- sinusitis

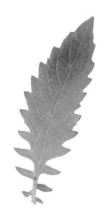

Gypsywort *Lycopus europaeus*

From an apparently disreputable past, gypsywort has now become a valued medicinal. Along with its American cousin, bugleweed, it has the specific ability to treat hyperthyroidism, or Graves' disease, safely and reduce the associated racing heartbeat and anxiety. Other benefits also repay a second look.

Lamiaceae
Deadnettle family

Description:
Perennial, to 1m (3ft); erect stature, with opposite jagged-toothed leaves; in summer bears tiny white flower whorls, with purple spots, in the leaf axils; grows in massed colonies.

Habitat: Wetlands, whether ditches, pond sides, riverbanks, damp woodland.

Distribution: Native to Europe and Turkey; common in England and Wales south of Yorkshire, western Scotland, and scattered elsewhere. Introduced in North America.

Related species: Other Lycopus species, native to North America, include Virginia bugleweed (*L. virginicus*), American bugleweed (*L. americanus*) and 'Chinese' bugleweed (*L. lucidus*).

Parts used: Leaves, which are stronger medicinally than the roots, and above-ground parts.

Gypsywort seems to have always been an outsider. In ancient times its deeply serrated leaf was likened to a wolf's foot (literally *Lycopus*) – hinting at transgressive as well as fanciful. And does the 'gypsy' in the plant's common name signify uncertain fears and prejudices about 'others'?

The first English account, in Henry Lyte's herbal (1578), describes how *the rogues and runagates, which name themselves Egyptians* [Gypsies], *do colour themselves blacke with this herbe*. The charge was elaborated in later accounts that travelling Romanies would dye their faces with the herb to look more exotic and then proceed to con the locals with magic and fortune-telling.

A more generous, but unrecorded, scenario would be that the Gypsies might have used the dye for their clothes rather than their faces, or perhaps have been the first to use and convey the health-giving properties of the plant (and hence give it 'wort' status).

English herbalist Julian Barker notes that in North America the

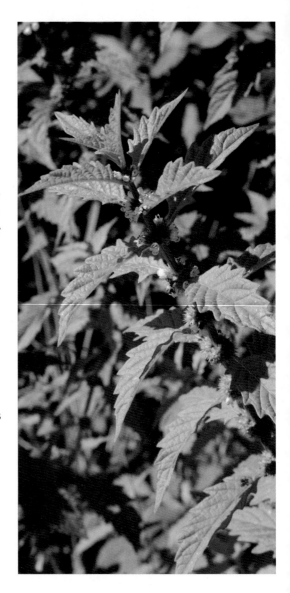

Native American peoples used their local Lycopus species as medicine and ate the roots.

Gypsywort's closest medicinal relative is the Virginia bugleweed (*Lycopus virginicus*) of the eastern US, which is thought to be slightly more bioactive, and has another common name, gypsyweed, that suggests similarity. This is the species most often used today on both sides of the Atlantic.

Two other American species are valued herbally, namely American bugleweed or water horehound (*Lycopus americanus*), and 'Chinese' bugleweed (*L. lucidus*). All the Lycopus species are perennials, need a wetland habitat and have comparable medicinal uses.

Gypsywort has little aroma and only two stamens, though it does share the square stems, opposite leaves, bunched flower whorls and running stolons of its mint cousins like lemon balm and motherwort with which it is often prescribed.

Use gypsywort for...

Bugleweed is the form of *Lycopus* most used commercially by herbalists on both sides of the Atlantic, but rather than importing it, British herbalists might well reconsider their native gypsywort.

Bugleweed itself was far from an outsider, and was mainstream medicine in 19th-century America, being included for a while in the *U.S. Pharmacopoeia*.

It was recommended at that time as nerve-calming and sedative, anti-haemorrhagic, anti-tussive (for coughs and lung problems), for urinary problems and as a mild narcotic that was safer than foxglove (digitalis). Such uses remain valid.

But what made *Lycopus* specifically valuable was the early 20th-century extension of its therapeutic range to include overactive thyroid and the associated racing heartbeat. Today bugleweed and gypsywort are the go-to herbs for treating hyperthyroidism, usually caused by Graves' (or Basedow) disease.

Graves' is an auto-immune condition that largely affects women from middle age onwards. Sufferers experience raised levels of iodine and thyroid-stimulating hormone (TSH), which the plants safely lower while also maintaining thyroid gland health.

Graves' is typified by accelerated heart rate, palpitations and related anxiety, along with goitre of the eyes, sometimes called 'wild staring'. Bugleweed and gypsywort taken as leaf tea or tincture can reduce these alarming symptoms, often given with lemon balm and motherwort to deepen the soothing and sedative effect.

Note that while small and regular doses of the plants improve the symptom picture for hyperthyroidism, its fundamental

... one of the mildest and best narcotics in existence. It acts somewhat like Digitalis, and lowers the pulse, without producing any of its bad effects nor accumulating in the system.
– Rafinesque (1828)

... one of the precious few thyroid inhibitors.
– Holmes (2006)

Traditional herbal treatment for hyperthyroidism provides us with one of the best examples of a condition for which a definite specific exists. This is Lycopus virginicus *or* L. europaeus, *commonly known as bugleweed.*
– Hoffmann (2003)

Caution: Bugleweed and gypsywort are safe to take long-term, but pregnant and lactating women are advised to suspend their use. Prolonged hormone imbalances, including TSH, should be referred to a practitioner.

Where there is pre-existing thyroid gland enlargement or weak thyroid function, *Lycopus* is contra-indicated. In one case in the literature high levels of *Lycopus* caused thyroid enlargement.

Gypsywort tincture
- overactive thyroid
- palpitations
- rapid heart beat
- coughs
- anxiety

The mint-like character of gypsywort's flowering tops

causes may be much harder to treat. Some authors describe the condition as genetic and incurable. Yet the plants have much to offer Graves' sufferers in quality of life. The same could be said for other herbal virtues the plants have been shown to possess, in reducing internal bleeding, such as heavy menstruation, calming tubercular and bronchial spasms, and being excellent relievers of indigestion.

Modern research

There has been experimental confirmation on Lycopus for its thyroid effects (2006) and the reduction in TSH levels (1994). Chinese research (2013), using *L. lucidus* on rabbits, showed cardiotonic effects, confirming traditional uses. Korean research on the same plant (2008) showed its leaves suppress high glucose-induced vascular inflammation.

Gypsywort tincture

Pick gyspywort when it is flowering in late summer. Chop it into one inch pieces, and place in a jar. Pour in enough vodka to cover it, then put the lid on and shake to release any air bubbles, topping up if necessary.

Put the jar in a dark place for about a month, shaking every few days. When the colour has gone out of the leaves, strain off the liquid and bottle it.

Dosage: half to one teaspoonful 3 times a day. It may be necessary to take a dose more frequently initially.

If you have an overactive thyroid, it is a serious condition requiring professional help and advice from your GP and a practising herbalist.

Gypsywort is often used in combination with lemon balm (*Melissa officinalis*) and motherwort (*Leonurus cardiaca*) for palpitations and over-active thyroid.

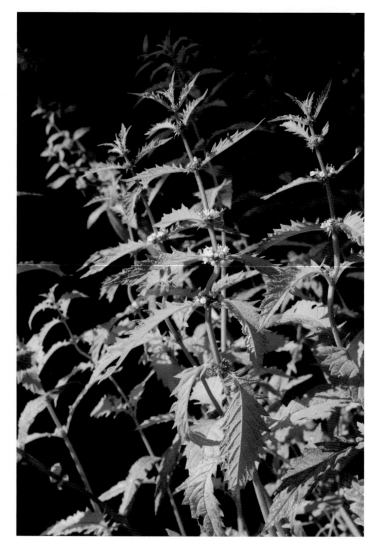

Heather, ling *Calluna vulgaris*
Bell heather *Erica cinerea*

Heather is much more than a pretty moorland scene on a Scottish shortbread tin. Historically, the two main species were a vital part of everyday life in many acid-soil upland areas, especially Scotland, and still have a significant economic role. Never accepted as 'official' medicine, heather's popular herbal uses have largely disappeared, but research is confirming traditional knowledge and opening up intriguing possibilities.

As well as the heathers themselves, the heather family contains many useful and decorative acidic soil-loving shrubs and smaller plants, such as rhododendrons, azaleas, vacciniums (including the fruitful cranberry, bilberry, blueberry and cowberry), bearberries and one tree, the strawberry tree.

The main heather species are subdivided into one Calluna species – ling or heather (*Calluna vulgaris*) – and at least ten Ericas, or heaths, including bell heather (*Erica cinerea*) and cross-leaved heath (*E. tetralix*).

Ling and bell heather are dominant in their heathland habitats; indeed they give their name to it. There are minor botanical variations, but the difference between them is observed best when they grow together: the swathes of magenta-purple flowers are bell heather, and the delicate mauve is ling.

Herbally, they have seldom been distinguished and have overlapping medicinal uses. Bell heather, however, makes for a stronger, darker honey, while ling honey is more viscous.

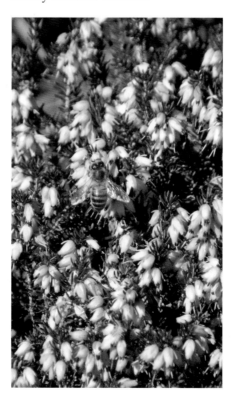

**Ericaceae
Heather family**

Description: Both species are evergreen shrubs growing to about 60cm tall. Heather or ling, *Calluna vulgaris*, has small purplish pink flowers appearing in late summer; bell heather or heath, *Erica cinerea*, has larger, brighter magenta pot shaped flowers over a slightly longer season, from May to October.

Habitat: Heath, moor, open woodland and bog, mainly poor acid, peaty or rocky soils.

Distribution: Widespread in the upland and moorland British Isles, especially to the north and west, and in the south. *Calluna vulgaris* is introduced in US.

Related species: Cross-leaved heath (*E. tetralix*) is the third main species, with similar distribution to bell heather but prefers wetter soils. Dorset heath (*E. ciliaris*) and Cornish heath (*E. vagans*) have restricted local habitats.

Parts used: Medicinally, the flowering tops, gathered in summer, used fresh or dried.

Heather or ling

Heather, from Anna Sophia Clitherow's Watercolour Sketchbooks, c.1804–1815, John Innes Historical Collections, courtesy of the John Innes Foundation

Scottish heather ale, after centuries of neglect, is currently back in favour, sold under the Gaelic name *fraoch*. The heather takes the hops role in brewing, mixed with malted barley and bog myrtle.

The Victorian botanist Anne Pratt noted that *those who have few resources learn to make the most of them*. This applies aptly to the way heather was an indispensable part of moorland life. It was a foundation for roads and tracks; it made walls and thatch, ropes, baskets and fish traps; it could tan leather; it was a food for domestic animals in winter; it made springy but comfortable bedding.

Calluna, interestingly, is not classical but from an 18th-century reclassification of the heathers. The name means 'brush', and may refer to bunches of ling made into besoms or informal brushes; or it might reflect medicinal use for the digestive and urinary tracts.

'Ling' is thought to derive from an Anglo-Saxon term for 'fire'. The young shoots of ling are the red grouse's favourite food. In modern economic terms, 'grouse moors' are valuable assets – ironically, just as moorland, the former symbol of a poor but self-sufficient peasantry, is being lost to various forms of 'development'.

The traditional communal reliance on heather may reflect a bygone age, but can be adapted by today's camping buff. Heather bunches make a good base for a sleeping bag; dead stems can fuel a campfire and young plant tips flavour tea – sweetened with heather honey. After your meal, clean your enamel plates with strands of heather. If it's raining, sit dry in your tent making a heather basket for ripe bilberries!

One final tip for wet walks is to follow the magenta clumps of bell heather as a marker of dry ground, which it prefers, amid more boggy areas preferred by cross-leaved heath (also known as bog heath).

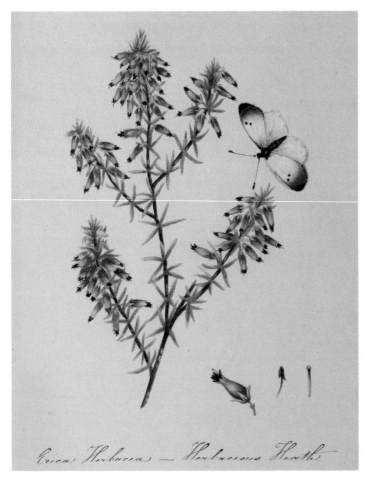

Erica Herbacea — Herbaceous Heath

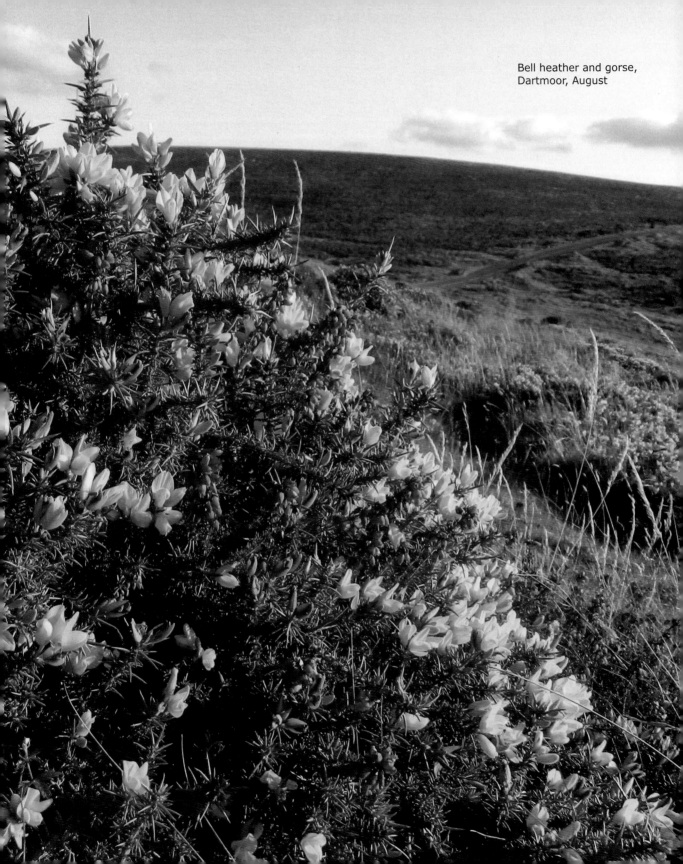

Bell heather and gorse,
Dartmoor, August

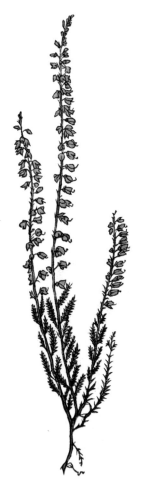

Heather, painting by
Rudolf Koch and Fritz
Kredel (1929), John
Innes Historical Collec-
tions, courtesy of the
John Innes Foundation

Use heather for …

As a medicinal, heather has classical origins in the 1st- and 2nd-century AD writings of Dioscorides and Galen, and the Erica family has been long known for its effectiveness in treating conditions of the urinary tract.

Bearberry, *Uva ursi*, is a close relative, found in Scotland, and is currently prescribed by herbalists for cystitis, prostate issues, inflammatory bladder and urinary stone or gravel. Heather could be a local, plentiful alternative.

Heather is antiseptic and diuretic for the digestive and urinary tracts, and takes these actions into easing the pain of nephritis, gout, arthritis and rheumatism.

Heather tea can be made from dried or fresh plants. Robert Burns called it 'moorland tea'. Heather tincture and distilled water are equally effective medicinally, and any of these forms can be applied in heather poultices or liniments. A heather bath can ease chilblains.

The original name *Erica* was linked in classical writings to 'breaking' in the sense of an internal stone. Parkinson reported the Italian botanist Matthiolus (1501–77) as writing that heather tea twice a day for 20 days would 'absolutely' break the stone.

Despite its classical heritage, however, heather has never been part of 'official' medicine. Perhaps its long association with areas of peasant poverty was against it?

Parkinson also noted the botanist Clusius (1526–1609) as claiming a heather flower oil helped cure 'the Wolfe in the face' or 'eating canker of the face'. This startling description could be an accurate word picture of the auto-immune disease lupus (the Latin for wolf).

Lupus is characterised, among many other symptoms, by a 'butterfly effect' of a rash that resembles bite marks. Where this becomes intriguing is in new evidence that heather protects for photosensitivity (see right).

Another Parkinson hint is that the distilled water can help dissolve tumours on the face – a potential marker for cancer research.

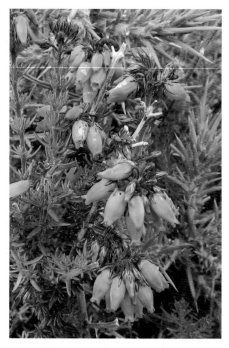

Modern research

2014 research confirmed the traditional antibacterial role of *Calluna vulgaris* tea or tincture in treating urinary tract infections. *E. coli* and *Proteus vulgaris* were controlled by the heather triterpinoids, including the newly named ursolic acid.

Similar findings emerged in 2013 for *Erica hebacea* (spring or snow heath) in neutralising *Proteus vulgaris*, a bacterium of the human intestinal tract. Earlier Scottish research (2010) had demonstrated that *Calluna vulgaris*, juniper and bog myrtle were all effective in treating the tuberculosis mycobacterium, again confirming old popular practice.

Most intriguingly, 2011 research indicated that *Calluna* is potentially photoprotective for the skin against UV rays.

Homemade heather ale

This is our own simplified recipe:

Take 28g (1oz) dried **heather tips** (we'd had ours in the airing cupboard for four months), and place in a large ceramic or glass bowl. Now add 200g (7oz) **local honey** (heather honey would be perfect) and 2 litres (3.5 pints) **warm water**. Sprinkle with ¼ teaspoon of **baker's yeast**.

Cover with a clean cloth, and leave in a warm place for a day or two until it starts to bubble. Strain into bottles and leave for another day to build up fizz, then refrigerate. Drink chilled.

It tastes 'yeasty' but refreshing, and will last up to a week if kept cold.

A fermented heather tea

Adapted from a modern Scottish recipe:

Pick **heather tips** and dry for at least a day. Liquidise to increase the surface area, and spread the mash onto a baking tray. Let it brew for three hours at room temperature. Then heat in the oven at 100°C until the contents are dry and crispy. Make as a tea on its own or mix with ordinary tea.

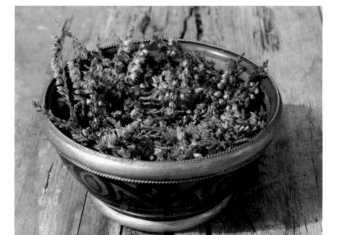

The Heather Bell
Away, away, ye roses gay!
The heather bell for me;
Fair maiden, let me hear thee say
The heather bell for me.
Then twine a wreath o' the heather bell
The heather bell alone;
Nor rose, nor lily, twine ye there;
The heather bell alone;
For the heather bell, the heather bell.
Which breathes the mountain air,
Is far more fit than roses gay
To deck thy flowing hair.
— Spittal (nd)

Heather ale
- refreshing
- nutritive

Heather tea
- cystitis
- prostate issues
- gout
- rheumatism

Herb robert *Geranium robertianum*

Herb robert is a familiar wild and garden plant that is almost too pretty to be called a weed. It has a rich folk history, with a perhaps surprising range of forgotten medicinal applications, which clinical research is now exploring and recovering.

Herb robert is the commonest and among the best-loved of the European wild cranesbills or geraniums. Both family names refer to the beak-like appearance of the seed heads, as do the related storksbills (*Erodiums*).

Herb robert bears small bright pink flowers almost year-round in milder areas, and the attractive lacework of dark green leaves and pale moist stems with their characteristic nodes often turn bright red in summer and later.

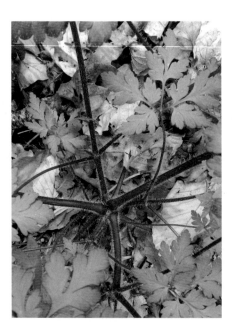

The redness is a key to the plant's place in folk memory and its long-held reputation as a herb connected to blood. The origin of the English name is elusive, and some commentators point to the Latin term *rubra*, for redness, as a possible source.

The first proper name associated with the plant is actually Rupert, probably St Rupert, a 7th-century Austrian bishop; a number of medieval, saintly Roberts, even a pope, have been linked with it, and then there is fairy tradition of 'robin' names (itself a diminutive of Robert).

Robin the bird, herb robert the plant and Robin Goodfellow – otherwise called Puck, the mischievous household sprite or hobgoblin – were intimately connected. In sympathetic magic their redness represented blood and life, but carried a darker meaning too, as a sign of ill luck or death: do not kill cock robin, do not uproot herb robert and do not cross Robin Goodfellow!

A multitude of common names for a plant suggests familiarity, affection, medicinal or foraging value, regional spread and long usage or wariness. The best British guide remains Geoffrey Grigson's pioneering book, *The Englishman's Flora* (1958). Grigson lists 110 British regional names for herb robert, and only one of these, death comes quickly, from Cumbria, refers to death as such. Nearly a quarter, 25 names, are variants on robert or robin; six are related to the plant's smell, and four to kissing. Most of the rest are descriptive rather than attributive.

Let us turn, then, to the matter of the plant's smell. The sweet-scented, large-flowered geraniums of the garden and house are actually Pelargoniums, hybridised from Southern African introductions in the seventeenth century. Pelargoniums are used in the perfumery industry and to make essential oils.

By contrast, crushed leaves of herb robert – one widespread name is stinking bob – have a musky smell that has been called disagreeable, foetid, mousy, foxy. John Pechey in 1707 was kinder: the smell was like parsnips, he thought.

Herb robert has hairs, but the scent is its main defence against predation. We can take advantage by crushing the leaves and rubbing them on the skin. This remains an effective repellent for midges and biting insects; maybe we should rename it 'herb rub it'! Crushing herb robert leaves

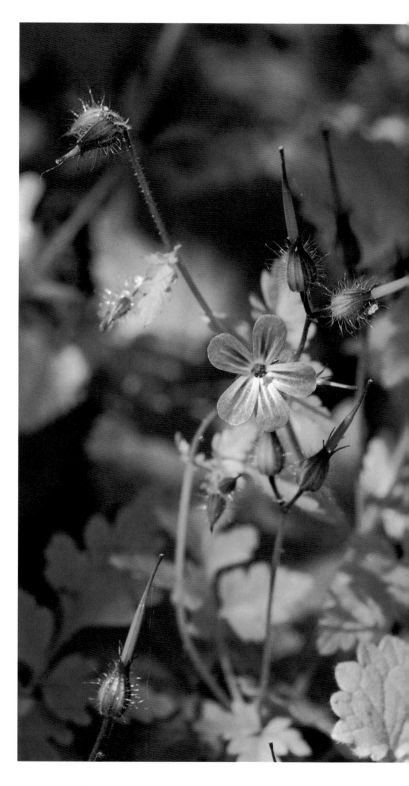

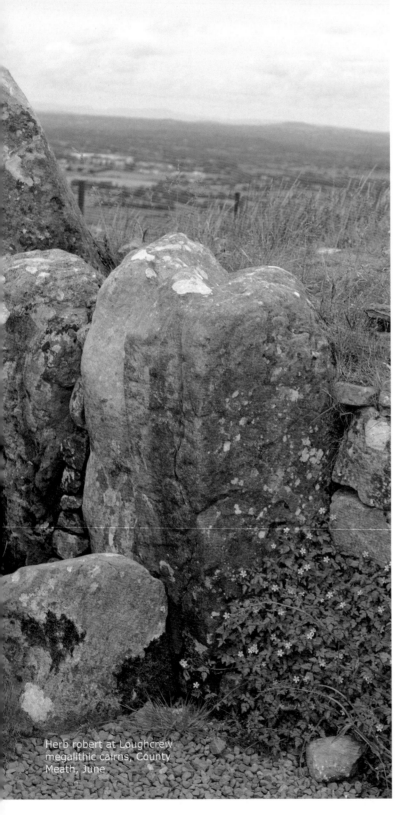

Herb robert at Loughcrew megalithic cairns, County Meath, June

is an always available and easy medicine for gardeners, and it will also staunch everyday cuts.

Use herb robert for …

Herb robert has a North American herbal counterpart, the wild geranium or alum root (*Geranium maculatum*), which is widely used and commercially available. Herb robert by contrast is now a largely forgotten herb, but has similar medicinal virtues.

These two geranium cousins are astringent, being high in tannins (*G. maculatum* has up to 30%), and vulnerary. As with other astringent plants, they have long been used for wound-healing and drying or clotting blood and other discharges.

In terms of blood-staunching, herb robert has been used in treatments for haemorrhage, metrorraghia, nosebleed, haemorrhoids and ulcers, especially peptic and gastric. In Ireland the plant was a favoured remedy for red-water fever, a disease of farm cattle.

'Other discharges' includes treatment for diarrhoea and dysentery, leucorrhoea, and excess breast milk and mucus.

In Southern Africa, a herb robert relative, *Geranium incanum*, is known as *Vrouebossie*, or woman's bush, and its tea is used in country areas to treat bladder infections, venereal diseases and menstruation-related ailments.

Another area of effective action of herb robert is for eruptions of the skin, including skin ulcers, tumours and eczema; Pechey in 1707 had already noted its value in treating erysipelas. A decoction of above-ground parts has been used as a mouthwash, for gum disease and for sore throat.

The kidneys are a site of traditional herb robert treatment, again in Ireland. The plant is mildly diuretic and cooling, and was used externally, in Ireland, for backache, eg as a compress soaked in herb robert tea.

Herb robert has juicy stems and is hard to dry – we found it resistant even to a dehydrator – so is most readily taken as a whole-plant fresh tea or tincture; the musky smell may not appeal to everybody, as we have seen.

A distilled water of herb robert has the same range of uses, as does a flower essence; its essential oil is worth consideration.

Finally, going back to the 'kissing' names, herb robert has a forgotten reputation as a mild aphrodisiac.

Modern research

Pharmacological research into herb robert is ongoing, and tends to confirm older uses. For example, work in 2010 found that a decoction of herb robert reduced blood sugar levels in rats with type 2 diabetes, supporting French folk tradition.

Herb robert has long had an underground reputation in treating cancers, especially of the skin, and tumours. Research (2004) into its high levels of the antioxidant germanium sesquioxide (organic germanium) supported such uses, but human clinical trials are still awaited and needed.

Additionally it has been shown that herb robert has antimicrobial potential, in treating *E. coli* infections (2012), and has been proposed as a possible AIDS treatment.

Finally, as an anti-inflammatory, an essential oil made from a combination of herb robert, clover and lavender proved effective in treating otitis, a painful ear inflammation (2014).

… though its scent is so disagreeable that the name of stinking crane's-bill is commonly applied to it, yet it is very pretty.
– Pratt (1866)

The herb bears closer investigation as a remedy. According to one authority it is also effective against stomach ulcers and inflammation of the uterus, and it holds out potential as a treatment for cancer.
– Chevallier (2016)

Harvesting herb robert
Herb robert is easy to harvest, but is so moist it is difficult to dry. We usually use it fresh. In mild areas the plant is available year round.

Herb robert tea
Put a sprig or two of **herb robert** per person in a teapot and cover with **boiling water**. Allow to steep for 5 or 10 minutes, then strain and drink, or allow to cool for use as a mouthwash or on the skin.

Herb robert tea
• mouthwash
• wash cuts & grazes
• antioxidant
• drink after X-rays
• drink after dental work

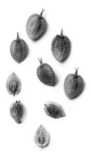

Hogweed *Heracleum sphondylium*

**Apiaceae
(Umbelliferae)
Carrot family**

Description: A common tall wayside plant flowering from summer into winter. Hairy stem and leaves.

Habitat: Waysides, damp meadows, waste ground, field margins.

Distribution: Throughout the British Isles, common in Europe across to Asia. Introduced to North America.

Related species: Giant hogweed (*H. mantegazzianum),* the other species found in Britain, mainly near rivers, is phototoxic. Cow parsnip (*H. maximum)* and other species are used in North America very much like hogweed.

Parts used: Young shoots, flower buds, roots and seeds are eaten and used as medicine.

Warning: Do not confuse with giant hogweed, *H. mantegazzianum,* which can grow to 3m tall and causes severe skin damage in sunlight.

Hogweed's abundance tends to obscure its virtues. Foragers prize its delicious celery-like shoots, farmers have long fed it to stock (yes, including pigs), and herbalists of old valued it, particularly Native Americans using the related cow parsnip.

Hogweed has been described as the *commonest tall wayside white umbellifer of the* [British] *summer and autumn.* The North American equivalent, the cow parsnip (*Heracleum maximum*), is equally well distributed, a common sight along highways, in fields and on waste lots.

The vigour of the Heracleum genus is honoured by reference

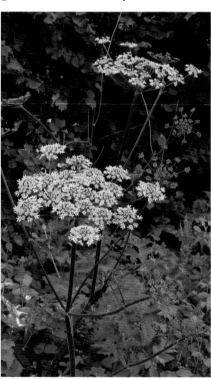

to the hero Heracles (in Greek) or Hercules (Latin). The common name hogweed is a little less heroic, reflecting the old use of the plant for feeding pigs and other livestock. As a modern forager points out, the flowers also smell foetid, which is rather 'unglamorous' to humans but appealing to insect pollinators.

Hogweed shoots, buds and seeds (both green and brown when mature) are favourites with foragers, and are enjoyed in traditional Baltic food and drinks culture. Hogweed also has long-established – if forgotten – herbal uses and potential new ones.

But there's another side we should address first, that of identification. Many people associate the word hogweed with the closely related giant hogweed (*Heracleum mantegazzianum*), a huge and impressive plant that can soar to 3 metres (14 feet) in a growing season. It prefers riverbanks, and is luckily much less widespread than its edible cousin.

It is wrong to say, as is sometimes seen, that giant hogweed is

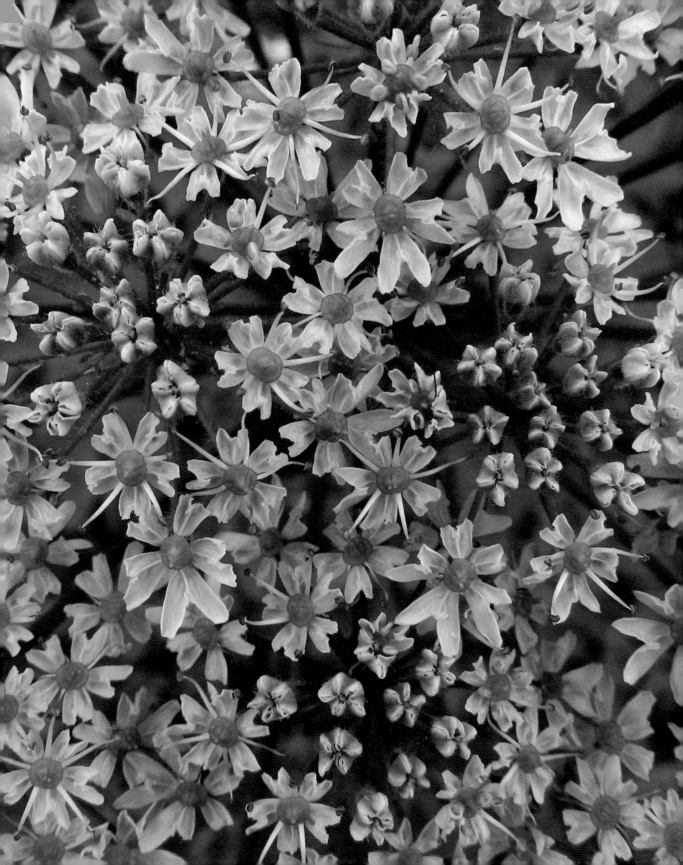

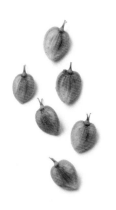

poisonous, but it is phototoxic. As its defence mechanism against predators the plant secretes furanocoumarins in its sap and bristly hairs. In the presence of sunlight these phytochemicals can cause contact dermatitis, with severe blistering and possible long-term purpling of the skin.

In hot sunny weather, hogweed can have a similar but much less severe phototoxic potential. If weeding or strimming hogweed, do wear gloves. Strimming shreds the stems and scatters the sap far and wide, so goggles too are a good precaution. Watch for your children picking hogweed stems for making blowpipes or toy boats, especially in the hot sun, and keep them away from giant hogweed.

Use hogweed for…

In North America cow parsnip was one of the most used Native American and First Peoples' wild herbs, as was hogweed in pre-revolutionary Russia and the Baltic states.

The medicinal range of both herbs was administered by root decoctions or tinctures. In North America cow parsnip root tea eased colic, cramps, headaches, colds, flu and tuberculosis, while poultices externally went on sores, bruises, stiff joints and active boils. In European herbalism Linnaeus knew hogweed as a sedative in 18th-century Sweden, while two centuries earlier in England Gerard advised it for headache and lethargy; in the mid-17th century Culpeper proposed it for epilepsy and jaundice. In modern French herbalism hogweed root is a male aphrodisiac and for high blood pressure (hypertension).

The European experience is interesting since it encompasses both stimulant and sedative roles for hogweed. The inference is that it works at neurological level, depending on dose and patient constitution, as an amphoteric, ie capable of opposite actions, or normalising function.

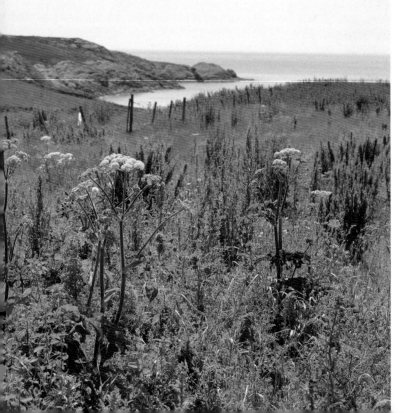

Hogweed above the cliffs, Anglesey, June

Contemporary American herbalist Matthew Wood draws attention (in discussing cow parsnip) to the work of the late William LeSassier, who found that chewing some seeds of *Heracleum* was 'revelatory', heightened sensitivity and conferred psychic benefits. We found the green seeds of hogweed to have a similar effect. This area suggests a line of further research, as do the older traditional uses.

Modern research

Research in 2008 identified novel uses for the Heracleum genus as an anti-asthmatic, and for memory and 'alertness-improving' effects.

Hogweed was used (2013) in tests of rat thoracic aorta to produce the first evidence for its vasorelaxant properties, supporting traditional anti-hypertensive therapies. Octyl butyrate, a component of the essential oil of hogweed, was shown (2014) to be cytotoxic to certain human melanoma and carcinoma cells.

Webster et al (2010) isolated anti-mycobacterial constituents in cow parsnip root, including several furanocoumarins, supporting former use for treating infectious diseases, specifically tuberculosis.

In addition to anti-fungal and anti-mycobacterial properties, the root of cow parsnip (2006) demonstrated antiviral actions, by means of immunostimulation.

This study demonstrates that aqueous extracts of the roots of H. maximum [cow parsnip] … possess strong in vitro antimycobacterial activity, validates traditional knowledge, and provides potential for the development of urgently needed novel antituberculous therapeutics.
– Webster et al (2010)

Harvesting hogweed

Hogweed provides several harvests through the year. The young **leaf shoots** are picked in the spring, and have a pleasant taste. Our favourite wild vegetable is the **flower buds**, picked while they are plump but still encased by the leaf base, making a neat little packet for steaming. The **seeds** can be nibbled green, when they have a strong smell of mandarin orange, or gathered when they mature and turn brown, then having a more complex spicy citrus flavour. **Roots** are best harvested from young plants in the autumn or the following spring.

[Hogweed shoots are] … unequivocally one of the best vegetables I have eaten.
– Phillips (1983)

Hogweed flower buds

Lightly steam **hogweed flower buds**, then fry them gently with **butter** and **garlic**.

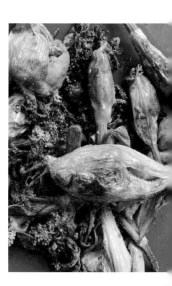

Well-being tea

Per cup of boiling water, use a teaspoon of **green hogweed seed** and a couple of leaves of **ground ivy**. Cover and leave to infuse for 10 or 15 minutes, then strain and drink.

We find this tea clears the head and relaxes the body. It makes a good evening tea.

Lesser celandine *Ranunculus ficaria* syn. *Ficaria verna*

Once you identify lesser celandine correctly (it's not greater celandine and not figwort), you have an effective, old but also modern remedy for the painful condition of haemorrhoids. External use of the plant is safe, but it is potentially toxic if taken internally – not that this discourages braver foragers, who appreciate the young leaves.

Ranunculaceae Buttercup family

Description: To 30cm (12in) tall, with rosettes of long-stalked, glossy and heart-shaped leaves, usually with paler inner markings; bright star-like yellow petals, 7–12, often 8 in number, with three green sepals; both fibrous and whitish tuberous roots.

Habitat: Damp woodland, waysides, gardens; invasive, often forms massed colonies.

Distribution: Abundant in Great Britain, except for north Scotland and parts of Ireland; throughout Europe, temperate Asia; introduced to North America.

Related species: Several subspecies, some of which spread by seed and others by bulbils; these subspecies can be used interchangeably for medicine.

Parts used: Whole plant, especially the tubers.

One of the earliest spring plants is the lesser celandine. It has such a pleasing combination of stars and hearts: the flowers are star-like, golden, almost shiny-enamelled; and the leaves are glossy green, heart-shaped, low to the ground.

By looks it should be, and is, of the buttercup (Ranunculus) family, but it is the only species of 600 or so with a safe external herbal use. In general, buttercups are acrid and toxic, causing blistering of the mouth and gastro-intestinal tract in cattle and humans alike, and are best avoided.

In Britain lesser celandine grows in colonies, forming swathes of yellow in damp woodland, by ditches and in gardens from February to May. Coming from winter gloom, you need all the light you can get, and this plant is a pleasure to behold.

In some areas of the northern USA and Canada, though, the proliferation of introduced lesser celandine is an alien invasion, swamping native plants like trilliums. It holds its own against ground elder in our own garden!

Poets and novelists have been engaged, entranced by this early brightness. Wordsworth preferred it even to his beloved daffodils. It was a shame, then, that Wordsworth's memorial in Grasmere has the wrong celandine, the sculptor repeating a common confusion with the unrelated greater celandine, but this time permanently in stone.

DH Lawrence had his character Paul Morrel in *Sons and Lovers* describe lesser celandine as *scalloped splashes of gold, on the side of the ditch*. Like Wordsworth, Lawrence enjoyed the way the flowers open and close with light, and *press themselves against the sun*.

Anonymous country-dwellers also joined in the fun: among names recorded for it are butterchops, crazy bet, cups, gentleman's cap and frills, golden guineas, spring messenger and starlight.

But all this spring profusion relies on what is underground, a root system that has fibrous roots and attached small tubers – *a broom handle festooned with potatoes*, as one modern writer calls it.

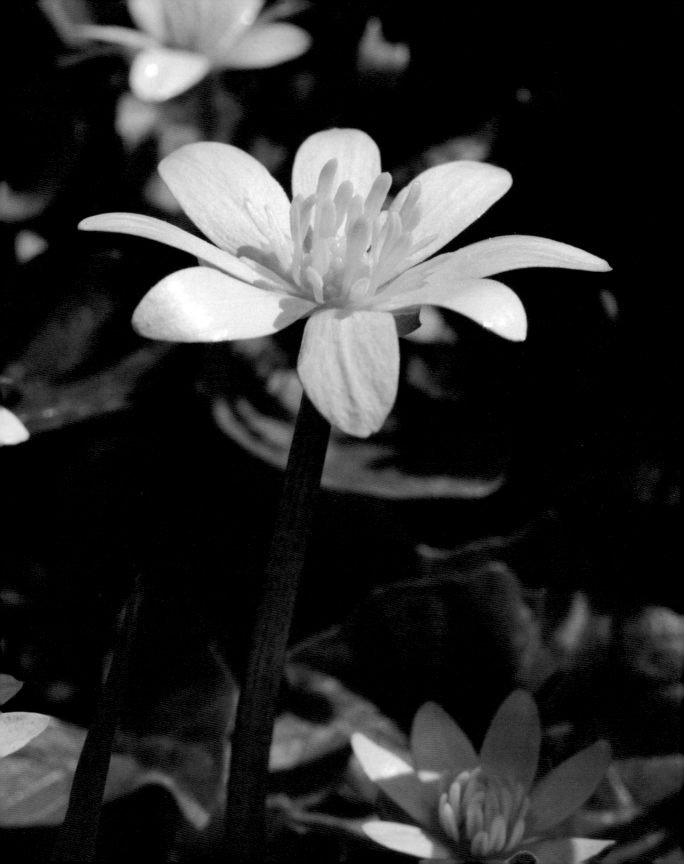

Each tuber is a storehouse from which a new plant emerges, and the tubers are the medicinal part, gathered in spring or autumn.

These white tubers were the 'figs' that gave rise to the plant's generic name *Ficaria*; another old European name, again confusingly, is figwort (the true figwort is *Scrophularia nodosa*). In the USA lesser celandine is also called a fig buttercup.

At one time, notably in Germany, the earliest-appearing leaves of lesser celandine were collected, as a remedy for scurvy. They do contain high levels of vitamin C, but also become toxic as the season progresses, owing to rising amounts of protoanemonin.

On the other hand, some contemporary foragers regard the leaves as safe and, with cautions, recommend them in stir fries and, in small amounts, in wild salads. The cooked tubers resemble potatoes in taste; these are recorded as a survival food in parts of Scotland.

But everyone knows the tubers for another reason. They are also termed 'piles' for their resemblance to haemorrhoids, and the plant is still called pilewort.

Haemorrhoids are a painful condition of dilated veins and swollen, protruding tissue at the anus. The piles can be internal or external. The condition often occurs in pregnancy or after childbirth.

Lesser celandine is an effective treatment, with its saponins soothing the inflamed tissue and its tannins toning the veins. A decoction is made into an ointment or a hot compress.

Nicholas Culpeper, in 1653, went further: it worked *by only carrying it about one, (but if he wil not, bruise it and apply it to the grief).* In other words, merely carrying the plant in some form would do, but if needed, apply it to the piles.

The medicine was and remains effective, but was it found by trial and error or by 'design', in that the plant's appearance gave a clue, a 'signature' for its ordained human purpose? Was lesser celandine a confirmation of the now long-discredited doctrine of signatures?

The modern consensus is that effect probably preceded cause; in the words of one commentary, *As in other cases, however, this may well be merely a post-hoc rationalisation.* Parkinson (1640) agrees that usage came first: *it is certaine by good experience.* The salient fact is that lesser celandine genuinely works in treating haemorrhoids.

It was also used to treat scrofula, or King's evil, a tubercular complaint of swollen glands in the neck, and for lumps and corns (the true figwort has similar uses).

… doth wonderfully help the piles or hemorrhoides, as also kernels by the eares and throate, called the Kings Evill, or any other hard wennes or tumors.
– Parkinson (1640)

Outwardly applied, 'tis a Specifick for Execrescencies in the Fundament and is much commended.
– Pechey (1707)

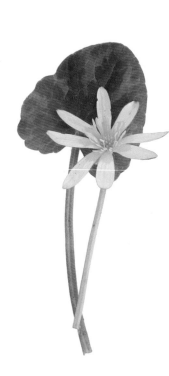

Modern research

There are no contra-indications for external use of lesser celandine, though a case report (2015) found that a 36-year-old woman suffered acute hepatitis after 'consuming' lesser celandine for haemorrhoids. Other factors such as alcohol or drug over-use were eliminated in this case. However, it seems she had been taking the plant internally as a tea, which is not a typical modern treatment regime for the plant.

Other haemorrhoid herbs

Anti-inflammatory (demulcent) and astringent (tannin-rich) herbs can be used in addition to or to replace lesser celandine in piles treatment. Rose family astringents, eg avens and agrimony, have been found effective, as are marigold, witch hazel (*Hamamelis virginiana*), horse chestnut or oak, in ointment or distilled water form.

Note that these are *topical* piles treatments. The *cause* of the piles, probably poor digestion and constipation, or liver dysfunction, should be addressed simultaneously; fibre, say, should be introduced to the diet gradually.

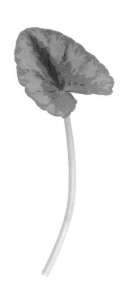

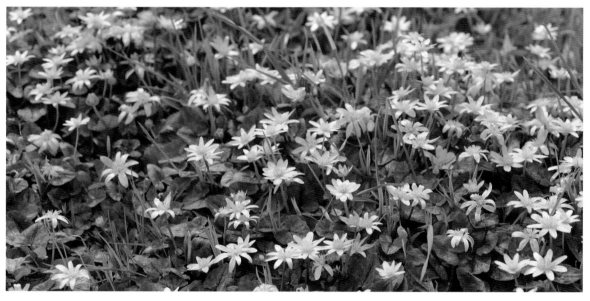

Lesser celandine ointment

Gather lesser celandine in early spring when they are in flower. If you are weeding them out of your garden, dig up the whole plant including the small tubers, but if you are harvesting wild plants you can just use the leaves and flowers.

Lesser celandine ointment
• haemorrhoids
• varicose veins

Cover the **lesser celandine** with **olive oil** in a saucepan. Simmer gently for about 20 minutes, then strain out the plant material and return the oil to the pan after measuring it. For every 100ml of oil, add 10g **beeswax** or 5g candelilla wax. Stir on low heat until the wax has melted. Pour into jars and leave to set before putting lids on and labelling.

Mouse-ear hawkweed *Pilosella officinarum*

**Asteraceae
Daisy family**

Description: Low-growing perennial, to 30cm (12in); *for detailed description, see adjacent text*.

Habitat: Drier short grassland and rough meadows, also rocky areas, sand dunes.

Distribution: Native to Europe and Western Asia; naturalised in USA and Canada, but an alien in some states and provinces; a notifiable noxious weed in Australia and New Zealand.

Related species: Other Pilosellas include shaggy mouse-ear hawkweed (*Pilosella peleteriana*); tall mouse-ear hawkweed (*P. praealta*); fox and cubs (*P. aurantiaca*); yellow fox and cubs (*P. caespitosa*). Each of these have subspecies, and hybridisation is frequent.

Parts used: Above-ground parts, as tea, tincture, juice, distillation.

Mouse-ear hawkweed is a useful but neglected herb, with specific actions for treating whooping cough and brucellosis. As these painful conditions have declined in the West, so has its own reputation. But it retains powerful antibiotic properties for home treatment of coughs, colds, bleeding, diarrhoea and fevers.

In early summer the bright yellow single flowerheads of the diminutive mouse-ear hawkweed twinkling by a ditch or on rocky soil are a pleasure to the eye, with forgotten medicinal benefits.

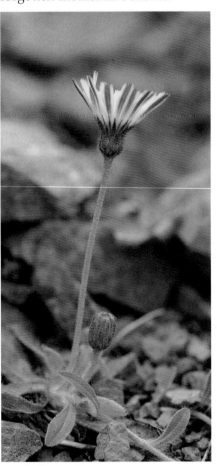

Sir John Hill in 1812 praised mouse-ear hawkweed as *an exceedingly pretty plant* [with] *scarce any smell but an austere bitterish taste.* He was outdone by Leo Hartley Grindon in 1859 (right).

Botanically, mouse-ear hawkweed occupies its own genus, the Pilosella, classified between the hawk's beards (Crepis) and the hawkweeds (Hieracium) of the Aster tribe. Until recently, it was called a Hieracium, specifically *Hieracium pilosella*.

It can all get very baffling, but the plant itself, fortunately, has clear distinguishing marks.

William Curtis's idealised portrait of the plant opposite shows the characteristic creeping stolons or runners, the cropped layers of sulphur-yellow florets on a single longish stem, the paddle-shaped and hairy 'mouse' ears in rosette leaves (green above and whitish below), and the alternating orange-red stripes under the calyx, like a medieval jousting tent.

The under-surface redness is an interesting feature of mouse-ear hawkweed, with its closest Pilosella relative being the russet-flowered fox and cubs (*P. aurantiaca*). There are other Pilosellas, listed left, plus various hybrids, which share medicinal properties with it.

It is worth clarifying that the plants known as *mouse-ears*, aka mouse-ear chickweeds, are unrelated members of the Cerastium genus, in the pinks or Caryophyllaceae family. We use the full English name mouse-ear hawkweed to avoid confusion.

We won't go into the further historical complications of the plants named *Myosotis* (Latin for mouse ear), which became the forget-me-nots (now in the Borage family) – John Parkinson in 1640 classified the blue forget-me-not alongside mouse-ear hawkweed as *Myosotis scorpioides repens*, the 'small creeping blew Mouseare'.

Use mouse-ear hawkweed for …
Mouse-ear hawkweed has a long history in treating respiratory disorders by soothing coughs, colds, asthma and bronchitis.

It is a herbal specific for whooping cough, a highly infectious disease generally treated by vaccination in developed countries. Epidemics still occur, and treatment is long and not always successful.

Mouse-ear hawkweed can be used alone in herbal whooping cough treatment or combined with other

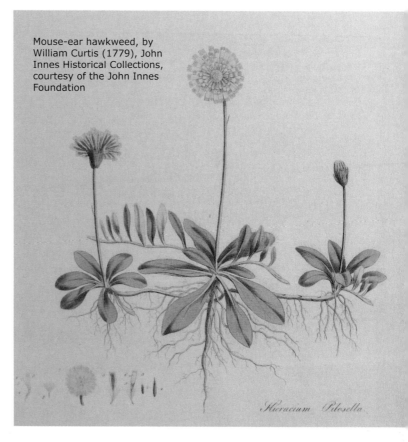

Mouse-ear hawkweed, by William Curtis (1779), John Innes Historical Collections, courtesy of the John Innes Foundation

recognised 'antitussives' such as mullein and coltsfoot.

The *British Herbal Pharmacopoeia* of 1983 gave a whooping cough mixture using mouse-ear hawkweed, white horehound, mullein and coltsfoot, although this recommendation had been dropped by the 1996 edition.

Mouse-ear hawkweed can be called a stimulating expectorant, which works by loosening stubborn phlegm and helps in ejecting it by increased salivation. It is also astringent and partly diuretic, which explains its action

It has been received into the [apothecary] shops under the name of Auricula muris, *and considered as possessing an astringent quality; but at present, in this respect, is but little regarded.*
– Curtis (1779)

[It grows in] *dry hedgebanks, delighting in the most sunny and drouthy conditions, where it can bask in the noontide ray … [the blossoms] in favourable seasons, and when in perfection, have the smell of raspberry jam.*
– Grindon (1859)

in toning inflamed muscle and in treating diarrhoea.

It was once a familiar wound herb, with its astringency also found useful in treating excessive menstruation or haemorrhaging. It was recommended for nosebleeds and piles, an action supported by its known antibiotic qualities.

Mouse-ear hawkweed is regarded as specific for treating brucellosis, a bacterial infection caught by people from infected livestock or milk. This presents as intermittent (sometimes called undulant or Malta) fever, which has been largely controlled worldwide.

Medicinally, the bitterish stem sap is swallowed or the plant boiled

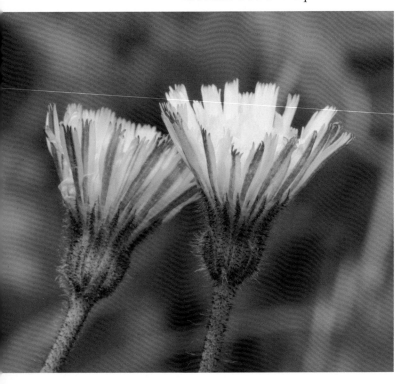

fresh as a decoction. A distilled water can be made, for either drinking or external application – used, as Pechey wrote, for *wound-drinks, Plaisters and Ointments*. Hill suggested boiling the leaves in milk for external use.

Some herbalists believe the fresh herb is more effective than the dried. Indeed, Julian Barker (2001) suggests a reason for the plant's fluctuating reception over time is the weak action of the dried form.

At one time mouse-ear hawkweed had a reputation for improving the eyesight, but this was based on a persistent belief that hawks (Greek *Hierax*, which gave the name Hieracium) would swallow the bitter sap to sharpen their own keen vision. Falconers were also said to feed their birds a tea made from mouse-ear hawkweed.

While a benign plant in its native Europe, mouse-ear hawkweed is condemned as an alien weed in some states and provinces of the USA and Canada, New Zealand, Australia and Japan. It can form impenetrable mats that crowd out native grasses grazed by stock. New South Wales's government, for example, classifies all hawkweeds as class 1 noxious weeds, which citizens must report for eradication; Hawkweed Alert is the online interactive program.

Modern research
A European Union herbal monograph on mouse-ear

hawkweed (2015) limits itself (citing lack of data) to use of tea or powder for urinary tract disorders.

Polish research meanwhile (2011) has identified a new isoetin derivative, a flavone, that was a strong antimicrobial, which reduced colon carcinoma cell line proliferation.

The Haudenosaunee people of New York state (2010 research) use yarrow and mouse-ear hawkweed, among other plants, as antimicrobials for treating diarrhoeal and stomach ailments, notably for forms of salmonella poisoning.

Serbian research (eg 2009), has confirmed mouse-ear hawkweed is high in umbelliferone, an antibiotic coumarin responsible for the anti-brucellosis action of the plant. Umbelliferone absorbs UV light, and has an application in sunscreen products.

Mouse-ear hawkweed relaxes the muscles of the bronchial tubes, stimulates the cough reflex and reduces the production of catarrh. This combination of actions makes the herb effective against all manner of respiratory problems, including asthma and wheeziness, whooping cough, bronchitis and other chronic and congested coughs.
– Chevallier (2016)

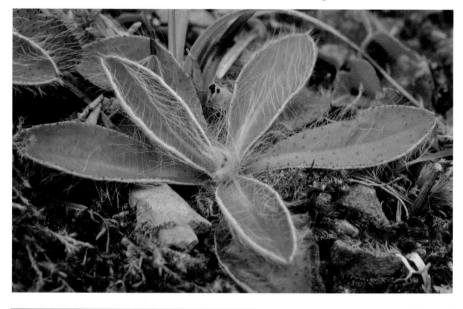

Identifying mouse-ear hawkweed: left, basal rosette; opposite, close-up of flowers

---

Syrup of mouse-ear hawkweed

Harvest when **mouse-ear hawkweed** is in flower. Put your pickings in a pan, cover with **water** and boil. Simmer gently for a few minutes, remove from heat. Cover pan, and leave overnight to infuse.

Strain off the liquid and pour into a clean pan. Add 200g sugar for every 250ml of liquid. Bring to the boil, stirring until sugar dissolves. Warm receiving bottles, pour syrup in, add cap and label.

Dosage: 1 teaspoonful 3, 4 or more times a day, according to need.

Syrup of mouse-ear hawkweed
• specific for whooping cough
• catarrh
• congested cough
• disorders of urinary tract

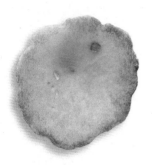

Navelwort *Umbilicus rupestris*

Navelwort is a common and attractive, almost alien-looking presence in shady West Country lanes and woodland edges, but its medicinal properties, as reflected in its various 'wort' names and ability to cool inflammation, are unduly overlooked.

A member of the stonecrop family of British succulents, navelwort or wall pennywort is a distinctive plant growing in colonies on sheltered walls, hedgebanks and tree roots, mainly in the west of the British Isles.

On paper at least, it might be confused with several other navelworts in unrelated families: blue-eyed mary or navelwort (*Omphalodes verna*) is a garden plant of the borage family; the marsh pennywort (*Hydrocotyle vulgaris*) of the pennywort family grows in wetlands and has pink flowers; and gotu kola (*Centella asiatica*), also called the Asiatic pennywort and Indian water navelwort, is an important Ayurvedic herb.

The English names of navelwort suggest an enduring popular esteem: a plant does not earn 'wort' status without proving itself medicinally (or for brewing). It has been known as navelwort since medieval times for the way its central dimple in the leaf resembles a belly button (it is named *umbilicus* in Latin). Another 'wort' name hinting at function,

current in both John Parkinson (1640) and Maud Grieve (1931), was kidneywort.

The name pennywort is a reference to the greenish-grey of the fleshy, round leaves, which look like an old silver penny; it has also been called moneypenny, penny cake, penny leaves and similar coin-related names.

Other common names hint at its herbal uses or virtues: it was cut-finger (wound-healing), corn leaves (applied to corns or warts) and coolers (probably for its value in relieving the pain of burns).

In classical terms, navelwort was *Umbilicus veneris*, the navel of Venus, to the Romans, and still to Parkinson. The name was not, however, matched by an equivalent aphrodisiac reputation, despite efforts by William Coles, in *The Art of Simpling* (1656).

If its names have been colourful and expressive, navelwort's distribution has been surprisingly stable, in always having a western bias in the British Isles. It was probably more widespread in

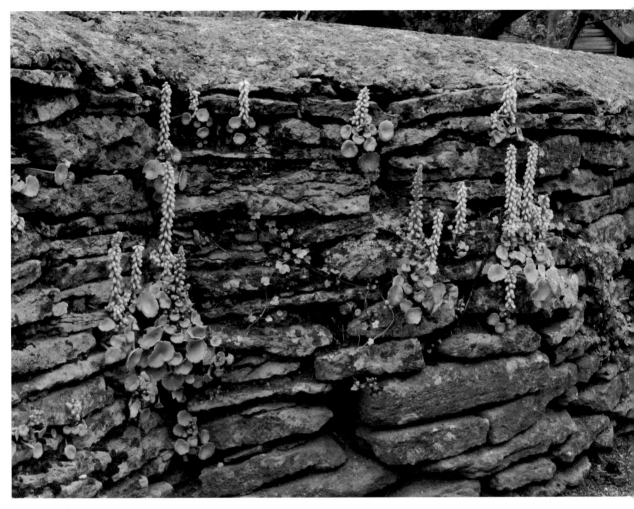

pre-industrial times – Parkinson said 'it groweth very plentifully in many places of this kingdome'.

As if to hint at the plant's gradually reduced distribution, the first edition of Gerard's *Herball* (1597) describes a navelwort plant growing on stonework in Westminster Abbey near to Chaucer's grave. The second edition, by Thomas Johnson (1633), omits this reference, no doubt because the plant had gone.

Use navelwort for …

Navelwort was once accepted in 'official' medicine: in Culpeper's English version (1653) of the *Pharmacopoeia Londinensis*, the reference book for physicians and apothecaries, it was recommended for 'kib'd heels [kibes were ulcerated chilblains], being bathed in it, and a leaf laid over the sore'.

It had been excluded from similar lists by the nineteenth century. Nonetheless it was once a

Navelwort on a wall in Gloucestershire, June

significant herbal presence, and it could be turned to much more by today's herbalists and first aiders.

It is the leaves that are used, for their watery, cooling sap – it is a close relative of the houseleek (*Sempervivum tectorum*), sometimes called the English *Aloe vera*, which has similar soothing uses.

The herbalist Julian Barker describes pulping navelwort leaves with a rolling pin and applying the mash to tired or sore eyes, to piles and chilblains. Using a compress or poultice will prolong the contact time.

Parkinson provides the most complete herbal perspective. The leaves, either in extracted juice or distilled water form, he

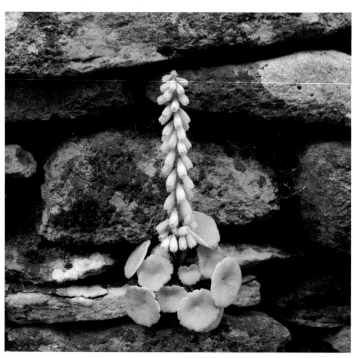

tells us, are 'very effectuall for all inflammations and unnatural heates'. He describes some of these: inwardly for 'a fainting hot stomacke' or hot liver, the bowels or womb; and outwardly, for pimples, redness, St Anthony's fire (the skin condition erysipelas), and for sore kidneys.

Navelwort leaves are also used to break stones in the kidney and liver, he says, to relieve 'wringing paines of the bowels and the bloody flux [dysentery]', and are 'singular good for the painefull piles or hemorroidall veines'.

Parkinson recommends an ointment, either of navelwort leaves alone or mixed with myrrh, for easing painful 'hot goute, the Sciatica and the inflammations and swellings of the cods [testicles]'. The plant is partly diuretic, and could relieve 'dropsie' (water retention or oedema), and would reduce 'the Kernells or knots of the neck and throate called the Kings Evill' (scrofula).

Navelwort was good for emergencies with 'greene' (fresh) wounds and burns: the skin of the leaves was removed, he said, and the juice or an ointment from it rubbed on the wound. The skin itself made a ready plaster for a splinter, and when left in place for a day or two would draw it out.

Parkinson does not advise the use of navelwort to treat epilepsy, which Mrs Grieve reported as an 'old reputation'; she said the practice was revived in the 19th century but added that the plant had no permanent reputation as an epilepsy remedy. The last reference to navelwort being considered for petit mal concerned flower essence developer Dr Edward Bach, who from 1930 to 1932 experimented with it as a flower remedy, but dropped it.

Navelwort leaves are edible, though John Pechey in 1707 was unenthusiastic: *The Leaves are fat, thick and round, and full of Juice, and taste clammy.* Contemporary foragers have proposed them for salads, stir fries and sandwiches.

Modern research
A 2012 ethnobotanical study found *Umbilicus rupestris* being used by a diaspora Slavic community in south-central Italy. They crushed the leaves, mixed in pork fat and soot, and put them on furuncles (infected hair follicles).

Showing there is nothing new under the sun, this is very close to a recipe in the Anglo Saxon *Old English Herbarium*, dating to about the year 1000, for *Cotyledon umbilicus*, the same plant. In this recipe equal quantities of the plant and pig's grease (the recipe specified using 'unsalted' grease for women) were pounded together and placed on a swelling, which would soon disappear.

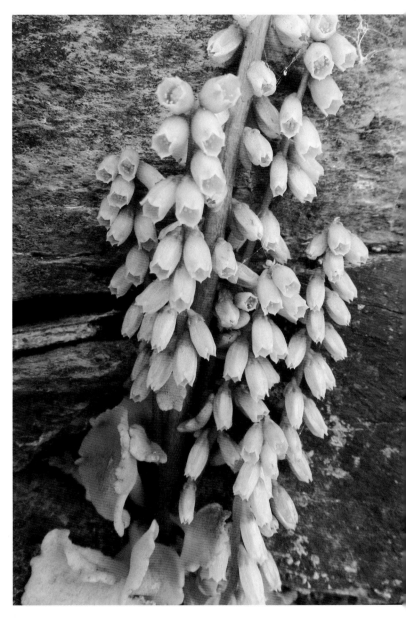

Fresh poultice
Use the fresh leaf as a poultice for burns and minor injuries as well as placing on hot swellings such as boils. Simply split the leaf and apply the wet side to the skin, or crush and apply, holding in place with a sticking plaster.

Fresh poultice
- burns
- boils
- haemorrhoids
- splinters
- cuts
- pimples

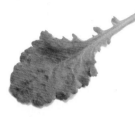

Ox-eye daisy *Leucanthemum vulgare*

**Asteraceae
Daisy family**

Description: A bright, sprawling meadow perennial of high summer, whose flowers consist of a large golden central disk, surrounded by numerous long white ray petals. Flowers borne on open, branching stems to 1m (3ft) high, flopping over as they age; short, stubby dark green leaves; roots shallow.

Habitat: Grassland, gardens, road verges, waysides, especially on rich soils.

Distribution: Across whole of British Isles but less common in Scottish Highlands; native in Europe, Middle East, north Africa; introduced to North America, Australasia.

Related species: A medium size between the much smaller native common daisy (*Bellis perennis*) and the larger Shasta daisy (*Leucanthemum* x *superbum*), sometimes a garden escape.

Parts used: Leaves, flowers.

Ox-eye daisy is a larger relative of the humble common daisy, and shares many of its medicinal virtues. In both cases modern herbalism has overlooked what these plants can offer, and the time might be right for a reconsideration.

The name 'daisy' derives from the Anglo-Saxon 'day's eye', from the way the flowers open up as the sun rises. Unlike the familiar common or lawn daisy, ox-eye daisy, its larger relative, stays open at night too, being almost luminescent in moonlight, and much the brightest plant presence on summer evenings.

This was noticed long ago – one of ox-eye's old names is moonflower. So here is a plant of both sun and moon, as its flowers symbolically indicate. The original scientific name given by Linnaeus in 1753, *Chrysanthemum leucanthemum*, ie 'gold flower, white flower', perfectly and euphoniously captured the plant's duality.

What a pity, then, that the current name, corrected in the 1990s, in Latin means only 'common white flower' – though in referencing ox-eye's abundance science is reflecting the problems ox-eye is posing for farmers, as we will see.

It is indicative of popular affection for a plant when it has a variety of common names, indicating local variations in appearance or use over time. Geoffrey Grigson's wonderful *The Englishman's Flora* (1958) certainly gives a long list for ox-eye daisy.

Among the regional names he notes are billy button, butter daisy, cow's eyes, devil's daisy, dog daisy, dundle daisy, fair maids of France, gools, grandmothers, horse blob, horse daisy, maudlin, midsummer daisy, mother daisy, open star, povertyweed, rising sun and white gowlan.

Another name for ox-eye is marguerite, long a familiar garden flower. It is said to be named for Margaret of Anjou, the French wife of King Henry VI. Strictly, though, marguerite is the large white daisy from the Canary Islands, *Argyranthemum frutescens*.

Its popular names do carry hints of a shadow side to ox-eye, as in 'devil's daisy'. What can be welcome in the garden might be anathema to the farmer.

Ox-eye growing unchallenged in a field could indicate that the land was being neglected, and in England Henry VI introduced

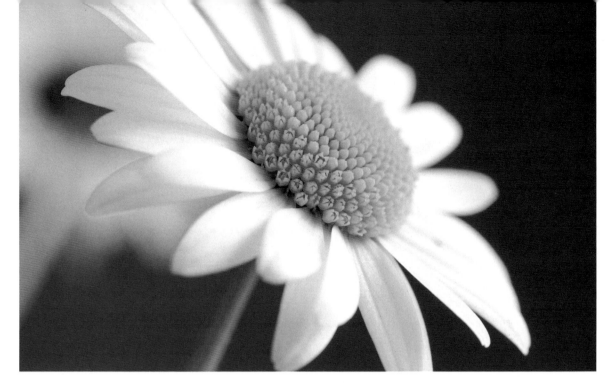

punishments for aberrant farmers. In medieval Scotland the presence of 'gools' in grassland led to fines of one wether [castrated] sheep.

In modern Australia there are records of their ox-eye daisies causing contact dermatitis in some people, and you find similar warnings in websites from the American West. Indeed, this beloved wild and garden flower in Europe is seen as a destructive alien weed in hotter, drier climates (purple loosestrife and St John's wort are among other examples).

What happens is that the plant's own protective mechanisms are exacerbated in more extreme conditions. Ox-eye stems develop a bitter, acrid juice that makes the plants unpalatable to grazing cows and pigs, as well as insects and most human foragers.

A close relative of the ox-eye is *Chrysanthemum cinerariifolium* – quite a mouthful in Latin, but better known in English as pyrethrum, the most effective natural insecticide – and ox-eye shares some of its qualities.

The website for Colorado State University highlights that ox-eye has no natural biological controls, that cows won't eat it and insects keep away from it. This leads to ox-eye pushing out other plants that stock animals prefer to eat.

In hot, dry conditions it only takes five days for the plant to set viable seed, which can lie dormant in the ground for some years. The plant has a shallow root system, as European gardeners know, but once the seeds are in the ground, it will come back again and again, no matter how often it is uprooted.

The characteristic disc (yellow) and ray florets (white) of ox-eye daisy

Flowers [of the Greater Wild White Daisie] *cast forth Beams of Brightness.*
– Pechey (1707)

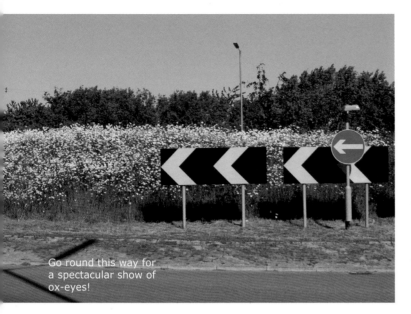
Go round this way for a spectacular show of ox-eyes!

Externally, ox-eye tea has an ancient reputation in lotion or compress form to relieve wounds and bruises; in Ireland it was used to bathe sore eyes. In these conditions its medicinal range is similar to that of chamomile, another distant relative.

Salmon (1710) advocates ox-eye distilled water for ruptures of the bowels and as a vehicle for other medicines. Likewise he maintains that its liquid juice heals any inward wound, spitting of blood and ruptures: take with *a glass of old Malaga or Red Port Wine.*

It consolidates and conglutinates the Lips of Wounds to a Miracle. – Salmon (1710)

The fresh leaves chewed, have a sweetish, but unpleasant and slightly aromatic taste, somewhat like parsley, but not hot or biting; they have been recommended in disorders of the breast, both asthmatic and phthisical, and as diuretics, but are now seldom called for. – Green (1820)

Use ox-eye daisy for...

Records of modern herbal use are sparse, which can lead to both 'bioprospecting' of older texts and also practical experimentation at a time when the plant is spreading. A herb does not lose medicinal power when it goes out of fashion – it is still there, particularly in wild strains, and available to try out for yourself.

The herbals suggest that ox-eye has a history as an antispasmodic, especially for whooping cough and asthma. It is tonic and sweat-inducing, the boiled root being effective in reducing night sweats.

The flowers made into an infusion are recorded as helping relieve chronic coughs and bronchial distress. Sir John Hill's *Family Herbal* of 1812 mentions that the 'great daisy' is 'balsamic and strengthening' for the lungs.

We found making an ox-eye flower essence to be wonderful. One recent year, early June marked Julie's birthday, a full moon and a lunar eclipse all at the same time. Julie began her moon essence at sunset, around 9 pm, and left it overnight from moonrise to moonset. Then on the summer solstice she made an all-day ox-eye sun essence. Both were profound in their effect, but markedly differing: the moon essence was predictably cooling and calming, the sun essence warming and stimulating.

Modern research

Research has been sparse and focused on the plant's physiology, speciation and cases of contact dermatitis, but a 2015 report found the plant had potential in crude oil phytoremediation, surviving exposure to the oil and enhancing reduction of crude oil in soil.

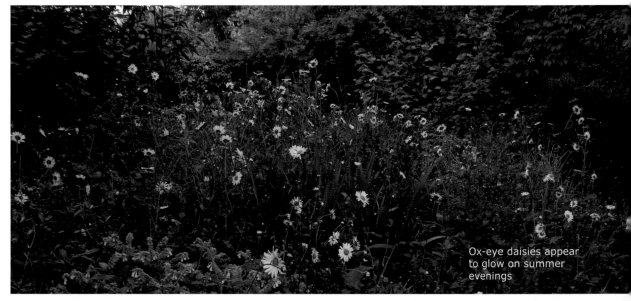

Ox-eye daisies appear to glow on summer evenings

Ox-eye daisy oil

Pick **ox-eye daisies** on a dry day. Spread out on a cloth or some paper and allow them to dry for a day or two, then fill a jar with them. Pour in **extra virgin olive oil** to fill the jar, stirring to release any air bubbles. Cover the jar with a piece of cloth or gauze held in place with a rubber band or string. This allows any moisture to escape. Leave in a warm sunny place for a few weeks.

Strain off the oil, which will have a peculiar daisy smell, into a bottle and label. You can add a few drops of essential oil to perfume the oil if you wish – choose oils that enhance the therapeutic use of the oil, such as eucalyptus, lavender or chamomile. Use as a chest rub for stubborn coughs, or on muscles for bruising or aches and pains.

Ox-eye daisy oil
- chest rub
- difficult coughs
- bruises
- aching muscles

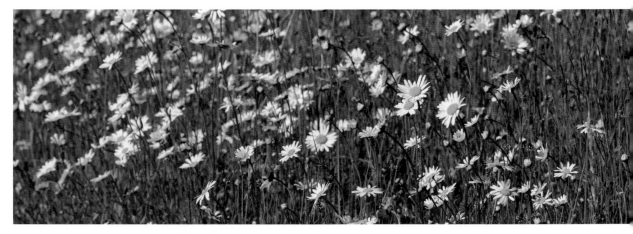

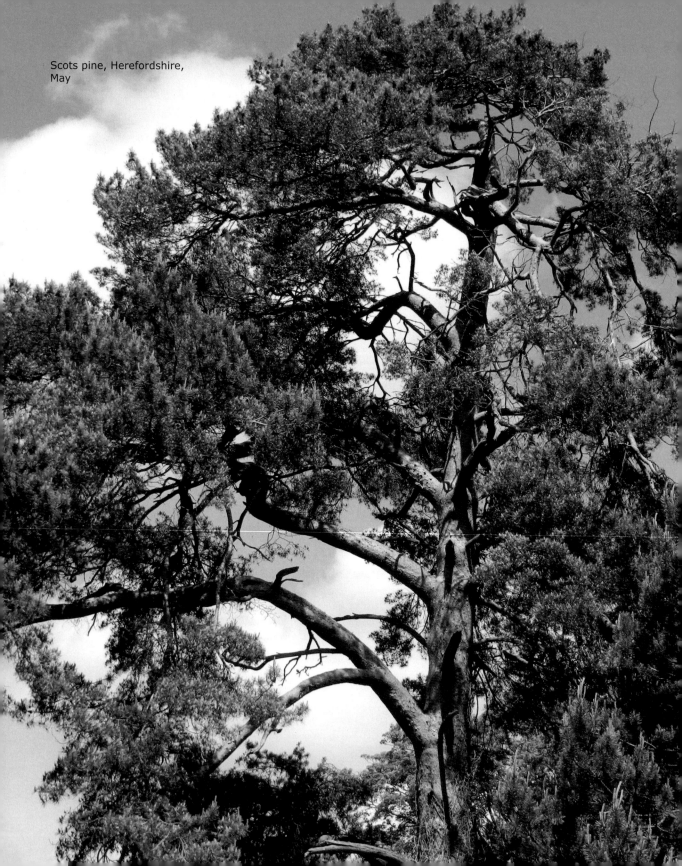

Scots pine, Herefordshire,
May

Pine *Pinus* spp.

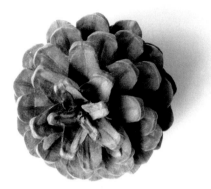

Pine has multiple human uses, providing pitch, tar, timber, kernels, sap and resin. It is a specific for respiratory issues, a disinfectant and antiviral.

Scots pine, also known as Scotch pine (or fir), is a conifer (cone-bearing) evergreen tree that has similar uses to other pines, but is one of only three British native conifers, with juniper and yew.

Pine has multiple uses, much like the date palm or coconut in their own cultures. It was prized first as a timber, for ships' masts, pit props, telephone poles and railway sleepers; in the First World War pine forests were felled for ammunition boxes and trenching.

The tree itself gives tar and turpentine, used in paints and varnishes, and a volatile oil for cosmetics and perfumes. Pine resin went into glues used in boat-building and for sealing wax and, when ground into powder, as rosin for violin bows.

Pine pitch was the oil of pine, widely used as an antiseptic and a preservative: amber, or fossilised pine resin, preserves insects from as long ago as 125 million years. In Traditional Chinese Medicine amber is called *hu po*, and was once used in urinary tract infection and for stones.

Although native Scots pine disappeared from most of Britain some 5,000 years ago through climatic warming, stumps and branches were preserved in many peat bogs. These pine remnants were resinous and provided free fuel and (unreliable) lighting until the early 19th century when oil lamps became popular.

Pine sap produces a potent wine; the roots could be used for ropes, and the cones give a brown dye. The 16th-century herbalist Pietro Andrea Matthiolus noted that distilled green 'apples' (cones) yielded a face wash much used to remove wrinkles.

At about the same time as Matthiolus, the first Spanish travellers to North America saw that inner bark of pine was a survival food of the native Americans; Linnaeus also describes it, mixed with flour, for a similar purpose in the Sweden of his time (mid-18th century).

More palatable of course are the silky-smooth pine kernels, which have long been a basis of Mediterranean food, including

Pinaceae
Pine family

Description: (Scots pine) height varies with soil, wind and other conditions, from dwarf to 30m and more (100ft); takes irregular pyramidal shapes, often with broken branches; fissured red-brown bark near the crown, greyer below; thin needles in pairs, grey-green; buds sticky with resin; male flowers yellow, female pink; cones green, grey-brown to brown.

Habitat: Scots pine are native only in small areas of the Caledonian Forest, but much planted in woods, heaths, shingle throughout Britain.

Distribution: The family is largely forest trees of the cool/cold temperate north; Scots pine is native to northern Europe; in North America by 1600.

Related species: The conifers include firs, spruces, larches and cedars as well as pines; the only other British native conifers are the threatened juniper (*Juniperus communis*) and yew (*Taxus baccata*). Some 100 pine species worldwide have similar uses.

Parts used: Bark, needles, resin, distilled water, tar.

in Pharaonic Egypt. Parkinson in 1629 noted their various use by *Apothecaries, Comfit-makers, and Cookes*. He said medicines made from pine kernels were *good to lenifie* [soothe] *the pipes and passages of the lungs and throat, when it is hoarse.*

Parkinson added the 17th-century truism that pine kernels *stir up bodily lust and encrease sperme*. We offer a recipe mixing pine nuts into an electuary with liquorice and cardamom to test his words.

That pine kernels are reputed to be aphrodisiac seems appropriate for a tree once sacred to Artemis, the moon goddess who presided over childbirth. The pine cone was a symbol of virility. This isn't all myth: our culture still chooses pine trees for Christmas celebrations and the yule log.

The scent of pine is distinctive – refreshing, clean, masculine (or so the advertisers want us to believe). It has been thought therapeutic in itself, and this belief underlay the siting of tuberculosis sanitaria within the pine woods of the Swiss Alps in the 20th century.

The scent is disinfectant, as we all know from commercial air fresheners that use pine scent. But this isn't new: Parkinson in 1640 wrote of *our ordinary Francumsence* [pine resin] *that is usually burned in houses and chambers, to aire and perfume them.*

Pine steam inhalations are a specific treatment for respiratory problems, using the bark or essential oil, along with drinking pine needle tea. Pine essential oil can be added to hot baths. Herbalist Peter Conway recommends 10 drops of pine oil with 5 ml of almond oil (carrier) poured into a hot bath as it fills; he says it is *wonderfully penetrating and relaxing, helping to release muscular tension.*

The famous Vicks Vaporub was originally made from cedarleaf and turpentine oils, among other ingredients. Patented in the US in 1894, it is now called Vicks and manufactured from petroleum-based products. It is well known for easing bronchial congestion, but any form of pine rub or massage oil will actually have similar value.

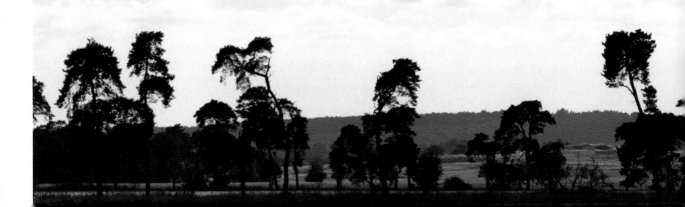

The sound of pines, as the wind eases through their tops, is comforting. The lovely old words soughing and susurrating are onomatopoeic efforts to capture this quality, while Keats said *pines shall murmur in the wind*.

So, pine is a tree that both smells and sounds special. It was also planted in special places – British examples include on warrior graves in Scotland, as landmarks along old droving routes and along beaches, and to form a row of windbreaks in the Norfolk and Suffolk flatlands.

All the same, as writer Charlotte du Cann argues, most conifers in Britain *stand unrespected in suburban parks and plantations*, whereas in America, in *a citadel of conifers*, in her words, the pine remains *a wild and ancestral tree, a world tree that grows in forests of great power and resonance*.

But modern research may be changing this picture, with pine gaining reputation as a 'functional food', that is, a medicinal food, and its traditional herbal uses being scientifically authenticated.

Use Scots pine for...

Not surprisingly, pine has a particular affinity for the respiratory system for conditions ranging from coughs to tuberculosis, strep throat and asthma. It is excellent in both early and late stages of colds to eliminate mucus (expectoration) and control infection.

Ireland-based herbalist Nikki Darrell points out that pine is particularly valuable for treating asthmatics who have been on long-term steroids. Steroids have been connected with adrenal insufficiency, and pine acts as an adrenal restorative.

The late American herbalist Michael Moore has a useful ascending scale for pine actions.

He rates a tea of pine needles as pleasant-tasting, mildly diuretic and expectorant. The inner bark used as a tea and sweetened with honey is stronger, and valuable in the later stages of a chest cold. Pine pitch, the size of a currant, chewed and swallowed, makes for stronger expectoration again, with the softening of deep mucus.

Backround scene: planted rows of Scots pine, near Mildenhall, Suffolk, October

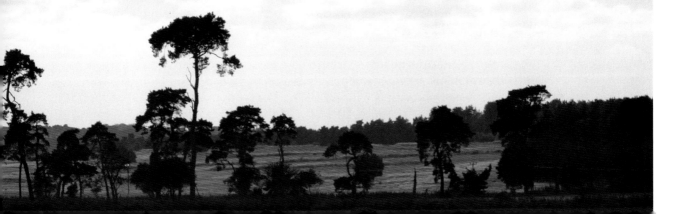

Pine Needle Tea, made by pouring 1 pint of boiling water over about 1 ounce of fresh white pine needles chopped fine, is about the most palatable pine product I have tasted. With a squeeze of lemon and a little sugar it is almost enjoyable.
– Gibbons (1966)

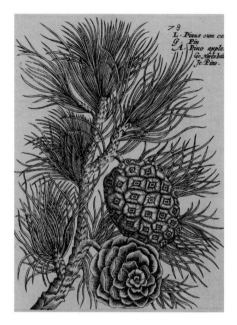

Another American herbalist, Matthew Wood, characterises pine as a stimulating antiseptic. It is used externally in the form of baths, poultices (for sores and burns) and for direct placement on wounds.

Native Americans are among many pine-based cultures to find that pine sap will prevent wound putrefaction, and help eliminate splinters and even bullets.

Pine's stimulating / antiseptic qualities extend further into proven efficacy for promoting blood circulation, as a laxative and an astringent, for relieving colic and headache, for soothing rheumatism, arthritis and oedema, and as an aphrodisiac. Finally, Pycnogenol is a commercially made extract from the bark of *Pinus pinaster*.

Modern research

Pine contains a category of flavonols called oligomeric proanthocyanidins (OPCs). These serve to protect the body's collagen against cell damage and thereby have a role in cancer prevention; moreover OPCs have been shown to slow the accumulation of fat in the arteries and reduce risks of heart disease.

Hence pine may have a supportive role in counteracting two of the major life-threatening conditions. What else is research showing?

More initials for one thing! Research on mice (2009a) indicates that pine's polyphenyl propanoid-polysaccharides complex (PPCs) inhibit allergic IgE reactions, notably in asthma. Asthma treatment costs $8 billion annually in the US.

Pine has been shown (2005a) to be more effective than resveratrol in inhibiting growth of yeast infections *Candida albans* and *Saccharomyces cerevisiae*. It is also effective against the bacteria *Staphylococcus aureus* (2000).

Drug-makers are taking note of these potentials, including Pycnogenol, in an extract of French maritime pine bark (2002), as also the possible role of pine as a 'functional food', namely one that contains bioactive compounds that have been shown to help relieve chronic health problems (2005b, 2009b).

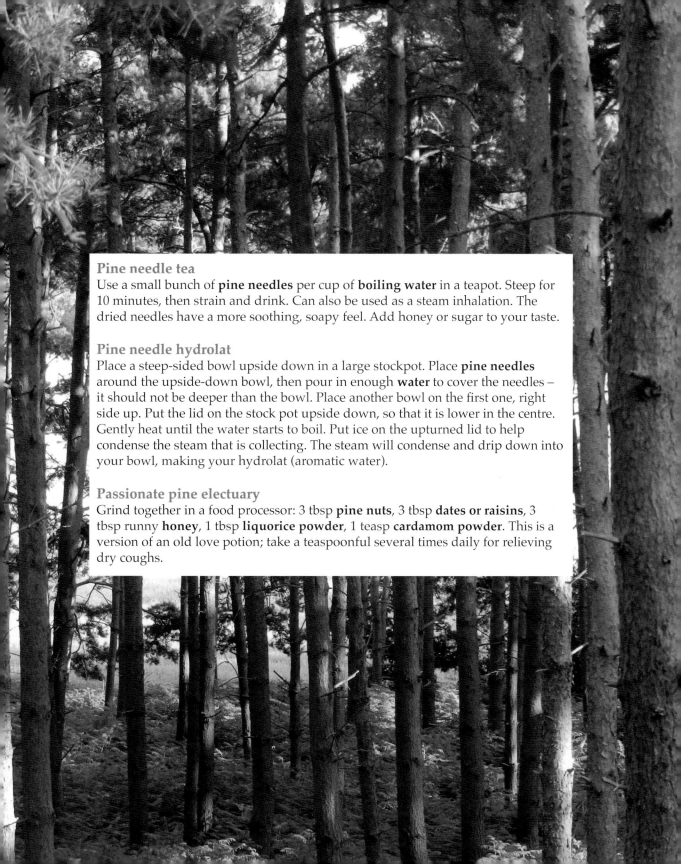

Pine needle tea

Use a small bunch of **pine needles** per cup of **boiling water** in a teapot. Steep for 10 minutes, then strain and drink. Can also be used as a steam inhalation. The dried needles have a more soothing, soapy feel. Add honey or sugar to your taste.

Pine needle hydrolat

Place a steep-sided bowl upside down in a large stockpot. Place **pine needles** around the upside-down bowl, then pour in enough **water** to cover the needles – it should not be deeper than the bowl. Place another bowl on the first one, right side up. Put the lid on the stock pot upside down, so that it is lower in the centre. Gently heat until the water starts to boil. Put ice on the upturned lid to help condense the steam that is collecting. The steam will condense and drip down into your bowl, making your hydrolat (aromatic water).

Passionate pine electuary

Grind together in a food processor: 3 tbsp **pine nuts**, 3 tbsp **dates or raisins**, 3 tbsp runny **honey**, 1 tbsp **liquorice powder**, 1 teasp **cardamom powder**. This is a version of an old love potion; take a teaspoonful several times daily for relieving dry coughs.

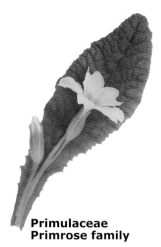

Primrose & Cowslip

Primrose, *Primula vulgaris* & Cowslip, *Primula veris*

These bright spring flowers cheer the spirits after long, dark winters, and are among Britain's favourite wild plants. They were once important medicinals, but could well be used again as safe remedies for treating insomnia, migraine, catarrh, arthritis and rheumatism, among other historic uses.

**Primulaceae
Primrose family**

Description: Perennials with large crinkly green leaves and pale yellow flowers in spring.

Habitat: Old woodland, ditches, hedgerows, banks, grassland and churchyards. Cowslips prefer more open grassy areas.

Distribution: Primrose is widespread through the British Isles, cowslips less common in north and west. Native to Europe and temperate Asia. Cowslip introduced to north-eastern US.

Related species: Oxlip (*P. elatior*) is a separate, rare species. The hybrid of primrose and cowslip is known as false oxlip, *P. x polyantha*. Bird's eye primrose (*P. farinosa*) and Scots primrose (*P. scotica*) have violet or purple flowers and a localised distribution.

Parts used: Roots, flowers, leaves.

Cowslip is an under-used but valuable plant.
– Chevallier (2016)

Primroses are one of the earliest spring wild blossoms – the name comes from 'prima rosa' or first flower (*primavera* in Spain and Italy). They are often still blooming when the taller cowslips join them a few weeks later.

It is the spring flowers that people love most. A survey carried out by the charity Plantlife in 2015 showed that bluebells were the nation's most popular flower, with primrose second and cowslip fifth. Perhaps it is their colour and freshness charming us after the long, dark winter, and no doubt these are the plants we loved in childhood, with early memories of woods and meadows.

Primrose attracted approving names, such as darling of April and ladies of the spring. But cowslip was from Old English 'cow-slop', or a plant springing up where cows in meadows deposited their dung.

If that was rather down to earth, cowslip was also known as bunch of keys or St Peter's keys, a name

inspired by the hanging flowers. These resembled the bunch of keys that St Peter metaphorically carried and could open the kingdom of heaven to a believer.

Interestingly, this name was a deliberate Christianising takeover of an earlier pagan (Norse) name: cowslip was once dedicated to the goddess Freya, the virgin of the keys. The keyflower plant or cowslip would open her own sexual kingdom. Such a myth had to be reconfigured!

The nodding head of cowslip may also have suggested a palsy (paralysis), and other ancient names included palsywort, paralytica and arthritica, the latter for the use of the roots for rheumatic and arthritic pain relief.

Coming up to date, cowslip has made a gratifying dramatic recovery from centuries of overpicking for making the popular cowslip wine or syrup. This practice has fallen into decline, and meanwhile local councils have widely planted cowslip on British roadsides as part of a meadow mix, ensuring that highways and waysides are an opportunistic new habitat for this much-loved flower.

Use primrose and cowslips for...
Primrose and cowslips have similar medicinal properties, though cowslips are more often used and have a deeper healing profile.

One abiding reputation of cowslip has been as a 'nervine', a plant that benefited the nervous system, in this case as a relaxing sedative. Hildegard of Bingen (1098–1179) was among the earliest European commentators on cowslip, which she recommended for melancholia, in the form of a compress of tea made from the plant, held over the heart while sleeping – in modern terms, an antidepressant remedy.

Both plants have been used to treat insomnia. Austrian naturopath Maria Treben (1982) met a man

... to ease paines in the head [primrose and cowslip are] *accounted next to Betony* [Stachys officinalis], *the best for that purpose. Experience likewise hath shewed, that they are profitable* [effective] *both for the Palsie, and paines of the ioynts, ... which hath caused the names of* Arthritica, Paralysis, *and* Paralytica *to bee giuen them.*
  – Parkinson (1629)

A basket of primrose and cowslip flowers

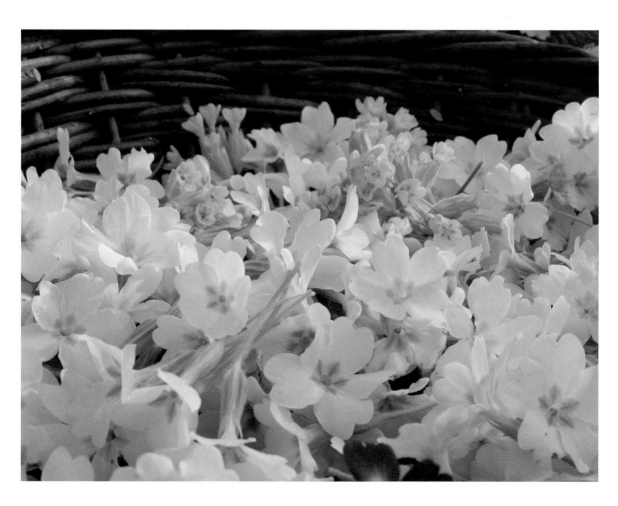

who could not sleep despite taking strong sleeping pills. Her remedy for him was a tea of dried plants: 10 parts cowslip, 5 of lavender, 2 St John's wort, 3 hops and 1 valerian root. A powerful mixture, it cured his sleeplessness within a week.

Cowslip wine was a well-liked method of adding a sedative effect to the pleasant alcoholic buzz, and it was extended to pacifying unruly children, if the Tulliver children in George Eliot's novel *Mill on the Floss* (1860) are drawn true to life.

The plants' profile also includes relief of headaches and migraines, panic attacks and nervous tension in general. Pechey in 1707 approved eating cowslip flowers and leaves as potherbs and in 'sallets': they were 'very Agreeable to the Head and Nerves'. They remain good to eat. Pechey also noted cowslip as anodyne, or pain-relieving, which science confirms through its salicylate content.

Cowslip has an antispasmodic quality too, with its saponin-rich roots proving to be strongly

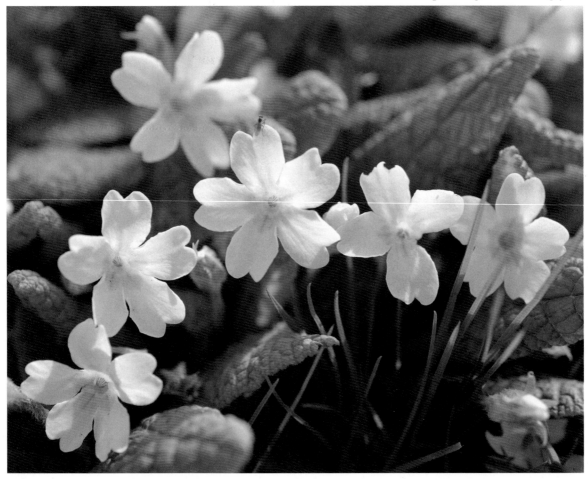

expectorant. A decoction of cowslip roots was once a familiar remedy for clearing phlegm and congestion, whooping cough and bronchitis. It is 'official' in Germany for catarrh, and may well have an unexplored value in asthma treatments.

In terms of 'palsy', as mentioned, one former use of the plants was to treat vertigo or loss of balance. John Wesley's herbal (1753) suggested for this: ... *drink Morning and Evening, half a Pint of Decoction of Primrose-root.* The other older uses for arthritis and rheumatism are explained by the salicylates in the roots having anti-inflammatory properties.

Cowslip also has a diaphoretic or sweat-inducing quality that underlies its fever-breaking and detoxifying potential.

It is a safe remedy for babies, children and the old. The flower essence-maker Saskia Marjoram sums up her experience of the flower as offering *a safe mothered feeling that enables you to skip with joy.* Avoid both plants, however, if you have a known intolerance to aspirin or salicylates.

Modern research
Polish research (2012) indicated the mechanism of the flavone zapotin as a chemopreventive and chemotherapeutic (anti-cancer) agent. First named in 2007, zapotin is extracted from the leaves of *Primula veris* (cowslip).

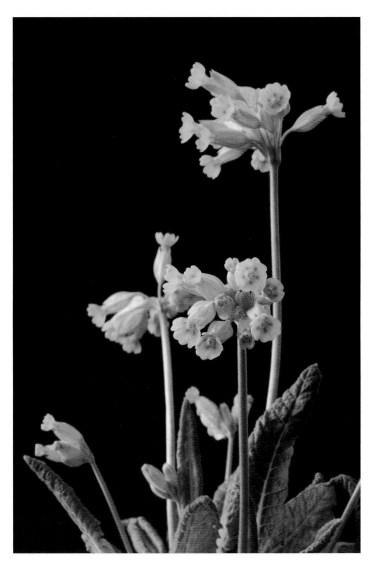

Cowslips (above) and primroses (left) by a country lane in Norfolk

Placebo-controlled, randomised double-blind trials (1994) into the German-made tablet, Sinupret, confirmed its decongestant effect in acute sinusitis. Sinupret contains extracts of *Sambucus nigra* (elder) flowers; *Primula veris* (cowslip) flowers; *Rumex acetosa* (sorrel) plant; *Verbena officinalis* (vervain) plant; and *Gentiana lutea* (gentian) root.

Caution: Avoid taking cowsip and primrose if you have a known aspirin allergy or salicylates intolerance.

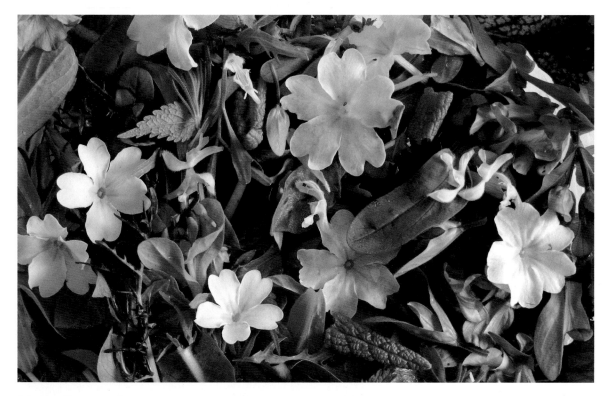

Primrose flowers and young leaves are a pretty addition to spring salads

Harvesting primroses and cowslips
Primroses flower for several months in the spring, with cowslips starting a little later. Only pick wild primroses and cowslips where they are plentiful. Garden varieties of primula can also be used.

Primrose or cowslip tea
Pick a few **primrose and/or cowslip flowers** per cup of **boiling water**. Infuse for about 5 minutes for a lovely golden, soothing cup of tea.

Primrose tea
- coughs
- anxiety
- insomnia
- colic

Primrose conserve
- dry coughs
- sore throats
- insomnia
- colic

Primrose or cowslip conserve
Fill a small jar with **primose and/or cowslip flowers**. Pour in **runny honey**, stirring to remove any air bubbles. Leave in a warm place for a few weeks, until the flowers have faded.

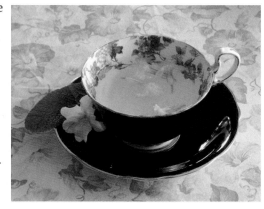

Strain out the spent blossoms. Take a teaspoonful for sore throats or digestive upsets.

Purple loosestrife *Lythrum salicaria*

Purple loosestrife is the old water-loving 'long purples' but is also called a 'purple plague' in parts of the USA where it is seen as an unwanted invader. Remarkably, it has a toxin-leaching role in land-healing or phytoremediation that is paralleled in a range of traditional and novel medicinal applications.

Purple loosestrife is a striking and glamorous British wild plant whose tall magenta flowerheads add delight to summer wetlands or wayside ditches. Gardeners too have taken to it – one notes how *its reliable drama has led many of us to grow it in damp spots in our gardens.*

Purple loosestrife stands tall and strong, as the old country name 'long purples' suggests. Its vigour can also be problematic for humans. In Fenland dykes it was once known as 'iron hard' for its impenetrable root system, which broke farm workers' shovels. It has become 'purple plague', the 'poster plant' of invasives in parts of the US.

Lythrum is thought to be from a Greek term for blood because the plant has an old medicinal reputation as a blood stauncher.

Salicaria is 'willow-like', for the plant's thin, tapering leaves; it was once called purple willowherb. Salmon (1710) hedges his bets: he says the name was given *because it grows among willows, or … has willow-like leaves.*

And 'loosestrife' itself? Refer to an old herbal, such as Salmon's, and you will find the yellow and purple loosestrifes described together in the same genus, the *Lysimachia*. It was only in the later 20th century that the two plants

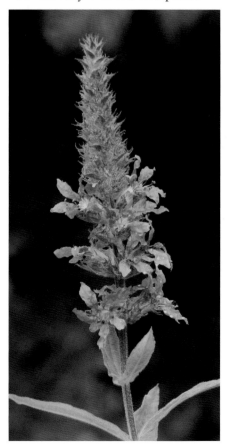

**Lythraceae
Purple loosestrife
family**

Description: A highly attractive perennial and vigorous coloniser, to 1.5m tall (5ft), with many erect, angular stems; bright magenta-purple flowers, whorled, with typically 6 floppy petals; leaves narrow, lance-shaped, untoothed; deep taproot and lateral roots.

Habitat: Forms colonies in watersides, whether wetlands, fens, ponds, rivers or ditches; can persist when soils dry out.

Distribution: Native to Europe, but also SE Asia and east/south coasts of Australia; naturalised in North America, and considered invasive in east, midwest and far west.

Related species: Perhaps surprisingly, not the yellow loosestrife (*Lysimachia vulgaris*), which is a Primula; the water purslane (*Lythrum portula*) is the closest relative, along with the rare grass poly (*L. hyssopifolium*).

Parts used: Above-ground parts.

were separated, with the yellow reassigned to the Primulaceae (but keeping the name *Lysimachia vulgaris*) and the purple given its own genus, *Lythrum*.

Lysimachus was a fabled king of ancient Sicily, and his name consists of two elements meaning 'undo' and 'war' – or 'loose strife'.

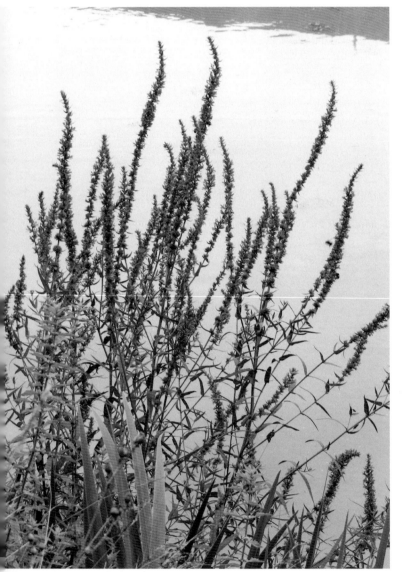

He is said to have been the first to use the plants to calm tetchy oxen in ploughing teams. When placed under the yoke, resting on the oxen's shoulders, the plant deterred the biting insects that abound in marshy areas. The oxen were duly pacified and their 'strife' brought to an end.

Names can only take us so far, of course, but early European colonists in North America seem to have used the plant to good effect with their own fractious oxen, and both forms of loosestrife made smudge sticks or incense to keep insects away from humans.

The first record of the plant in North America was in 1814, in an eastern port, following a presumed accidental introduction via a cargo of ballast from Europe. Lacking soil and plant predators of its native habitat, the plant prospered, spreading through river systems west and north, becoming larger and massier as it did so, reaching Alaska by 2001.

The charge is that it overshadows and outperforms native wetland plants, such as the bulrush-like cattail (*Typha latifolia*), and creates impenetrable colonies or disturbs irrigation channels. Purple loosestrife is well equipped to be a coloniser, with one plant putting up 30 to 50 stems and, in a recent calculation, some 2.7 million tiny seeds a year. Unavailing clearance efforts are said to cost upwards of $45 million annually in the US.

But American herbalists, notably Timothy Lee Scott and Jim Mcdonald, have raised counter-arguments to the conservation orthodoxy. They say purple loosestrife can work to rehabilitate wetlands by absorbing excess nitrogen and phosphorus from fertiliser and pesticide runoff.

In fact, the plant has remarkable powers of phytoremediation or land-healing, Mcdonald notes. That is, like other so-called 'green liver' plants, purple loosestrife can neutralise chemical contaminants such as lead or the banned polychlorinated biphenyls (PCBs).

Use purple loosestrife for ...
Purple loosestrife is astringent and tannin-rich enough to have been used to tan leather, but its astringency is mitigated by a high mucilage content that eases inflamed tissue as it tones it.

This unusual combination of properties underlies the plant's reputation in both Western and Chinese medicine for treating diarrhoea, dysentery ('bloody flux'), leaky gut, irritable bowel and many forms of discharge with blood and inflammation. It was found effective in the 19th century for use in epidemics of infant cholera and typhus, and its role in treating epidemic infection is as yet under-researched.

The plant was a wound herb, and John Parkinson among other herbalists recommended an ointment made with butter, wax and sugar for 'wounds and thrusts'. Another aspect of purple loosestrife's affinity for blood discharges is its historic role in treating excessive menstrual bleeding, via a vaginal douche.

The distilled water, Parkinson wrote, *likewise clenseth and healeth all foul ulcers and sores wheresoever, and stayeth their inflammations, by washing them.* The water, he added, was also effective as a gargle for painful inflammations like quinsy (throat abscess) and the king's evil (scrofula, a tubercular swelling of the lymph nodes). Applied externally, it also helped remove spots and scars, such as those from smallpox and measles.

Parkinson also noted that *the distilled water is a present remedy for hurts and blowes on the eyes, and for blindnesse,* provided the vitreous humour was not damaged.

Parkinson's biographer, Anna Parkinson (a probable descendant), had a remarkable confirmation of this assertion. She told us she once had something painful in her eye, and remembered what Parkinson had written about purple loosestrife.

She didn't panic, but calmly made a water distillation of the plant. When it was ready, she applied the liquid to her eye, which gave ready relief – this seems to us a courageous example of faith in a mentor!

Purple Loosestrife offers great potential as a valuable and practically useful medicinal, possessing an admirable balance of astringent and mucilaginous properties.
– Mcdonald (2013)

[The liquid juice is] *of an exceeding binding Quality ... Dioscorides says it is good to stay all manner of Bleedings at Mouth or Nose, or of Wounds, or any other Bleeding whatsoever. ... [It stops] all fluxes of the Belly, even the Bloody-flux* [dysentery] *it self.*
– Salmon (1710)

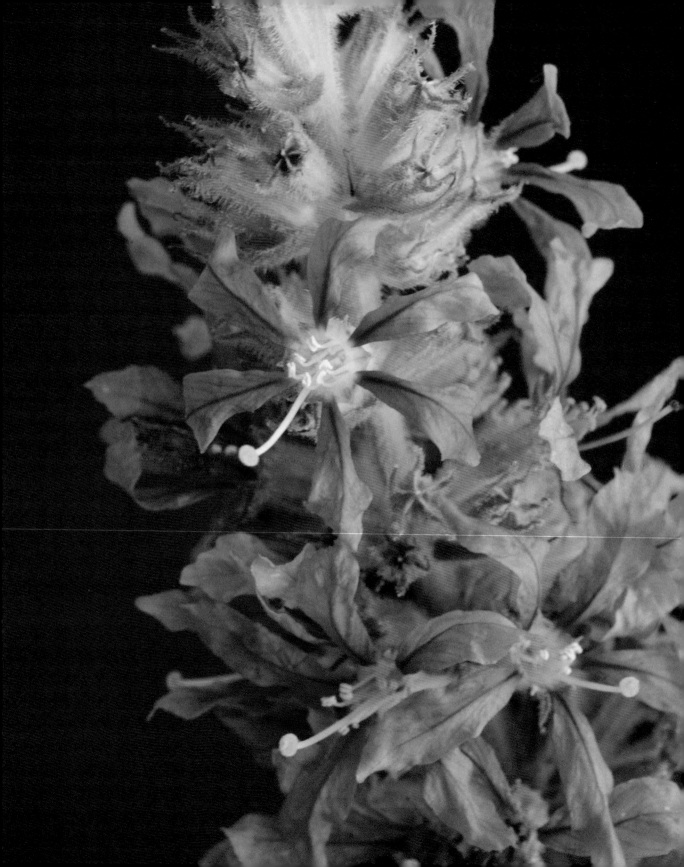

Purple loosestrife is 'superior' to eyebright in preserving the sight, said Mrs Grieve, and Timothy Lee Scott points out that it offers a widely available alternative to this plant, which has been over-harvested in the wild in the US.

The distilled water can also be used as a poultice for drying/toning any painful external condition, and is safe for children.

Another area of growing interest in purple loosestrife's actions is as a powerful antibacterial, antifungal and antimicrobial.

Modern research

Writing in 1931, Mrs Grieve commented that purple loosestrife is *Scarcely used at present medicinally, but once esteemed.* Things have changed, and there is now a growing body of recent research that has identified some of the active principles of purple loosestrife's wide range of pharmacological actions.

Work by a European team (2010) showed that *in vitro* purple loosestrife has 12 types of glycoconjugates; three of these showed complete inhibition of plasma clot formation, but two others were pro-coagulant. This suggests that, like yarrow, purple loosestrife is amphoteric with respect to blood flow, that is, it can act both as a coagulant (the traditional use) and an anti-coagulant at different times.

The plant's glycoconjugates were also demonstrated (2012) as having greater antitussive and bronchodilatory effects than the drug salbutamol.

The anti-inflammatory properties of purple loosestrife were shown (2015) to result from tannins identified as ellagitannins, and specifically dimeric salicarinins.

Earlier research (2005) supported purple loosestrife's effectiveness against the pathogenic fungus *Cladosporium cucumerinum* and the bacteria *Staphylococcus aureus*. The ester vescalagin was isolated as the active principle of the antibacterial activity. Purple loosestrife is definitely a plant worth using.

A quick purple loosestrife ointment

Pick **purple loosestrife** while in flower, or leaves whenever available. Chop up and cook gently in enough **ghee** (clarified butter) or **coconut oil** to cover for about 15 minutes, then strain out the plant parts and pour into clean jars. Note that coconut oil will be liquid in hot weather.

Purple loosestrife tea

Put a sprig of **purple loosestrife** per person in a teapot, and cover with boiling water. Steep for 5 to 10 minutes. Strain and drink, or cool for external use on the skin or as an eyewash.

Purple loosestrife ointment

- fungal infections
- bacterial infections
- cuts & grazes
- blemishes

Purple loosestrife tea

- loose bowels
- fungal infections
- bacterial infections
- cuts & grazes
- blemishes

Rowan *Sorbus aucuparia*

A handsome tree through the seasons, rowan is far more than a city ornamental. The name rowan stands for protection, and it was used across northern Europe as a charm against witchcraft for livestock, homes and the individual. Herbally a rose family astringent, it is made into a tea and tincture, the famed jelly and an ancient form of ale.

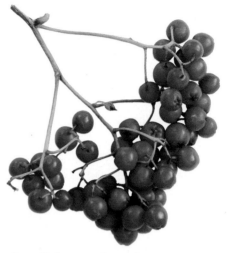

Rosaceae
Rose family

Description: A small deciduous tree, growing to 15m (50ft); slender and elegant in form: silvery-grey trunk in winter, bright green pinnate, ash-like leaves in spring, frothy white flowers in summer and bright orange-red berries in autumn.

Habitat: Woodland, wayside, mountain and marginal land; grows at higher altitudes than any other native British tree.

Distribution: Northern and western parts of British Isles; native to temperate Asia, Europe; naturalised in North America.

Related species: Whitebeam (*Sorbus aria*), wild service tree (*S. torminalis*), the American mountain ash (*S. americana*).

Parts used: Berries, bark.

Rowan's common names attest to its ancient importance as a tree evocative of fresh life (quicken, wicken or wiggen, quickbeam) and magic (witchbane, witchwand, witchbeam). It is both enchanting to behold and protects against enchantment.

More prosaic is its descriptive name mountain ash (often used in North America). True, it thrives on poor mountain soil, but it is no ash, merely having ash-like leaves.

The Latin species name *aucuparia* hints at rowan's attractiveness to birds in the autumn and winter, when migrant fieldfares, redwings and waxwings descend on berry-rich British rowan trees, gobble the fruit and spread the seeds. An *auceps* was a fowler, who used rowan's berries as a lure; hence an old name, fowler's service tree.

'Rowan' itself, as befits a plant whose association with man goes back to prehistory, has various suggested origins: a Norse word similar to 'rune', protection; a

Swedish term for redness; or a reference to a spinning wheel, for which rowan wood was often used. The genus name *Sorbus* is for the service trees and beams.

A beautiful and compact tree, rowan is beloved of civic planters as a quick-growing ornamental for roadsides, parks and churchyards. This is the tamed version, though, and rowan remains at heart a wild pioneer tree, growing in dwarf forms at higher elevations and latitudes, fighting for a foothold in inclement weather, and coping with browsing deer or sheep, or moose in Scandinavia.

Protection is the keyword for rowan's role, for stock and homes as much as people. But carrying pieces of rowan loose or wrapped in red twine as charms has never appealed to authority. Take the book *Demonologie* (1598) where King James VI of Scotland (and I of England) condemned *such kinde of Charmes as commonlie dafte wives uses … by knitting roun-trees … to the haire or tailes of the goodes.*

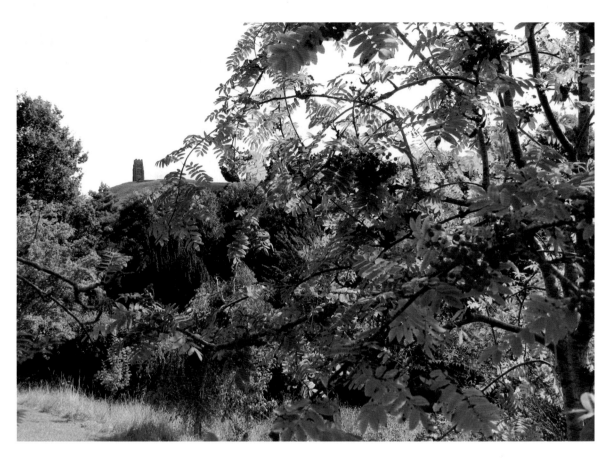

Use rowan for ...

Rowan is a rose family astringent, and the bark is tannin-rich. It is a traditional tea or tincture for treating diarrhoea, piles, vaginal discharge and menstrual pain. The bark is also a dye (black and orange) and once used in tanning.

The fruit is nutritive, if tart. It has only a little pectin, which is why crab apple is added in making the famous jelly to help it set. A decoction of the berries with added apple and sugar is a country remedy for whooping cough. A rowan gargle is used for sore throats. Its diuretic quality helps in strangury (inability to urinate), and it is used for rheumatism and arthritis. It is a useful anti-inflammatory for sore kidneys.

Cooking rowan alters its irritant parasorbic acid to the more tolerable sorbic acid, which underlies the general advice to avoid taking it in raw forms.

Modern research

The service tree (*Sorbus domestica*) inhibits aldose reductase, which may be useful in diabetic complications (2008), and the related *Sorbus commixta* has potent anti-inflammatory effects (2010).

Fruiting rowan in the Chalice Well garden, under Glastonbury Tor, August

Their spells were vain. The hags return'd To the Queen in sorrowful mood, Crying that witches have no power, Where there is Rown-Tree wood.

– The Laidly Worm of Spindleston Heugh, *a tale of a Northumberland dragon (13th century or earlier)*

Rowan jelly
- digestive upsets
- diarrhoea

Rowan syrup
- coughs
- colds
- sore throats

Rowan elixir
- colds
- rheumatism
- diarrhoea

[Diodgriafel, rowan ale, is] *made of the berries of* Sorbus Aucuparia, *(Roan Tree) abundant in most parts of Wales; by pouring water over them and setting the infusion by to ferment. When kept for some time, this is by no means an unpleasant liquor; but necessity obliges these children of penury to use it, without waiting for the fermentative process.*
– Evans (1798)

As a soft fruit it is ... something of a failure, but, of course, it has one use which rescues it from foraging oblivion – Rowan jelly.
– Wright (2010)

[The berries] *are, however, terribly bitter but, as a Scottish friend once pointed out, they're our version of cranberry jelly, perfect for roasted meats.*
– Fowler (2011)

Rowan jelly

A traditional jelly, but nobody seems to agree on the balance of rowan berries and apples. We like equal amounts, and prefer crab apples to cooking apples. The apples or crab apples lighten the piquancy and their pectins help in the setting process.

Pick over and wash your **berries** and **apples**, quartering the latter; put both into a large pan, add **water** to cover and boil for some 20 minutes to a pulp. Allow to cool. Pour through a jelly bag and allow to drip over-night. Next day, measure the juice into a pan, and add 400g or 1lb **sugar** for each 500ml or 1 pint of **juice.** Heat slowly, stirring the sugar in until dissolved. Boil for 10 minutes or so, until a drop of the liquid solidifies when dribbled onto a cold saucer. Skim off the scum. Now pour into sterilised jars (heat in the oven for 10 minutes), cover and label.

Rowan syrup

Put 1kg (2.2lb) **rowan berries** into a pot, add **wate**r to cover and sim-mer until soft, about 25 minutes. Strain off the liquid, return berries to the pan and repeat with fresh water. This second boiling needs less time, roughly 15 minutes. Strain the liquid into a clean pan, add about ¾ caster (superfine) sugar to liquid (750g to 1 litre liquid). Boil hard for 5 minutes, then bottle in sterilised bottles. Label.

Rowan elixir

This heady elixir is made of equal parts of **vegetable glycerine** and **vodka** or **brandy**. Simply fill your jar with fresh-gathered and picked-over rowan berries, add the liquids, cover and leave in a dark place for at least six weeks. Strain off when the berries look bleached out.

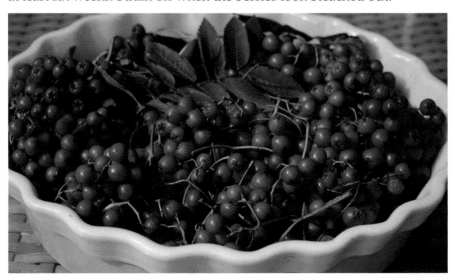

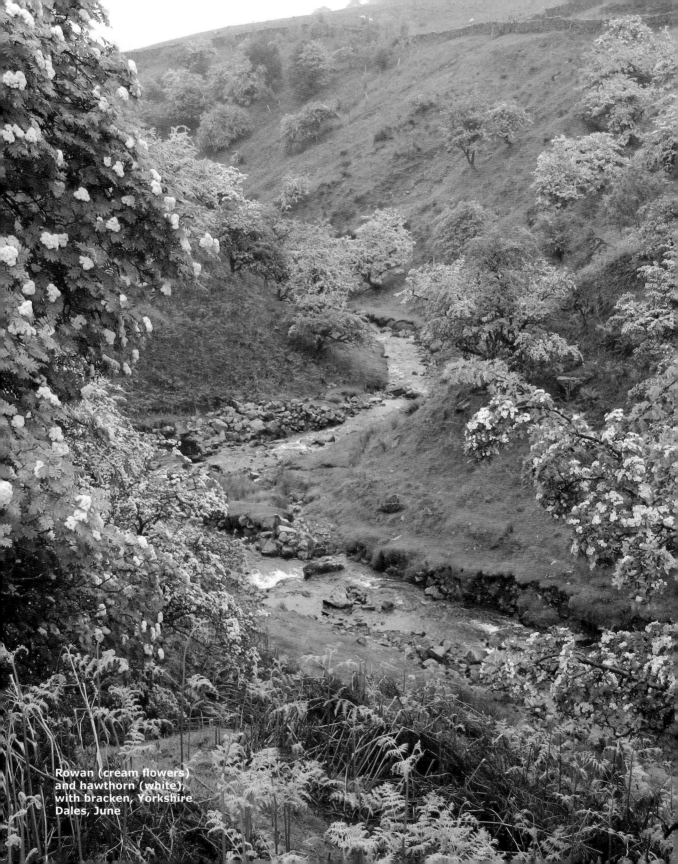

Rowan (cream flowers) and hawthorn (white), with bracken, Yorkshire Dales, June

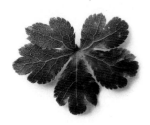

Sanicle *Sanicula europaea*

**Apiaceae
Carrot family**

Description: A hairless perennial, some 60–70cm (2ft) high, with basal, palm-shaped, dark green 3- to 5-lobed leaves; the small puffs of white/pink flowers sit atop long stalks, often grouped 3 x 3, with a tenth central flower; fruit has hooked spines.

Habitat: Deciduous woodland, especially beechwoods on chalk, in colonies.

Distribution: Widespread in British Isles, Eurasia. *Sanicula marilandica* in North America.

Related species: Among the large Apiaceae family, sanicle is within a subfamily that includes masterwort or astrantia (*Astrantia major*) and sea holly (*Eryngo maritimum*). Common North American species are Canadian sanicle (*Sanicula canadensis*) and black sanicle or snakeroot (*S. marilandica*).

Parts used: Above-ground parts.

Sanicle is an easily overlooked woodland plant that was once regarded as a panacea, a cure-all, for healing wounds and uncontrolled bleeding, ulcers, tumours, and diseases of the mouth, throat, chest and lungs. It deserves to be better known for these uses and for its growing repute as an antiviral remedy.

Sanicle (or wood sanicle in older herbals) is a forgotten and often overlooked plant of temperate deciduous woodland. It is one of those herbs that you never notice until it is pointed out to you, and then you see it everywhere.

When flowering in early summer sanicle's white/pink blossoms sit like ten or so pom-poms on top of a hairless stalk, more Allium than Apiaceae. Plantswoman Sarah Raven likens it to *a molecular model in a chemistry lab*.

A useful identifier is sanicle's preferred habitat – damp shade in old and usually coppiced woodland. Woodland authority Oliver Rackham (2006) includes it among 80 plant/tree indicators of ancient British woodland.

This habitat is under threat, as coppicing is in decline (which affects the shade regime) and as woodland is lost to development. The good news for sanicle fans is that, as we have found, it will grow readily in the garden, and make a good ground cover for shady areas.

Use sanicle for...

The common name has a connection with the Latin term 'to heal', and sanicle has a distinguished past as a medicinal, chiefly as a wound herb and anti-inflammatory for the chest and mouth. A medieval French saying summarises its reputation in ten words: *Celui qui Sanicle a / De plaie affaire il n'a* [who the Sanicle hath / At the surgeon may laugh].

Sanicle is one of the traditional European 'consounds' or wound herbs, and often linked with bugle (*Ajuga reptans*) and self-heal (*Prunella vulgaris*), both members of the deadnettle (Lamiaceae) family. Each of the three has been called 'self-heal' at some time. Comfrey is another 'consound'.

Geoffrey Grigson (1958) cites a 15th-century wound drink using leaves of sanicle, yarrow and bugle, crushed in a mortar and 'tempered with wine'. Each component had a subtle, complementary role: *This is the vertu of this drynke: bugle holdith the wound open, mylfoyle* [yarrow] *clensith the wound, sanycle helith it.*

Self-treatment for wounds was much more familiar in the past than now, but we believe it is valuable to know that herbs such as these (classed as vulneraries) can still be used as first aid. Sanicle works well for bruises and other minor injuries – simply chew a leaf to soften it, then apply to the injured area. If you are at home, you could also use a compress soaked in cooled sanicle tea and apply it to the skin.

Among other vulneraries or wound-healing herbs, including several common wild plants, are aloe vera, ashwagandha, burdock, calendula, comfrey, elder, garlic, plantain, St John's wort, thyme, woundwort and yarrow; tea tree essential oil can be added to this list, as can honey.

Sanicle is astringent and bitter, and had a long-standing reputation for dealing with irregular 'fluxes' or flows of bodily fluids. This extended from the blood, whether menstrual bleeding or ulcers, to disturbed urine or stool and upset stomachs. Sanicle tea is pleasant and can be drunk regularly to help heal internal ulcers.

Above all, sanicle was known as a treatment for the respiratory tract, as a gargle and mouthwash, for gum and throat problems, and for the lungs, including for tuberculosis. In North America, the local sanicle, *Sanicula marilandica*, was famed for treating sore throats and fevers.

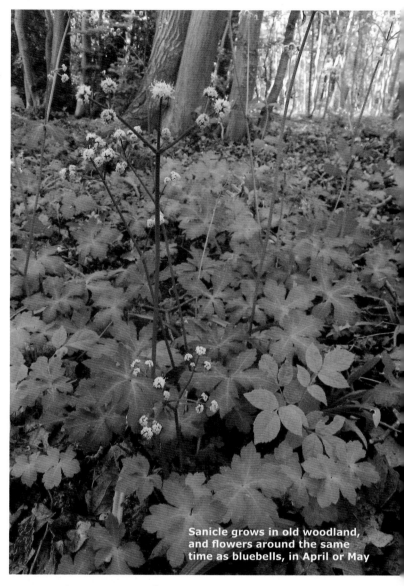

Sanicle grows in old woodland, and flowers around the same time as bluebells, in April or May

But sanicle's reputation has declined, particularly in the 20th century. We'd say this reflects broader medical changes (as in the standard treatment of tuberculosis) rather than any fault of the plant. The last great champion of sanicle was English herbalist Richard Lawrence Hool in the 1920s.

... there is not found any herbe [other than sanicle] *that can give so much present helpe, either to man or beast, when the disease falleth upon the lunges or throate, and to heale up all the malignant putride or stinking ulcers of the mouth, throat, and privities.*
– Parkinson (1640)

Hool's 1924 book features a sanicle tea to soothe ulcerated lungs or stomach. He suggests two parts sanicle to one part each of marshmallow and mullein in boiling water. The dosage is one or two glassfuls every three hours.

Hool also mentions a report in *Dr Skelton's Botanic Record* (1852) that a man had cured himself of consumption (tuberculosis) by drinking a pint daily of a tea of sanicle mixed with ginger, and then sweetened.

We propose that it is time that sanicle was not only identified in its woodland setting but also harvested, grown in the garden and used once again in medicine.

Modern research

A 1999 article confirmed antiviral effects for sanicle tea, with plaque inhibition shown in human parainfluenza virus type 2 (HPIV-2). An alcohol tincture of the plant did not have the same effect.

This complemented studies in 1996 by the same research team, which found that some kinds of influenza virus were disabled by sanicle extracts, without toxic effects on the subjects.

Research using the VOLKSMED database of traditional Austrian plant remedies (2013) found that sanicle was among 67 plants (of the 71 tested) to show anti-inflammatory activity *in vitro*, with 'moderate' to 'strong' effects.

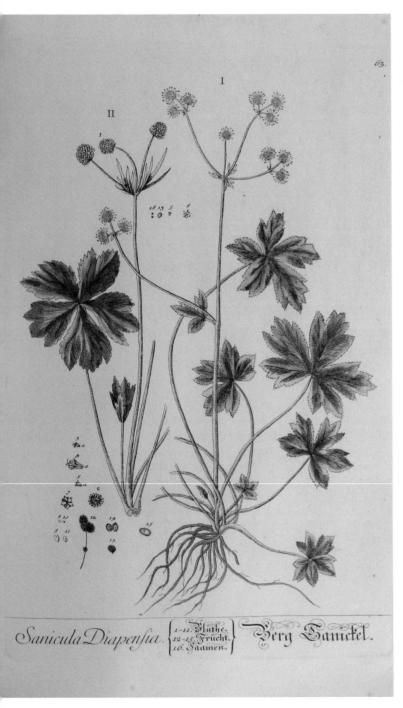

Sanicle, painted by Elizabeth Blackwell (1750), courtesy of the Wellcome Library

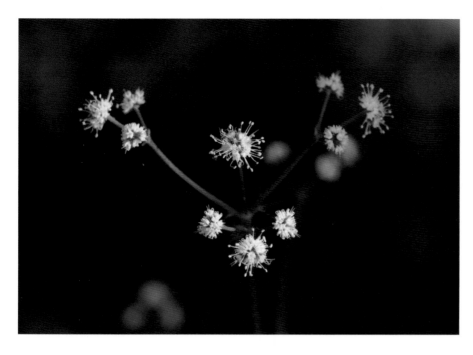

Sanicle tea à la Parkinson

We tried John Parkinson's 1640 recipe for a sanicle tea. He states that the plant is astringent and bitter in taste, and suggests boiling fresh leaves and roots together, as a decoction, with 'a little hony put thereto'.

Two or three **sanicle leaves** per mug of **water** makes a good strong brew, with 10 or 15 minutes of gentle simmering until it turns golden. Then strain and add **honey** to taste. The honey not only makes the tea taste better, but adds to its effectiveness. The liquid can be bottled while hot or allowed to cool first, and keeps in the fridge for some weeks.

We found the initial effect to be relaxing, changing after a few minutes to stimulating. The energy is accompanied by a feeling of clarity, so you can decide what jobs need doing and then go ahead and finish them.

Sanicle flower essence

Julie made this essence with a shamanic friend, near the edge of an ancient woodland where there was a ploughed field just beyond. Sanicle strengthens our connection with the ancient magic of the forest, while providing strength and protection from external influences. It is both grounding and uplifting, and clarifies perception.

For full instructions on how to make a flower essence, see page 291 under forget-me-not.

In cases of diseases of the chest and lungs, spitting of blood, scrofula, ulcers and tumours, or internal abscesses and ulcerations, there is no plant superior to Wood Sanicle.

– Hool (1924)

Wood sanicle has powerful medicinal properties and many uses. This is one of the herbs that could well be called a 'cure-all,' because it possesses powerful cleansing and healing virtue, both internally and externally. ... It is a powerful herb to heal both internal and external wounds and tumors [as a tea].
– Kloss (1939)

... vies for consideration as one of the most important but completely forgotten woundworts of the Middle Ages.
– Wood (2008)

Sanicle tea
- relaxing
- energising
- diarrhoea
- stomach upsets
- ulcers
- mouthwash
- sore gums
- lung problems

Sanicle essence
- connection
- strength
- protection
- intuition

Scabious

Field scabious, *Knautia arvensis*; Devil's bit scabious, *Succisa pratensis*

**Caprifoliacae
Honeysuckle
family**

Description:
Perennials, to 1m/3ft
high (small scabious
about half as tall);
'pincushion' purple-
range flowerheads;
devil's bit and sweet
scabious are more
rounded.

Habitat: Roadsides,
woodland clearings,
meadows; small
scabious follows the
chalk; devil's bit prefers
damp, also heaths,
fens.

Distribution: Europe
and Middle East; devil's
bit locally abundant
in British Isles; field
scabious common
except for most of
Scotland, central
Wales, western Ireland;
small scabious locally
common, England only,
mainly south and east;
sweet scabious rare but
for Kent and Cornwall.
Field scabious is a
widespread introduced
species in the US.

Related species: Over
650 worldwide; many
garden-bred.

Parts used: Whole
plant, roots having
strongest medicinal
effect.

Scabious is perhaps best known as a garden border plant. Its pale lilac flowerheads are attractive to both humans and butterflies, it is easy to grow and has long stems that make it a good choice in flower arrangements. But did you know this was once a trusted wild-gathered plague herb?

'Scabious' covers a number of pretty lilac or blue-flowered meadow plants, the most common of which are not within the Scabiosa genus. It's confusing!

In fact, the most frequently found scabiouses across the British Isles have other genus names: devil's bit scabious, or devil's bit, is *Succisa pratensis*, and field scabious, *Knautia arvensis,* is named for the German botanist Christopher Knaut (1638–94).

The true scabiouses – best known are the small scabious, *Scabiosa columbaria*, and the sweet scabious, *S. atropurpurea* – are at best locally common in the British Isles.

All four species are part of the wider scabious grouping for botanical and indeed medicinal purposes. Sheep's bit scabious, or sheep's bit (*Jasione montana*), however, is not a true scabious, despite its appearance. It is a *Campanula*, and not medicinal.

Modern reclassification has re-allocated the Scabious genus from the teasels to the honeysuckles. Field botanists might well hearken back to Linnaeus, who, in the mid-18th century, could name both *Knautia* and *Succisa* as *Scabiosa*!

As for 'scabious' itself, history offers two versions. First, the name comes from the Latin root-word *scabo*, meaning rough, as the hairy stem of field scabious might be described. More likely, perhaps, is the meaning for scab, mange or itch, describing some of scabious' medicinal properties. Perhaps the rough stalks were once used to rub the itch of scabies?

Geoffrey Grigson, for one, was unhappy with the English name. He wrote in 1958: *Scabious from the scab is a sad name for one of the most obvious, abundant, and pretty weeds of the cornfield. Perhaps one might abandon Scabious for 'Gipsy Rose'.*

No such luck yet, but there are other pleasing descriptive names from the past, for *Knautia* and *Succisa*: pincushion flower, blue bonnets, billy buttons, lady's hatpins and clodweed.

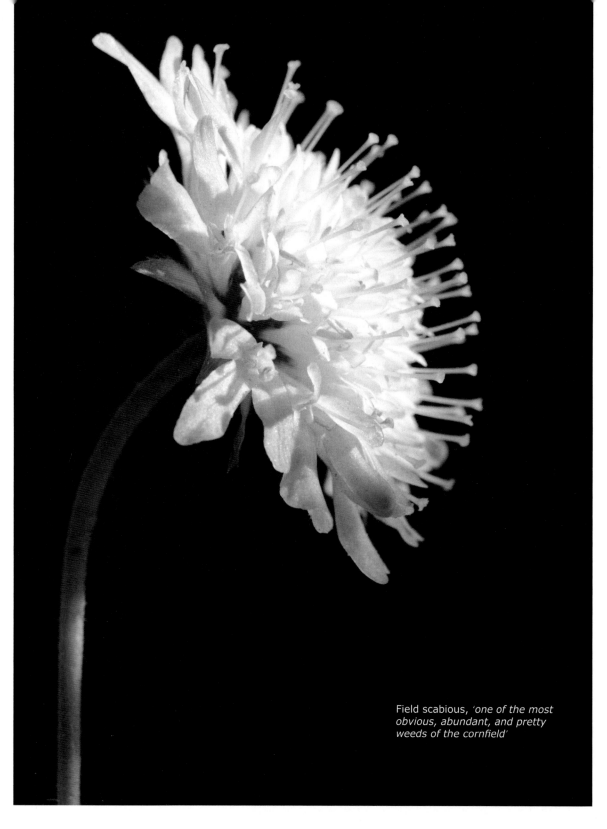

Field scabious, 'one of the most obvious, abundant, and pretty weeds of the cornfield'

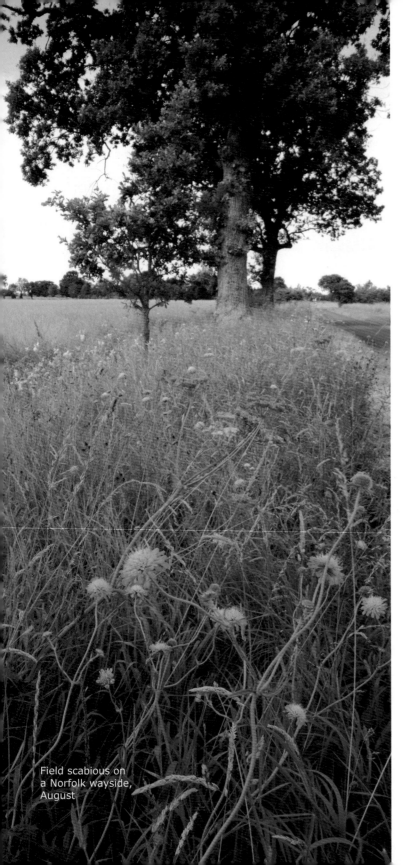

Field scabious on a Norfolk wayside, August

But there is one more name to mention, a remarkable one at that – devil's bit. This refers to the small truncated rootstock of the plant, which gave its former name *Morsus diaboli* or devil's bit(e). The story went that the root was so strong and good a medicine that the devil, 'envying the good that this herbe might do to mankinde', bit it off to destroy it.

Use scabious for…
Given this background, it will hardly be surprising that scabious root was a serious (if unavailing) treatment for plague and pestilence. The root was boiled in wine and the brew drunk, regularly, as a preventative. Its diaphoretic property helped patients sweat and break fevers.

The same remedy was used to treat bruising, dog bites and other blood wounds. The first book on distillation, the German alchemist Hieronymous Brunschwig's *Vertuous Book of Distillation* (1500), said an ounce of scabious water, drunk in the morning before food *is good for the pestilence*.

Additionally, the above-ground parts were crushed and laid on carbuncles, sores and itches, including scabies itself, to ripen and heal them. John Parkinson (writing in 1640) was confident that the bruised green herb of scabious, applied to a carbuncle or plague sore, *is found certaine by good experience* to dissolve or break it within three hours.

Parkinson's leading use for scabious, however, was as an expectorant for respiratory relief. He noted that devil's bit was the more bitter and stronger-acting of the scabious species. Both herbs could be made into syrups, decoctions or a distilled water.

By 1812, however, Hill's *Family Herbal* signposted the declining appeal of scabious. No longer a herb to fight the devil or the plague, for Hill it was a strong infusion for asthma, a syrup used for coughs and a juice applied on 'foulnesses of the skin'. Mrs Grieve in 1931 said much the same. But by 1979, Malcolm Stuart could write it off: *The herb* [Devil's bit scabious] *is not very effective medicinally and is rarely used today.*

But that marked a nadir, not an end. American herbalists like Matthew Wood and Peter Holmes are looking afresh at scabious. Wood, for example, in a workshop that Julie attended, reported herbalist Bernadette Dowling's finding that a long-brewed scabious tea was effective for relaxation. Holmes finds scabious has 'excellent topical applications', as in swabs, compresses and ointments; is good for bronchial issues and for various skin conditions. It's the sound of a wheel turning, not one halting.

Modern research
A scabious cousin, *Scabiosa arenaria*, in Tunisia (2015), was shown to inhibit α-glucosodase, a finding useful in type 2 diabetes treatment. Research on the same plant (2012) found its essential oil had antibacterial and anticandidal properties, comparable to those of thymol (the control).

In an ethnobotanical survey in rural Peru (2010), *Scabiosa atropurpurea* flowers were being used fresh orally or inhaled for menstrual regulation.

Scabious was in the past considered one of the finest remedies available for treating conditions affecting the skin. Like Plantain, Scabious addresses a large range of external conditions from wounds and abscesses to skin infections. … Clearly this is another plant that deserves more widespread use in respiratory and topical applications.
– Holmes (2007)

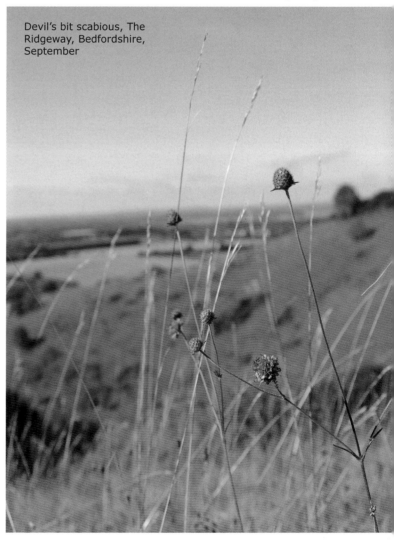
Devil's bit scabious, The Ridgeway, Bedfordshire, September

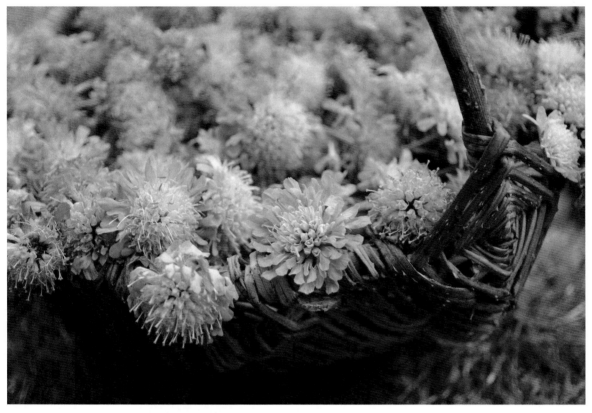

Scabious syrup

- coughs
- asthma
- respiratory infections

Scabious syrup

The inspiration for this recipe came from John Parkinson, who published his magnum opus, *Theatrum Botanicum*, in 1640.

Put a handful or two of **scabious** above-ground parts, fresh or dried, in a saucepan with 2 tablespoons chopped **liquorice root**, 2 tablespoons **fennel seed**, 1 tablespoon **aniseed** and 6 **dates**, chopped.

Add enough **water** to cover the herbs. Put the lid on the saucepan and bring to the boil, then remove from heat and cool overnight. The next day, strain the liquid into a clean saucepan, and gently simmer until reduced by about a third. Pour into a warmed sterile bottle. It has a rich, sweet flavour that masks any bitterness from the scabious.

Dose: Take 4 or 5 teaspoons a day, for respiratory issues.

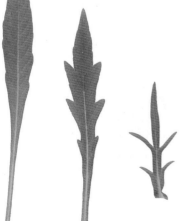

Leaf progression of common scabious, from basal (left) to topmost leaves (right)

Sea buckthorn *Hippophae rhamnoides*

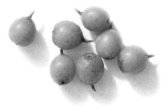

Sea buckthorn is a 'modern' herb, with an ancient Himalayan reputation but large-scale contemporary commercial exploitation. It is planted, especially in Central Asia and China, as a defence against desertification and erosion, and to fix sandy shores in Britain. Its vitamin- and antioxidant-rich orange berries are a superfood favourite; as well as skin and common cold treatments they have significant potential in elder health.

One recent September we picked and photographed the bright orange berries of sea buckthorn at Overstrand on the north Norfolk coast, and a few days later walked among the sea buckthorn specimens in the Mediterranean area at Kew Gardens.

Kew has many subspecies and cultivars of *Hippophae rhamnoides* (*Elaeagnus rhamnoides*) on show. Some were bushes and some trees up to 10m (33feet) high; they variously had thinner or thicker glaucous, willow-shaped leaves, and mostly bore smallish yellow or orange berries.

We agreed, after sampling and comparing as many berries as we could, that the most complex and satisfying taste came from the wild bush by the coast. Cultivation usually sweetens and simplifies flavour, and in this case the wild berries were larger and tangier.

Sea buckthorn berries are not easy to gather, because of the thorns and their squishiness if left too late, but are so well worth the effort. Choose your moment, and prepare for an experience that is intensely sweet, mixed with sourness, astringency and depth.

Winter migrant birds have always known the nutritious value of sea buckthorn berries, as did the ancient Greek, Chinese and Mongolian peoples. But no one knows whether the 'horse' element of the generic *Hippophae* name really refers to horses being given the berries to make their coat lustrous, as the original names suggest ('shining horse').

No matter, it is highly valued, and not only for the berries as food or medicine. Its roots grow fast and deep, stabilising sand and river banks, and are a first-line erosion and run-off defence in China. It is planted against desertification.

Moreover, the roots are also nitrogen-fixing, helping transform salty, sandy or acid soil into more fertile land for later crops. The density of the interlocked

**Elaeagnaceae
Sea buckthorn family**

Description: Spiny deciduous shrub, to 3m (10ft) tall, spreading vigorously by suckers, forming impenetrable thickets; narrow curling silvery leaves; flowers small, green, inconspicuous; they form plentiful green, later translucent orange berries, up to 1cm diameter, staying on the branch over winter.

Habitat: Sand dunes, sea shores as a rare British native; more commonly grown by roads, riverbanks, as an ornamental and to stabilise ground. Planted in deserts and mountains in Central and East Asia.

Distribution: Native in Europe, Russia, China. Introduced to Canada where it is called seaberry.

Related species: Spreading oleaster or autumn olive (*Elaeagnus umbellata*) is the only other British member of the family. Buckthorn (*Rhamnus cathartica*) and alder buckthorn (*Frangula alnus*) are in the unrelated Rhamnaceae, buckthorn, family.

Parts used: Berries, leaves.

branches and the profuseness of the thorns also quickly produce sea buckthorn thickets that form barriers to stock or human access and make efficient windbreaks.

This can be what is desired, but without rigorous maintenance can also become a runaway problem on the seashore and more so in civic planting – a pleasing show of berries in the autumn may well turn into an out-of-control jungle.

Use sea buckthorn for...
The first medicinal mention of sea buckthorn appears to be in a Tibetan text of the 8th century, where sea buckthorn ('rGyud bzi') features in 84 recipes.

Sea buckthorn's fame is much more recent, however, dating from the late 20th century, as is

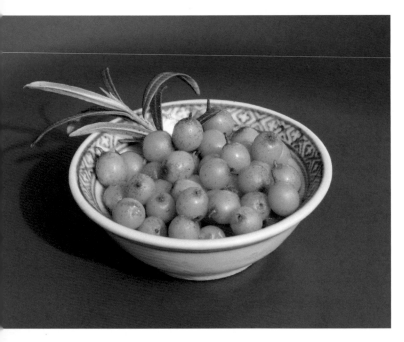

its separation from the buckthorn family and recognition as a separate genus. Buckthorn itself, *Rhamnus cathartica*, was formerly much more prized, as a purge. Parkinson's 1640 herbal, for example, scarcely mentions sea buckthorn or its berries.

But Parkinson does give an interesting recipe now long forgotten: *A decoction of the* [sea buckthorn] *leaves and inner barke thereof made in water whereunto a little allome* [alum] *is put is very good to wash the mouth when there is any inflammation or Ulcer or other disease therein.*

Modern emphasis is on sea buckthorn's rich resources of vitamins and minerals, in a heady cocktail of antioxidant benefits. The berries (and to a lesser extent the leaves) contain more vitamin C than oranges, more vitamin A (betacarotene) than carrots, high vitamin B2 and E; high omega 3 and 7; high potassium and quercetin; malic acid (giving the piquancy), flavonoids, unsaturated fatty acids, and so on.

The benefits are well advertised in many commercial products. We will pass by the claimed cancer and cardiovascular benefits, and highlight anti-inflammatory action and skin protection from UV radiation and free radical damage, via a sea buckthorn oil or sunscreen. The oil is said to have been used after the Chernobyl reactor disaster (1986) to treat radiation burns. It is more usually applied in the unsettling skin conditions psoriasis and eczema.

In this, there is a continuity here with older practice: Parkinson's list of skin conditions so treated in his time included *Saint Anthonies fire* [erysipelas] *and other fretting and eating Cankers* [cancers]… *pushes, wheales* [skin eruptions] *etc.*

Sea buckthorn oil – commercially made from the seeds, pulp or whole fruit – is easily absorbed by the skin, and the omega 7s strongly support mucous membranes and skin lipids. The berries' high vitamin C helps combat the common cold, in building resistance and as a prophylactic. Mixed with rose hips it is more palatable for children.

The benefit we will focus on, however, is sea buckthorn's dramatic end-of-options curative power and for convalescence. For example, an occasional whole berry helped Julie through six weeks of recovery and kept further infection at bay.

Regular use of the berries is said to protect against arteriosclerosis and improve the eyesight by assisting microcirculation. The berries are said to ease the menopause and to help maintain cognitive health. In other words, sea buckthorn should be promoted to the list of outstanding herbs, and wild ones at that, for elder health. Moreover it is a safe and long-term remedy.

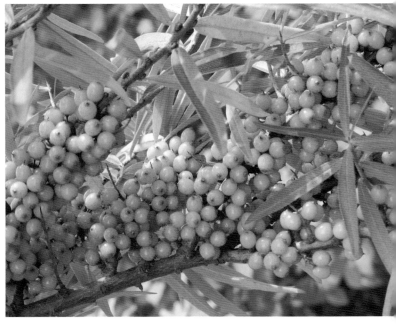

Modern research

Sea buckthorn capsules have become a well-known health supplement and superfood, sold online and in health shops.

The juice meanwhile has become a superfood trend. It was identified as an element of 'cutting-edge New Nordic cuisine' in a 2016 US press report. Expect to find it in 'healthy' cocktails and smoothies for a year or two yet. Perhaps the next taste will be a literal version of its old folk name 'Siberian pineapple'?

It has also been the subject of a surge of research in the present century, well summarised in a 2012 'remedial prospective'.

Among the more specific medicinal studies are a human trial in 2006 in which the oil eaten

The berries are very abundant, on short peduncles, ovate, or ovate-globular … red or yellow when ripe, succulent, smooth … gratefully acid, and are much eaten by the Tartars.
– Wilkes (1811)

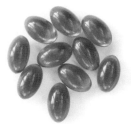

Sea buckthorn oil capsules

in porridge reduced risk factors of cardiovascular disease. A 2011 study on rats showed that the oil lessened cardiotoxicity.

The seed oil showed 'significant' wound-healing activity on rats with induced burns (2009), and it was a 'hopeful drug' for the prevention and treatment of liver fibrosis in other research (2003). A sea buckthorn wine intended to treat oxidative stress and hypercholesterolemia has been made (2013), and a herb tea from the leaves and twigs shows high rutin and antioxidative content (2016).

Harvesting sea buckthorn

What you need is the whole berries or their juice. Wear protective gauntlets against the thorns, and take care. It is easiest to collect by lifting the berries with a fork into a container, such as a plastic sandwich box. It will be messy, with unwanted bits of leaf and twigs, but these can be strained off at home. And think of the bracing sea air!

Some foragers advocate cutting off whole fruit-bearing branches and taking them home, until needed, but you should have express permission of the landowner to butcher the plant like this. It may be feasible where the thickets have overgrown and need clearing.

Store the berries or 'mush' in the fridge until needed; freezing will sweeten the overall taste (a process known as 'bletting').

Sea buckthorn kefir

Add 2 tablespoons **water kefir grains** and ¼ cup **light brown sugar** per litre of **water**. Leave to ferment for about 48 hours, then strain out the

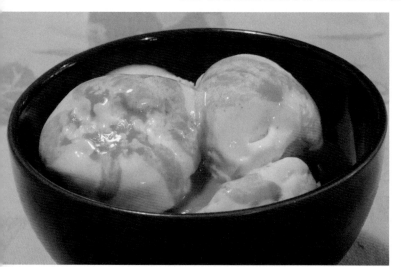

grains and pour the liquid into bottles. Fill each litre bottle ¾ full, then top up with **apple juice** and 1 to 2 tablespoons of **sea buckthorn juice**. It's ready to drink as soon as it becomes slightly fizzy, usually after 24 to 48 hours depending on the temperature and other factors.

Sea buckthorn with ice cream

One of the easiest and most delicious ways to use sea buckthorn is to pour the juice over your vanilla ice cream or glacé.

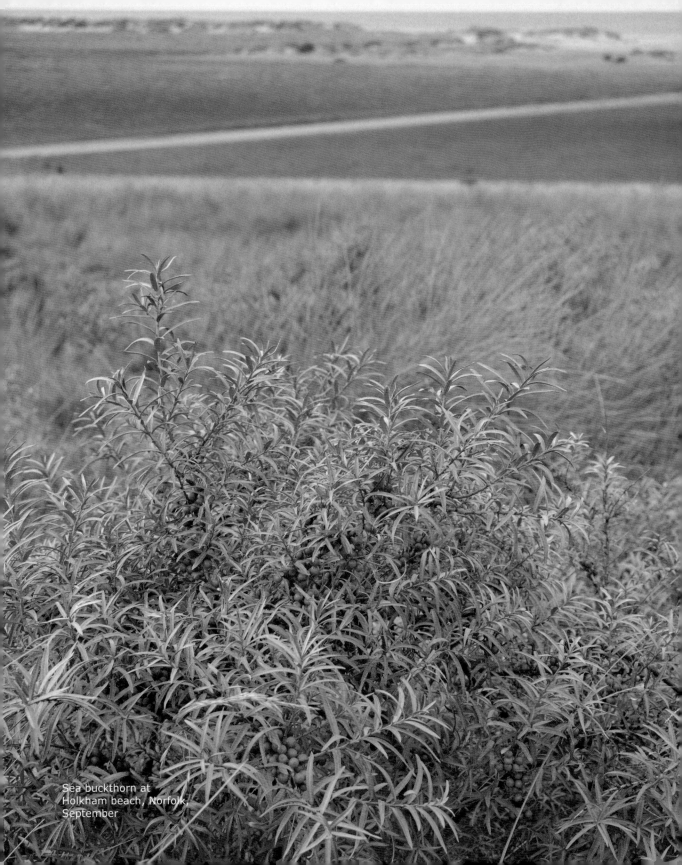

Sea buckthorn at
Holkham beach, Norfolk,
September

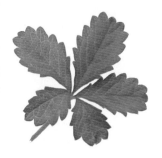

Silverweed, *Potentilla anserina*
Tormentil *Potentilla erecta*
& Cinquefoil *Potentilla reptans*

**Rosaceae
Rose family**

Description: Tormentil is generally erect, the other two are creeping; all have bright yellow flowers, with 5 petals, except for tormentil, usually with 4; silverweed leaves are distinctive; all have knobbly rootstocks, thickest, hardest and reddest in tormentil.

Habitat: All three similar: waysides, dunes, open woodland, while tormentil also favours heath and bog.

Distribution: All three widely distributed through the British Isles. Mainly in northern hemisphere; native to Europe and western Asia; silverweed native to North America, introduced to Australasia.

Related species: Near-relatives of agrimony and avens (also Rose family), with similar medicinal profiles as astringents.

Parts used: Leaves and flowers for silverweed and cinquefoil, roots for tormentil.

These three Potentilla species are the best-known medicinal plants in the genus, and have largely overlapping uses. Known since ancient Greek times for treating colitis, diarrhoea and mouth issues, they are strong astringents whose traditional but generally overlooked benefits are attracting new interest.

The Potentillas are a genus in the rose family, with some 17 species and subspecies in Britain, about 75 in Europe, and over 300 worldwide. The numbers are approximate because of the ease with which the Potentillas hybridise – a botanist's challenge, if not a nightmare – and with ongoing reclassification issues.

But those who practise wayside medicine are lucky in that the three leading medicinal Potentillas are readily recognisable. The genus name translates as 'little powerful one', and the reference is to medicinal potency, which we can now ascribe to high tannin content and resulting astringency.

Tormentil varies in height, being shorter in open heathland and taller in shaded woodland, but it is the one species that typically has four yellow petals. The other Potentillas usually have five, but silverweed is the only species to have silver-green foliage, especially noticeable below its

saw-tooth leaves. Cinquefoil or five-leaf grass has the usual five petals and leaves but also stretchy stolons, which can be a metre long.

Tormentil, *Potentilla erecta*, has also been known as blood root and tormenting root. The unusual English name is from medieval Latin *tormina,* meaning both colitis and the pain or torment it causes; some say it referred to the pain of toothache. Tormentil root, then, was taken to ease these unpleasant conditions – and still can be.

Julie's tormentil tincture is blood red, goes straight to the back of

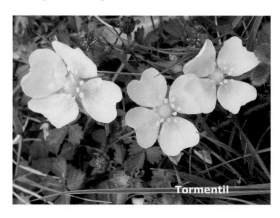
Tormentil

the throat and is very dry and astringent (Sir John Hill in 1812 called the effect 'austere'). It feels exactly right for treating throat and mouth issues.

The tannins are unusually high (sometimes over 20% of the physical constituents), enough to make tormentil roots useful in tanning leather, particularly in areas where oak trees are scarce.

Silverweed, *Potentilla anserina*, has other attractive names, such as prince's feathers, Argentina, fish bones, goosewort, goose tansy, bread and cheese, traveller's ease.

Most are explained by the leaf colour or plume-like form. *Argentina* is from *argent*, Latin for silver. *Anserina* means 'goose-like', for the way geese love to eat it (as do most stock animals, except for sheep). Traveller's ease is for an old use of leaves as a shoe lining.

Silverweed roots have been a significant famine food, from the Western Isles of Scotland to the Pacific Northwest of America. We love the tender, floury flavour of the boiled roots. The plant was so frequent in sandy shores that it was sometimes actively farmed, and dug up with ploughs.

As a source of starch, roots can be boiled or roasted and ground into flour, for bread or porridge. The 19th-century folklorist Alexander Carmichael called silverweed 'one of the seven breads of the Gael'.

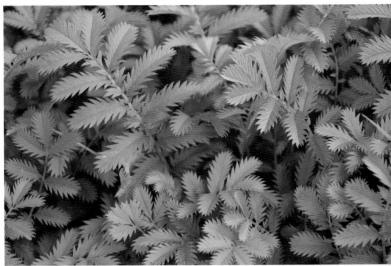

John Ray in 1670 thought they tasted like parsnips; John Wright in 2010 suggests chestnuts or Jerusalem artichokes.

Cinquefoil, *Potentilla reptans* (literally creeping cinquefoil), was also known as five-leaf grass – Mrs Grieve, as late as 1931, used this common name as her main heading. Other country names she reports include five-finger blossom, golden blossom and St Anthony's turnip.

Cinquefoil is aggressive, its reddish runners (stolons) making vigorous ground cover in bare ground, waysides and woodlands. It is an ancient companion of man. It seems that cinquefoil is the original Potentilla described by the Greek herbalist Dioscorides in the 1st century AD as *Pentaphyllon* (five leaves), and whose qualities as a fever remedy he espoused. Already in his time it was an anti-malarial herb in Egypt.

Silverweed leaves, above, and flower, below

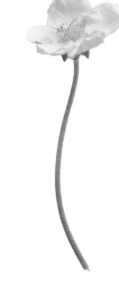

[Tormentil and silverweed] *... are two varieties of* Potentilla *and can be used interchangeably. However, Silverweed root ... is also an intestinal* relaxant/ spasmolytic, *and is also called Crampwort.*
– Holmes (2006)

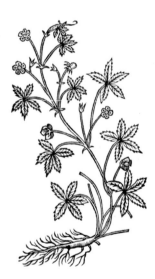

Cinquefoil, woodcut from Parkinson, *Theatrum Botanicum* (1640)

Use silverweed, tormentil and cinquefoil for...

The medicinal uses of these closely related species are largely interchangeable. French herbalist Jean Palaiseul calls them the 'potentil sisters'. Internally, the trio work effectively on 'tormenting' conditions such as acute diarrhoea and dysentery, colitis (both mucous and ulcerative forms), peptic and gastric ulcers, irritable bowel and Crohn's disease.

The astringent effect (most profound in **tormentil**) involves coating vessel membranes with a protective layer, being antiseptic to inflammation and helping stop discharges. John Pechey noted in 1707: *It dries, and is very astringent; wherefore there is no Remedy more proper for Fluxes of the Belly and Womb, than the Roots of Tormentil.*

Externally, a decoction or lotion of all three plants helps stop local bleeding in cuts and piles, or vaginal discharge; is soothing for sores, burns, sunburn or frostbite; and makes an excellent gargle for any throat or mouth-based inflammations. In addition to the tea as a drink, compresses soaked in it can be applied to sore places.

This broad range of treatment possibilities makes the Potentillas a very useful family to know for long-distance walkers and campers: whether facing sunburn or windburn, rucksack rash or saddle-sore pack animals, grazes, sore feet or gippy tummy, you are likely to have help at close hand. Chewing at the very hard root of tormentil or the other plants is good emergency relief for sore gums, toothache or mouth ulcers.

Specifically, **silverweed** is most used as a mouthwash, for sore gums and loose teeth, and is gentle enough (having more mucilage) for a baby's teething. Mixed with milk, it was popularly thought to remove freckles and lighten a sunburned complexion. A country name for silverweed, in Britain and the USA, is cramp weed, and the tea is excellent for a cramping stomach.

Supplementing its generic qualities, **cinquefoil** has a specialism as an intermittent fever remedy, as in ague or malaria.

All three plants are considered safe and non-toxic, but long-term use should be approached cautiously, especially for people suffering from persistent diarrhoeal-type issues.

Modern research

A 2009 study of *P. erecta* rhizomes on rats and mice showed no toxicity in strong dosages, confirming recent clinical human trials. These found no toxicity in using tormentil to treat ulcerative colitis in adults and rotavirus-induced diarrhoea in children.

In a major review (2014a), herbal treatments of ulcerative colitis (aloe vera gel, *P. erecta* extracts, wheat grass juice and curcumin) were assessed. Tormentil extracts at 2,400mg per day halved the clinical activity index and C-reactive protein levels of 16 patients, without side effects.

In 2003, 40 children, aged from 3 months to 7 years with rotavirus diarrhoea were given *P. erecta* drops, which cut duration of the diarrhoea to 3 days (placebo 5).

A study (2014b) found that four Potentilla species all showed free radical-scavenging effect (DPPH),

and influenced the viability and cytokine production of colon cell walls. Nine Potentilla species had proven antibacterial effects, notably against *H. pylori* (2008).

A 2011 study was the first to look at the *in vitro* inhibitory effects of *P. erecta* aerial parts extracts against cariogenic *Streptococcus* spp. strains in the human oral environment. Results suggested plant efficacy as a possible supplement for pharmaceutical products presently used for mouth care.

It [tormentil] is considered one of the safest and most powerful of our native aromatic astringents, and for its tonic properties has been termed 'English Sarsaparilla'.
– Grieve (1931)

Of all the many astringents available I find small doses of this one [tormentil] almost irreplaceable in the treatment of peptic, especially gastric ulcers.
– Barker (2001)

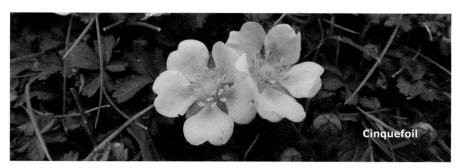
Cinquefoil

Potentilla root wine
We used cinquefoil root because it is our local abundant species, but tormentil or silverweed can be used the same way. Cinquefoil has a taproot with a swollen node at the top.

Pour 1 cup **white wine** into a small saucepan. Add a small handful of chopped cinquefoil **roots**, a couple of **cloves**, and a small piece of **cinnamon** stick. Simmer gently with the lid on for about 15 minutes, then remove from heat, add a teaspoon or two of **honey** and leave to cool. Bottle and label.

Take a small wineglassful three times a day for convalescence and weakness after an illness. It can also be used as a mouth rinse for gum problems.

Silverweed root sauté
Break off the swollen roots of **silverweed**, and simmer in a little **water** until tender. Sauté with butter or oil.

Potentilla root wine
- convalescence
- gum problems
- mouth ulcers
- loose bowels
- heavy periods

Sowthistle *Sonchus* spp.

**Asteraceae
Daisy family**

Description: Smooth sowthistle (*Sonchus oleraceus*) has smooth grey-green matt leaves and pale yellow flowers; prickly sowthistle (*S. asper*) is similar but with darker green and spiny 'thistly' leaves; perennial sowthistle (*S. arvensis*) is straggly with golden hairs and deep yellow flowers in late summer and autumn. Height depends on habitat.

Habitat: All three species like disturbed ground, arable fields, waysides; smooth sowthistle often found in gardens (and flowers in mild winters), perennial sowthistle on shorelines and riversides.

Distribution: All three species abundant across whole of British Isles except for the Scottish Highlands. Found worldwide, and classed as invasive in the US and Canada.

Related species: Marsh sowthistle (*S. palustris*) is a locally common fenland species in eastern England; can grow to 3m (10ft) tall.

Parts used: Stems and their latex, leaves, flowering tops; roots used in Asia.

The sowthistles comprise some 60 species worldwide, three of which are native to Europe and the Middle East, and have readily spread to temperate regions around the world. They are known, variously vilified or valued, as invasive arable weeds, foraged food and as a largely forgotten medicinal.

In terms of kinship, appearance and usefulness the sowthistles (genus *Sonchus*) lie somewhere between the dandelions and thistles. All are members of the vast Asteraceae or daisy family.

Julie remembers being made aware of the culinary possibilities of sowthistle by a passage from Margaret Roberts (1983) on its use in South Africa: *The Tswanas on our farm gather* [sowthistle] *from the mealieland* [corn] *edges and feed it to their pigs. In times of vegetable scarcity they make a mild and pleasant spinach-like dish from the young leaves and flowering tops, flavoured with chopped onion.*

But the reputation of sowthistles is mixed. Edible plant collector and grower Stephen Barstow points out they are classified as weeds in over a quarter of all countries (some 55 of 193 in the United Nations). Yet sowthistle is *just about the most useful vegetable in my garden* for most of his growing season.

Arthur Lee Jacobson, an American herb blogger, adds: *Sow Thistles are close cousins of lettuces, and the best*

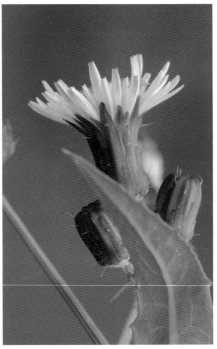
Smooth sowthistle

specimens are described more truly as wild salad herbs than as loathsome weeds. Taste the greens and maybe you'll agree.

The perennial sowthistle (*S. arvensis*) is an opportunist, pioneer plant and is thought to be an early coloniser after the retreat of the ice caps; it readily grows after fires, volcanoes, earthquakes and bombs; and in almost any soil, even in cracks in concrete. Modern farmers know it reproduces from root fragments after ploughing as well as from its seed parachutes.

The sowthistles are an ancient food and medicine, with British archaeological records from the Bronze Age in Derbyshire. It was certainly familiar in ancient Greece and Rome. Pliny tells a legend of Theseus, who was given a meal of sowthistle leaves by a poor peasant lady, Hecale, on his way to capture the Bull of Marathon.

It has not escaped modern commentators that this is akin to Popeye and his spinach, the leaves endowing the underdog hero with powers of courage and strength. As a green forage food sowthistle is found in most contemporary cultures of temperate regions, from *kucai* in China to *preboggión* in Italy, from *puwha* of the Maori of New Zealand to *morogo* or *imifino* in South Africa. This should hardly be surprising given that *oleraceus* (as in smooth sowthistle) means 'edible'.

It was noted by Pliny (1st century AD) as an everyday salad and vegetable item, and is still an ingredient in *insalata di campo* (field salad) in northern Italy, alongside chicory and dandelion. The related alpine blue sowthistle (*Cicerbita alpina*) is such a delicacy in the Trento and Veneto regions that its picking has had to be regulated.

Sowthistle is part of the Passover seder meal in Israel. Described as *maror* (bitter), it symbolises the bitterness of Jewish slavery.

In a less solemn context, American forager 'Wildman' Steve Brill says he can always count on sow thistles for the 'Wildman's Five-Boro Salad' featured at his mid-December annual Wild Party in New York. He comments that it is an appropriate dish for this event, since some guests eat like pigs!

So, is sowthistle animal or human food? It is both. It is sought out by pigs and fed to pigs, but has also been called dog's thistle, hare's lettuce and rabbit's meat. Various animals – chickens and cage birds too – know it is good for them.

The botanist John Ray had a view on this. He noted in 1690 that some people used sowthistle as a winter vegetable with salad, but *We leave it to be masticated by hares and rabbits.* That may be Ray's loss, because the cooked leaves taste sweetish, nutty and flavoursome.

Use sowthistle for...

The genus name *Sonchus* means hollow, referring to the stems. The stems of all species have a milky latex or juice, which has inspired popular names of milkwort, milkweed and milk thistle (all of these are distinct from milk thistle per se, *Silybum marianum*).

The juice is traditionally a wart medicine, as are most latex

[Common sowthistle] *is quoted as one of the world's worst weed plants and is said to be a pest in at least 55 countries. But to me, this is just about the most useful vegetable in my garden from late spring when the perennials are finished to late autumn. Do as I do, FEST ON PESTS!* – Barstow (2014)

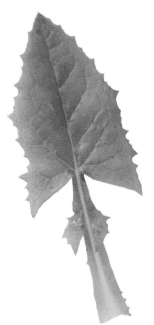

Smooth sowthistle leaf

Sow thistle may be a common weed throughout South Africa, but it is one with such healing properties that one is very pleased to see its appearance every year.
– Roberts (1983)

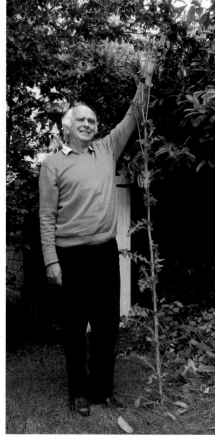

Matthew standing by a very tall prickly sowthistle in our garden, June

plants. It was seen as cooling in herbal action, and John Parkinson (1640) notes that *the herbe bruised or the juyce is profitably applied to all hot inflammations in the eyes, or wheresoever else.* It yielded a soothing salve applied on hot skin eruptions of various kinds, and can still be used in this way. The leaves were poulticed for the same purpose, and applied to wounds or to bring down fevers.

Parkinson adds another virtue now forgotten: *the juyce boyled is a sure remedy for deafnesse and singings and all other diseases in the ears.*

Coming closer to the present day, sowthistle was used by Chinese residents in early 1900s San Francisco, where it was said to benefit opium users trying to break their addiction. This finding requires modern examination, but sowthistle does have a reputation for treating addiction and anxiety in general.

Recent research explains sowthistle as protective for the liver and kidneys through its polyphenol content, with free radical-scavenging properties. This is reflected in a former reputation as a hepatitis herb. In Nepal the juice of the root is used to clear the bile ducts.

One traditional use that has modern support is for using the latex diluted in a liquid to treat cough, asthma and bronchitis. Parkinson again: *the milke that is taken from the stalkes when they are broken, given in drinke, is beneficial to those that are shortwinded and have a weesing withall.*

A final recommendation from Parkinson is that the distilled water of sowthistle is fit for 'the daintiest stomach' and is 'wonderfully good' as a face wash.

In China the local sowthistle is used by older people for maintaining vitality and virility; it has been used clinically for erectile dysfunction, and for 'strangury' (small quantities of urine) or dysuria (painful urination).

Modern research

If older uses of sowthistle are impressive and perhaps should never have been forgotten, white-coat research is adding some remarkable potential extensions.

In significant New Zealand findings Thompson & Shaw (2002) show that use of sowthistle (and/or watercress) in Maori diets may reduce their colorectal cancer levels, compared with non-Maori peoples. The figures per 100,000 people were 22.2 for Maoris and 43.7 for non-Maoris. Disadvantaged in most lifestyle indices, the Maori were nonetheless at lower risk of this form of cancer, and use of these plants in their diet appeared to be the decisive factor.

Research in Pakistan (2012) confirmed that *S. asper* was protective against potassium chromate ingestion that led to male sexual dysfunction in rats. Other findings by the same team (2011) demonstrated that the same plant had 'remarkable capacity to scavenge' and its antioxidant phytochemicals lent it potential as a medicine against free radical-associated oxidative damage, especially in the liver and kidneys.

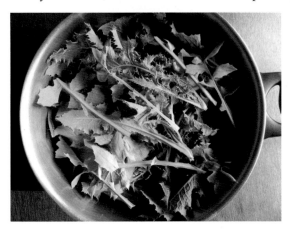 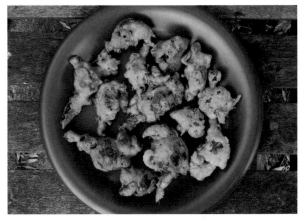

Harvesting sowthistle

Sowthistle can be harvested much of the year. We love eating the succulent flower buds, best picked when the first few flowers are opening. For eating the leaves, smooth sowthistle is best, but the leaves of prickly sowthistle can be used if the spines along the edges are trimmed off – easy with a pair of scissors. The pot above (left) contains both species.

Sowthistle pakora

Collect a few handfuls of sowthistle leaves or flower buds. Mix 250g/½ lb **gram** (chickpea flour), 1 teaspoon **baking powder** and ½ teaspoon **salt**, then stir in enough **water** to make a batter. Add your chopped-up **sowthistle**, and mix into the batter. Heat **vegetable oil** for deep frying. Drop tablespoons of the mixture into the hot oil and fry until golden, then drain. Eat while hot.

Speedwell

Veronica officinalis, V. beccabunga, V. chamaedrys, V. serpyllifolia

The speedwells look like tiny waifs and strays of the wayside flora, their bright blue flowers optimistic and pleasing. Actually they are tough wild survivors, once valued in mainstream European herbalism as a panacea and returning to favour for treating inflammations, nervous exhaustion and whooping cough.

**Plantaginaceae
Plantain family**

Description: Generally low-lying (to 50cm, 20in), mostly perennial herbs, usually with opposite leaves, round stems and attractive blue or violet spectrum four-petalled flowers either at tip or in leaf axils of the stem.

Habitat: Usually dry meadows, hedgerows and gardens, though brooklime grows in streams and some scarcer species are found in the Breckland heaths of East Anglia.

Distribution: Native to Europe, Western Asia, and naturalised in North America and Australasia.

Related species: The common wild British speedwells include brooklime (*Veronica beccabunga*) and the following speedwells: common field (*V. persica*), germander (*V. chamaedrys*), heath (*V. officinalis*), ivy-leaved (*V. hederofolia*), marsh (*V. scutellata*), slender (*V. filiformis*), thyme-leaved (*V. serpyllifolia*) and wall (*V. arvensis*).

Parts used: Above-ground parts.

The Veronicas or speedwells were once included in the figwort family (Scrophulariaceae) but are now classed as plantains (Plantaginaceae). Whatever their designation they remain small, eye-catching and sparky. As Mrs Grieve notes, the Veronica genus *contains some of our most beautiful native flowers, the speedwells*.

There are some 500 speedwell species worldwide, with about 27 in the British Isles, nine of which can be regarded as common (see related species). We focus on four: the 'official' or heath speedwell, brooklime, germander and thyme-leaved speedwell. We will treat them together, and propose that thyme-leaved speedwell should be added to the other more common species as a useful medicinal.

Our interest was piqued in a recent year when it seemed that speedwells were pursuing us. We were searching for heath speedwell, the official species used in medicine, but instead everywhere we went we found the similar but tiny thyme-leaved speedwell growing. We even returned home and found it abounding in our own garden, in plant pots and in the lawn, which hadn't been mown while we were away!

Why the nudges? To get in the mood to answer that we try out a spoonful each of a tincture of thyme-leaved speedwell made that summer.

First impression is of a light, aromatic, aniseedy taste, with a touch of sweet astringency. It goes straight to the third eye, leaving a euphoric, eye-cleaning sensation and a slight buzziness. After about two minutes the focus descends and spreads out, feeling like a spirit of goodwill that warms and wakens you up – not just in the heart, but the body as a whole.

It's rather wonderful, a calming yet uplifting sensation – maybe speedwells are to be understood as spiritual herbs operating on the UV spectrum, or have their physical uses just been replaced and forgotten? In any case we thought the plants were telling us something.

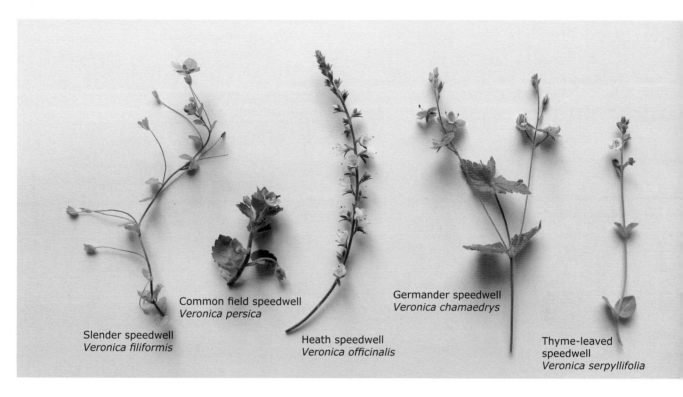

Slender speedwell
Veronica filiformis

Common field speedwell
Veronica persica

Heath speedwell
Veronica officinalis

Germander speedwell
Veronica chamaedrys

Thyme-leaved
speedwell
Veronica serpyllifolia

We did finally find heath speedwell growing, in Ireland, first in the Burren, then at Loughcrew on 2 July – the year's 182/183-day tipping point – there it was, official speedwell growing abundantly in the grass.

The common name 'speedwell' bears an old meaning of 'thrive' or 'get better', as in 'speed you well' or 'God speed'. The more formal 'Veronica' might derive from the Latin words *vero* and *eikon*, meaning 'true image'.

One story relates that a woman, later St Veronica, bathed the face of Christ as he carried the Cross, and the image left on the cloth resembled patterns on the flowers. This visage may not be clearly apparent, but do look at speedwell flowers with a hand lens. Observe their intricacy – the white border outside the deep azure blue of germander and its 'bird's eye' central white spot; the tiny leaves of thyme-leaved speedwell; the bright blue flowers and succulent, dark stems of brooklime; the pale violet petals with darker lines of heath speedwell, and so on.

Another rendering of 'Veronica' is from the Greek *phero* and *nike*, meaning 'I bring victory', referring to its plant's medicinal usefulness.

Take these name explanations for what they are worth, but there is no doubt that speedwells were cultivated in monastic gardens, and for centuries were

Identifying the most widespread British terrestrial speedwells

This little herb [Heath speedwell] *has wonderful healing properties seemingly out of all proportion to its size.*
– Roberts (1983)

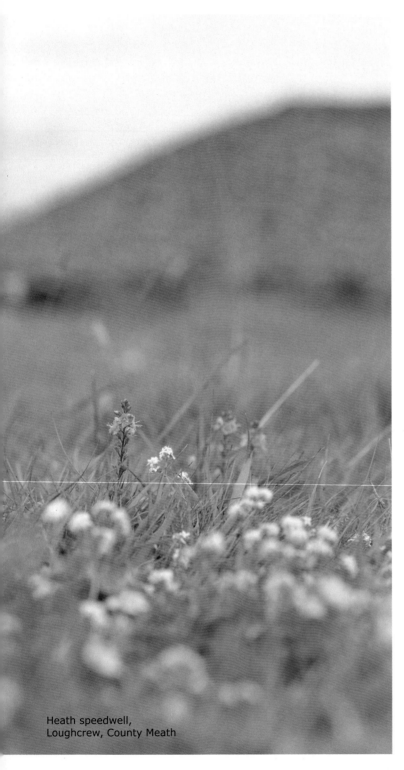
Heath speedwell,
Loughcrew, County Meath

part of mainstream European herbalism. The speedwells were valued, almost as a panacea, as expectorants for treating bronchitis and asthma, arthritis and rheumatism, for haemorrhages, for skin, liver and kidneys, and externally as wound herbs.

John Parkinson (1640) ascribed strong 'virtues' to the speedwell family, as *a singular good remedy for the Plague, and all Pestilentiall Fevers*, for leprosy, for *all manner of coughes and diseases of the brest and lunges*, for opening obstructions of the liver and spleen, for kidney stone and various tumours.

In 1690, heath speedwell was the subject of a 300-page monograph by Johannes Francke, the *Polychresta Herba Veronica*. Shortly thereafter John Pechey (in 1694, and a second edition in 1707) related how a *large Dose of the* [speedwell] *Decoction, taken for some time* expelled a kidney stone that a woman had had for sixteen years; a speedwell poultice removed the inflammation of 'an incurable Ulcer' in a man's leg; and the distilled water cured a woman's 'Fistula in the Breast'.

By the 19th century, however, speedwell had declined in medicinal regard and was mostly used as a tea substitute, known in France as *thé d'Europe*. The great Linnaeus in the previous century said he preferred this to black tea. We find it very restorative when we are feeling weary and tired.

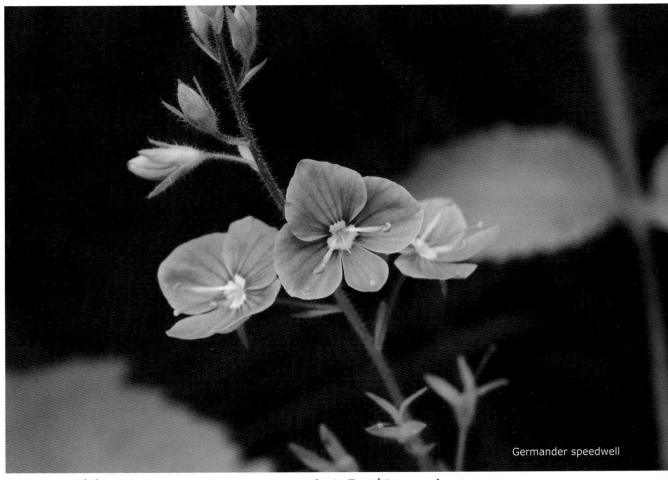

Germander speedwell

British herbalist Julian Barker summarises: *From its heady days of the 16th and 17th centuries where it was vaunted as panacea for all manner of digestive and respiratory troubles, including TB, it has slipped into the position, if remembered at all, of a good domestic beverage and digestive aid.*

This status was exacerbated in 1935 when the French botanist and systematiser of phytotherapy, Henri Leclerc, stated his opinion that speedwell tea was no more useful than the hot water used to make it. But this was a low point. Maria Treben in Austria and Margaret Roberts in South Africa, among others, have since championed speedwell and advocated its reintroduction into contemporary herbal medicine. We couldn't agree more.

Use speedwells for...
Treben points out that the Romans learned of speedwell from the Teutons, and it was a Roman compliment to say that someone has *as many good qualities as a speedwell.*

Only time and further research will tell whether it was right to drop this herb [Heath speedwell] *from our* materia medica.
– Hatfield (2007)

We suggest speedwells should be better regarded, for all-rounder status and for long-term, safe treatment of chronic but improvable conditions.

Try speedwell tea, distilled water or flower essence for yourself, and chances are you will experience similar sensations to those we had for the tincture.

It is as mentally clarifying as ground ivy tea but also feels nourishing in the body. The various speedwells we have tried have similar restorative effects, though with subtle differences eg slender speedwell lacks the grounding effect of germander speedwell.

In Ireland the plants were known as 'sore eyes', because an infusion was made into a lotion for tired eyes. At one time it shared the name 'eyebright' with *Euphrasia*, the better-known eyebright.

There is no reason why the tea cannot be used productively today for coughs or skin conditions, as it once was; similarly, a 'wound herb' does not lose its effectiveness just because it has gone out of fashion. Treben recommends speedwell compresses for *all inflamed, non-healing wounds*.

Interestingly, a Gaelic name for thyme-leaved speedwell translates as 'herb of the whooping cough', and modern research confirms that this plant contains scutellarin, a compound named from the calming herb skullcap.

The tea and other speedwell preparations can be considered whenever there is nervous exhaustion brought on by mental overload. Treben notes how two cups a day of equal amounts of horsetail and speedwell tea helped a priest remember the words in his sermons: he reportedly exclaimed: *my memory lapses disappeared surprisingly.*

<u>Brooklime</u> used to be eaten with watercress and oranges against scurvy. Modern forager John Wright doesn't much like the taste, but comes up with four reasons to write about brooklime: *it is edible, it's good for you, it's very common and the Latin name is fun.*

<u>Thyme-leaved speedwell</u> had a specific use for Native American Indians as a juice for earache, along with poultices for boils and a tea for chills and coughs.

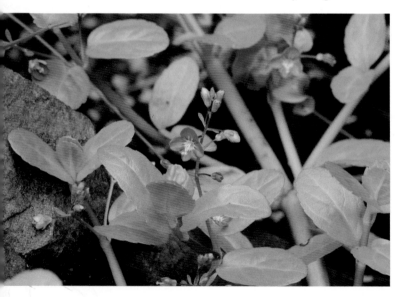

Brooklime, a non-terrestrial speedwell, with fleshy edible leaves and stems

Germander speedwell is mainly used for itchy skin and as a wound herb, while heath speedwell, the 'official' medicinal herb, shares the uses of the other species.

Modern research

V. officinalis had anti-inflammatory effects on human lung cells on a molecular level, but has yet to be tested in clinical trials. It was found to be a deinhibitor of COX 2 (2013). Another study of *V. officinalis* (1985) showed anti-gastric ulcer activity in rats and regenerated mucosa, seeming to confirm popular observation.

V. ciliata, a plant used in Traditional Chinese Medicine, showed (2014) strong antioxidant properties on the liver and was protective for acute hepatoxicity, as a free-radical scavenger.

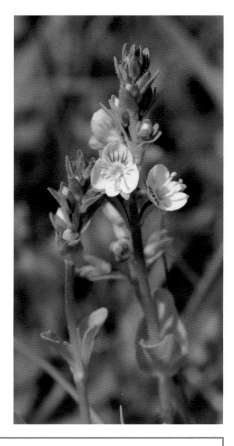

Thyme-leaved speedwell has tiny white flowers with delicate purple stripes

Speedwell tea
We usually choose germander speedwell, but use whichever species is common where you live. Put a few sprigs per person in a teapot and infuse in boiling water for about 20 minutes.

Speedwell foot bath
Use whichever species is common where you live – we have tried germander, field and ivy-leaved speedwells. Make a big pot of strong tea with your plants, then pour the plants and all into a basin large enough to put your feet in. Add warm water as necessary to top up. Soak your feet for about 20 minutes, adding new hot water if needed.

One of our students cycled home in record time after her speedwell foot bath, and said she felt energised all evening.

Germander speedwell flower essence
Follow the instructions for forget-me-not flower essence on page 291 to make your essence. Take a few drops on the tongue several times daily.

Speedwell tea
• restores
• energises

Speedwell foot bath
• restores
• energises
• refreshes tired feet

Germander speedwell flower essence
• clears the sight
• shifts awareness
• spiritual homesickness
• clarity of perception
• grounding

Sphagnum moss *Sphagnum* spp.

Sphagnaceae
Sphagnum family

Description: Dense colonies, with individuals up to 30cm (12in) high, with species varying from light green to red; branched, with stem leaves, inconspicuous flowers and brown, raised spore stalks.

Habitat: Peat bogs, a highly acidic, wet and anaerobic environment.

Distribution: Uplands of western and central Britain, especially Scotland and Ireland; northern Eurasia and North America, New Zealand, Chile.

Related species: The standard British and Irish field guide describes 34 species. These have similar medicinal and economic properties.

Parts used: Whole plant, dried and sorted.

[By using sphagnum] *Time and suffering are saved, as well as expense; the absorbent pads of moss are soft, elastic and very comfortable, easily packed and convenient to handle.*
– Grieve (1931)

Sphagnum moss (also peat or bog moss) has a spectacular capacity to absorb blood, is antiseptic, and easy to collect and transport. These properties made it a superb battlefield or foraging medicine; if you are cut while outdoors, yarrow or any astringent will stop bleeding and sphagnum can be the dressing.

Sphagnum moss is a denizen, and indeed creator, of peat bog habitats from tropics to poles, comprising some 120 species worldwide. In northern Eurasia and North America it was an early coloniser of the wasteland left by retreating ice caps. In effect it was a green bandage that healed the scars of the scourged frozen land under anaerobic pioneer vegetation that would become deep layers of peat.

The word 'bandage' is appropriate in human terms too, for sphagnum has been a wound dressing since prehistoric times; one Bronze Age warrior buried in Lothian had a chest wound packed with moss, while records of the Irish–Viking battle at Clontarf (1014) and the Scots–English encounter at Flodden (1513) refer to sphagnum dressings applied by field doctors.

Why is this plant so good as a natural bandage? The answer relates to sphagnum's structure. Its stem leaves consist of green or red photosynthetic cells and large, inert hyaline cells, which make up most of the plant's volume. The purpose of these dead cells is to absorb liquids and store them, which they do so well that some sphagnum species take in over 25 times their own weight in liquid.

A significant research finding is that pathogenic bacteria and human blood cells, as well as water, pass readily through sphagnum's hyaline cells. Hyaline cells have spiral thickening, which means they do not collapse if the moss dries out or is wrung out – that is, the moss is reusable.

Also the cell walls are rich in groups of pectic polysaccharides, known as sphagnan. These pectins ionise at low pH values (about 2, while the pH of blood is about 7.4). This means that sphagnum will lower the pH of its environment (ie acidify it) and inhibit pathogenic bacterial growth, which needs a more neutral-to-alkaline environment.

In practice, then, sphagnum will absorb astonishing quantities of water, blood, serum, pus and other liquids, while also being strongly antiseptic. In 1914–18 this made for a telling combination of life-supporting virtues in conditions

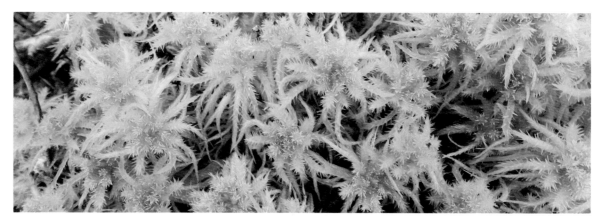

of trench warfare, where wounds easily suppurated and water soon became microbial-rich sewage.

Gathering of sphagnum for the British war effort owed much to an Edinburgh surgeon and RAMC lieutenant-colonel, Charles Walker Cathcart, who officially organised large-scale gathering, collection and forwarding to the battlefields.

Field surgeons found the moss superior to cotton wool for dressings: cotton was less absorbent, not antiseptic, less reusable and increasingly scarce as the war dragged on. Not only was the imported supply erratic but cotton was being diverted to the manufacture of explosives.

Meanwhile, crofters, girl guides and volunteers collected a cheap, endless supply of sphagnum from western Scotland and Dartmoor, and later Ireland. By 1918 one million dressings a month were sent to the trenches, including by then from Canada and the USA. One assistant in Edinburgh offered her thanks in verse (see right).

Garlic juice was routinely added to the sphagnum dressings as extra antiseptic. Many Allied lives were saved by such shrewd valuation of old herbal knowledge.

Other, civilian uses of sphagnum ought not to be forgotten: in various cultures, especially in Northern Europe, Canada and the Himalayas, it has made an easily gathered, free and soft material for nappies, menstrual pads and boot liners; it can stuff mattresses and pillows, and makes good insulation and animal bedding.

Solidified as peat, sphagnum was for long the traditional Irish fuel; New Zealand has a thriving trade in exporting the moss for hanging basket liners; it is used in potting soil mixes and is also a germination medium for orchids and fungi. It has been used to kill microbes and latterly to monitor air pollution.

Sphagnum is beautiful and eminently useful; it is, in the words of Simple Minds, a 'don't you (forget about me)' plant.

The doctors and the nurses
Look North with eager eyes,
And call on us to send them
The dressing that they prize.
No other is its equal –
In modest bulk it goes
Until it meets the gaping wound
Where the red life blood flows,
Then spreading, swelling in its might
It checks the fatal loss,
And kills the germ, and heals the hurt
– The kindly Sphagnum Moss.
– Mrs A M Smith, a member of the Edinburgh War Dressings Supply organisation, 1917

It is a good thing to know … when one is traveling in the wild, and needs to bandage a wound, because not only does the Sphagnum Moss act as an absorbent, but it seems to have antiseptic qualities. … one should not hesitate to use this moss.
– Coon (1957)

Sweet chestnut *Castanea sativa*

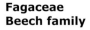

**Fagaceae
Beech family**

Description: Tall (to 30m, 100ft), deciduous tree, formerly coppiced; deeply fissured and twisted bark; longest leaves of any wild British tree (to 30cm, 1ft), deeply serrated, narrow, emerald green; long, beige male flower spikes and smaller green female flowers; sharply spiked cupules, each with 1 to 3 brown nuts with pointed ends.

Habitat: Usually planted in Britain, but self-propagates in south; nuts may not ripen in north.

Distribution: From Middle East, naturalised in Mediterranean and Northern Europe; also native to China, Japan; introduced to India, US, Australasia.

Related species: Not related to horse chestnut (*Aesculus hippocastanum*). *Castanea dentata* is the very tall (to 60m, 200ft) native North American species, decimated by blight in the first half of the 20th century, now being replanted; the Japanese sweet chestnut is *C. crenata*, and the Chinese form is *C. mollisima*.

Parts used: Leaves, nuts (fruit), buds.

Sweet chestnut is an ancient food crop of mountainous Mediterranean areas, the nuts often replacing grain as a source of flour. The leaves are a traditional medicinal treatment in respiratory conditions such as whooping cough and croup, for sore throat and diarrhoea, and the flowers are a Bach flower remedy. It is also in the news as a potential treatment for the 'superbug' MRSA that acts differently from antibiotics.

Sweet chestnut is an ancient food crop in the Mediterranean, being cultivated for over 4,000 years; older records exist for China, and in Japan it was used before rice.

The ground-up nuts are the source of an edible flour that has little protein or fat and no gluten, but twice as much starch as potato.

John Evelyn's pioneering book on trees, *Sylva* (1664), noted that *The bread of the flower* [flour] *is exceeding nutritive; 'tis a robust food, and makes women well complexion'd, as I have read.* He added the conventional wisdom that the nuts are liable to be windy, and could swell the belly and exacerbate colic.

But overall Evelyn was full of praise: the tree is *a magnificent and royal ornament* whose flour should be used by Britain's 'common people', rather than fed to pigs.

Sweet chestnut has long been used for animal fodder and litter, a timber and fuel, and the sweet Italian honey, *miele di castagno*.

Use sweet chestnut for...
Medicinally, says Thomas Bartram (1995), it is a *drying astringent, antirheumatic, antitussive*. It is best known for the last of these, as a leaf tea or tincture for dry and violent spasmodic coughs, such as whooping cough and croup, and as a gargle for sore throat.

Bartram suggests mixing 2 parts sweet chestnut and 1 part wild cherry bark for whooping cough. Pechey (1707) proposed a spoonful of the flour mixed with honey as 'a first-rate remedy' for coughs and 'spitting of blood'.

As a drying astringent the leaves and tincture remain effective for catarrh and diarrhoea. As an antirheumatic it has been found beneficial for muscular rheumatism, back pain and joints.

To complete its medicinal profile, sweet chestnut is one of the original 38 Bach Flower Remedies (taken to counteract despair and depression by faith and self-belief).

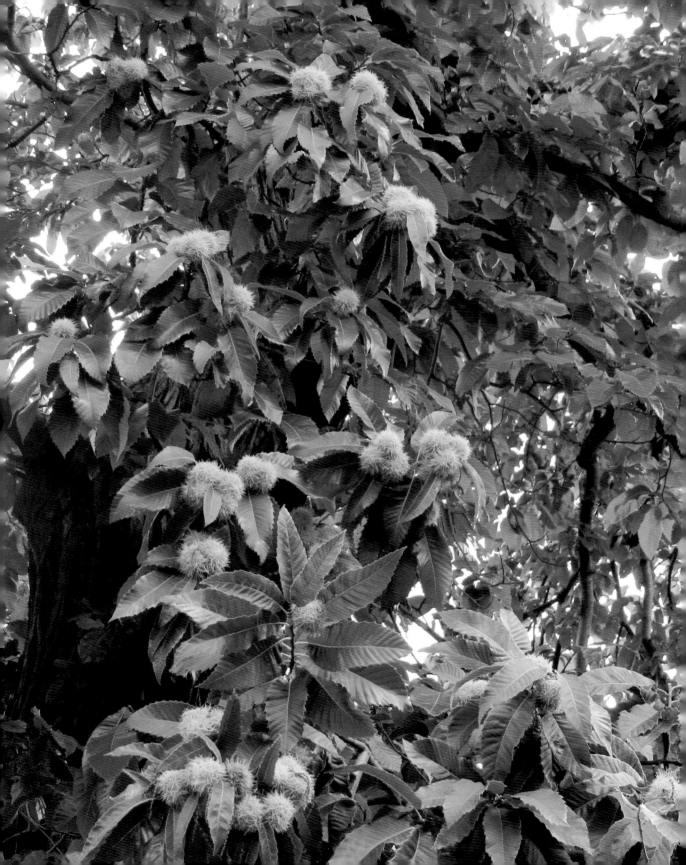

Sweet chestnut flowers, Norfolk, July

In conclusion, we have demonstrated that a folk-medical treatment [C. sativa] for skin inflammation and SSTIs that does not demonstrate 'typical' antibacterial activity (bacteriostatic or bactericidal) nevertheless shows great potential for development as a therapeutic due to its ability to specifically target and quench S. aureus virulence. The results of this study are important not only to future antibiotic discovery and development efforts, but are also vital to the validation of this previously poorly understood traditional medicine as an efficacious therapy, and not simply an unsubstantiated relict of folklore.
– Quave et al (2015)

The spring buds are a modern gemmotherapy treatment as a venous and lymphatic cleanser. Harvest the buds just before they open and extract in a mixture of alcohol, water and glycerine.

In rural southern Italy there is a current use of sweet chestnut leaves as a decoction for external treatment of skin infections, not found in British herblore.

Modern research
This empirically proven Italian method has been the focus of bioactive research by a team led by Dr Cassandra Quave of Atlanta's Emory University. The team tested over a hundred herbs used in Italian villagers' treatment of skin and soft tissue infections (SSTIs).

The study included the hospital 'superbug' MRSA (methicillin-resistant *Staphylococcus aureus*) as an SSTI, as it often presents as a skin infection.

Three herbs stood out powerfully: sweet chestnut, black horehound (*Ballota nigra*) and dwarf elder (*Sambucus ebulus*). A publication by Dr Quave and colleagues in August 2015 focused on sweet chestnut leaves, showing that ursene and oleanene derivatives (triterpenes) in the leaves inhibited quorum-sensing (QS) pathways, or cellular communication, in MRSA pathogens.

The process involved the leaf extract shutting off the QS ability of the bacteria to create toxins that usually cause tissue damage. Dr Quave commented: *At the same time, the extract doesn't disturb the normal, healthy bacteria on human skin. It's all about restoring balance.* A single 50 microgram dose of the chestnut leaf extract cleared up MRSA skin lesions in mice, preventing further tissue and red blood cell damage. The extract did not lose activity, or become resistant, even after two weeks of repeated exposure.

What is new here is that the 'disarming' of the communication channels of the pathogen offers an alternative to failing antibiotic methods that attempt to kill MRSA and eventually meet bacterial resistance. This is a significant step towards a post-antibiotic age.

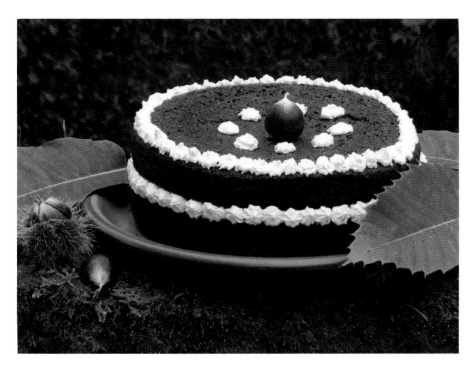

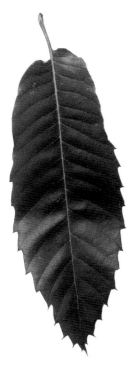

Sweet chestnut cake

John Pechey (right) would not approve, but we love this gluten-free cake, which can easily be vegan. Chestnut flour imparts a lovely flavour.

Preheat oven to 180°C. Sift into a large bowl: 2 cups **chestnut flour**, 1 cup **ground almonds**, ½ cup **cocoa powder**, 2 cups **light brown sugar**, 2 teaspoons **bicarbonate of soda**, 1 teaspoon **salt** and 3 tablespoons **linseed**, ground. Add 2 cups **water**, 2 tablespoons **vinegar**, 2 teaspoons **vanilla extract** and ½ cup melted **butter or coconut oil**.

Pour into two greased and floured 8-inch (20cm) round cake tins, and bake for 40 minutes, until a straw poked into the centre comes out clean. Cool, then chill in the refrigerator before removing carefully from the tins. Layer together with **whipped cream** or **coconut cream**.

Antibacterial ointment

Chop up a handful of **sweet chestnut leaves** and place in a small saucepan with enough **extra virgin olive oil** to cover. Heat gently for half an hour, then strain out the leaves, measure the oil and return to the pan.

Add 10g **beeswax** for every 100ml of oil. Heat and stir until the wax has melted, then pour the ointment into jars.

In some Places beyond Sea they make Bread and Frumenty of the Flower [flour] of the Nuts; but such sort of course Diet is in no way pleasing to the English, who (God be thanked) have Plenty of wholsom Food, and great Abundance of all things necessary.
– Pechey (1707)

Antibacterial ointment
- cuts
- grazes
- pimples
- boils
- skin infections

Thistle *Cirsium* spp.

Milk and blessed thistle are commercial-scale medicinal herbs, but other wild species, such as spear/bull, creeping/Canada and marsh thistle, have a traditional and potential healing reputation. Thistle's alkalinity in medicinal drinks and for treatment of joints and arthritis are exciting prospects.

**Asteraceae
Daisy family**

Description: Spiny biennials/perennials; with pink, purple or yellow flowerheads; often tall and erect; spear thistle (*Cirsium vulgare*) is downy, with single pink flowers, winged leaves; creeping thistle (*C. arvense*) has scented lilac flowers; marsh thistle (*C. palustre*) is reedy, with clustered flowers.

Habitat: Waste ground, hedgerows, waysides, fields; marsh thistle needs dampness.

Distribution: Widespread in Europe, Western Asia; naturalised in North America, Australasia, often termed invasive/noxious weeds.

Related species: Milk thistle (*Silybum marianum*) and blessed thistle (*Cnicus benedictus*) are commercial medicinals; others, eg musk (*Carduus nutans*), dwarf (*Cirsium acaule*), welted (*Carduus crispus*) and slender thistle (*Carduus tenuiflorus*), are similar medicinally.

Parts used: Roots, leaves, stems, flowers.

The thistle is the quintessential Scottish emblem, but 'Scotch thistle' is not native to Scotland – it is actually the cotton thistle (*Onopordum acanthium*), a white downy thistle from East Anglia.

We can even pin a date on the arrival of the symbolic Scotch thistle to its 'homeland'. It was the novelist Sir Walter Scott who, in 1822, masterminded the visit of George IV to Scotland, and quickly invented several 'traditions' for the monarch's pleasure, including restoring banned tartans / clans, and choosing a national thistle.

Oddly, there is a thistle that occurs almost wholly in Scotland – the melancholy thistle (*Cirsium heterophyllum*). But it is literally spineless, has soft flowers and is pretty rather than formidable – not at all apt for Scott's purposes.

If you want a wild native thistle for Scotland, or for any other part of the British Isles, look to spear thistle (*Cirsium vulgare*), creeping or field thistle (*C. arvense)* and marsh thistle (*C. palustre*). These are widespread members of the

Cardueae subgroup of non-latex-producing thistles, with burdocks, milk thistle, globe artichoke, knapweeds and cotton thistle.

For the record, the other subgroup of the true thistles is the Lactuceae, which do yield latex. Among these species are chicory, the lettuces, nippleworts, hawkbits, oxtongues, sowthistles, dandelions and mouse-ear hawkweeds.

Spines and latex are of course defensive mechanisms for thistles, making them unpalatable to animal browsers. For, as forager Miles Irving notes, if you have formidable defensive weapons like these you don't need additional bitterness as a deterrent.

This is why wild thistles make a good, sweet food source. This is additional to the cultivated eating thistles like artichoke and cardoon. So thistle roots, stalks, peeled stems and basal leaves are all targets for the forager, as they were in subsistence times before.

There are no poisonous thistles, for much the same reason, and

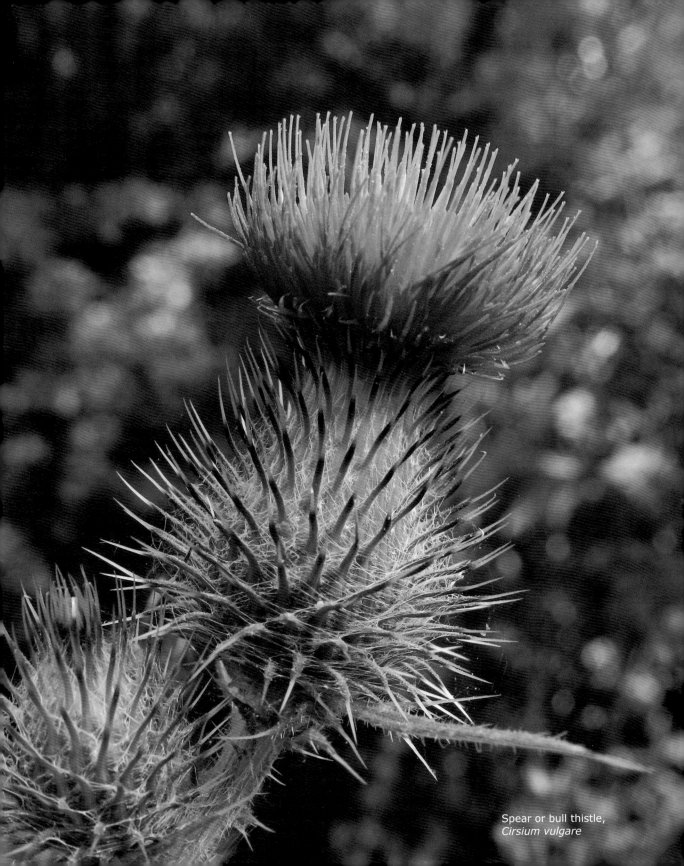

Spear or bull thistle,
Cirsium vulgare

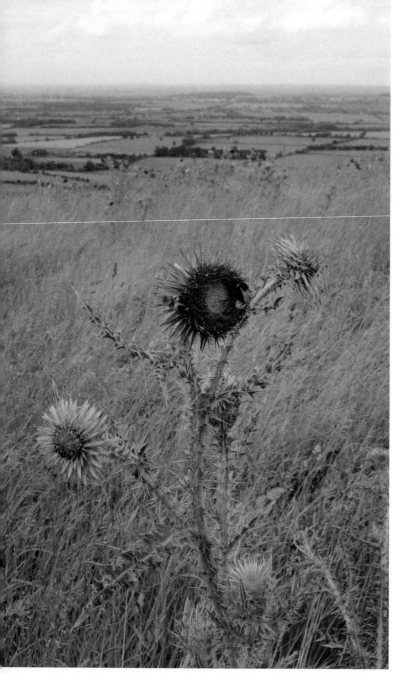

Musk thistle, *Carduus nutans*, White Horse Hill, Uffington, Oxfordshire, August

But these symbolic, edible plants also have a disreputable side in British farming. Spear thistle and creeping thistle are defined as injurious weeds under the Weeds Act 1959. This means that farmers must take steps to prevent their spread (along with three other plants: curled dock, broad-leaved dock and common ragwort).

Spear thistle is known as bull thistle in North America, and is noxious in nine US states. It has a similar status in Australia. Creeping thistle is called Canada thistle in the US, but is actually the imported European plant.

Use thistle for...
Milk thistle (*Silybum marianum*) and blessed thistle (*Cnicus benedictus*) are well-known and cultivated as herbal remedies, and can be found in any good herbal.

In 1812 Sir John Hill could state that milk thistle was *a very beautiful plant, common by roadsides.* Both thistles can still be found wild in the British Isles but now in insufficient abundance to consider them true 'wayside plants' and be included here.

Broadly speaking, the wild thistles share the hepatoprotective (liver-supporting) and cholagogue (bile-secreting) properties of the mainstream, cultivated thistles, but with lesser strength of action.

Milk thistle has the highest percentage of silibinin flavonoids,

indeed thistles will counteract strong poisons, including some fungi. The main downside for foragers, apart from getting behind the barrage of spines, is that perennial thistles, eg creeping thistle, become woody and tough.

which are the active constituent of the standardised extract silymarin. This is antioxidant, blocks damaging toxins in the liver and stimulates liver cell growth.

Silymarin is widely used in pharmaceutical products for liver cirrhosis, chronic hepatitis and prostate cancer treatment.

Spear thistle has an older reputation in cancer treatments, and as a cardiac tonic. In this light, herbalist Julian Barker suggests that cotton thistle *is perhaps deserving of the kind of investigation that Globe Artichoke has received.*

Creeping or Canada thistle was a leaf tea 'tonic' and diuretic, once used for treating tuberculosis internally and for skin eruptions, ulcers and poison ivy rash externally. Its root tea was for dysentery and diarrhoea. Another old country remedy, found in Scotland and various parts of England, was for a thistle tea for depression (as was melancholy thistle) or chronic headaches.

An altogether more modern take on thistle drinks is that of American herbalist Katrina Blair. She focuses on the alkalinity of thistle, as a juice or made into a chai, lemonade or tea.

Blair reminds us that almost all disease arises from over-acidity in the body. Modern life adds to this acidity via pollution, pesticides and preservatives, refined foods

and stress, among other toxic factors, but thistles can readily supply bioavailable alkalinity.

Julie can add another idea for improving alkalinity: regular deep breathing raises pH levels towards 7, the alkalinity threshold.

Modern research
There is a fascinating finding by American herbalist Matthew Alfs (2014) regarding potential use of bull (spear) thistle (*Cirsium vulgare*) tincture in treating spondyloarthropathy (SpA).

Alfs says clinical trials appear *to confirm a little-known, folk-medicinal tradition that* C. vulgare *supports the health of joints, tendons and ligaments in a most remarkable way.* Treatment was based on a tincture

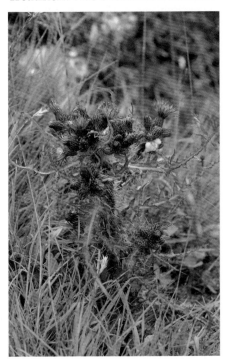

Marsh thistle, *Cirsium palustre*

[For] *A Chronical Head-Ach: ... take a large Tea-cup full of Carduus Tea, without Sugar, fasting for six or seven Mornings: Tried.* – Wesley (1765)

[For] *The Stone in the Kidneys: boil an Ounce of Thistle-root and four Drams of Liquorice in a Pint of Water. Drink half of it at a Time fasting.* – Wesley (1765)

Thistle stalks are a great source of mineralized, ... highly alkanized water, ... alive with the brilliance of the thistle plant. ... Thistle offers the body a true alkaline experience. – Blair (2014)

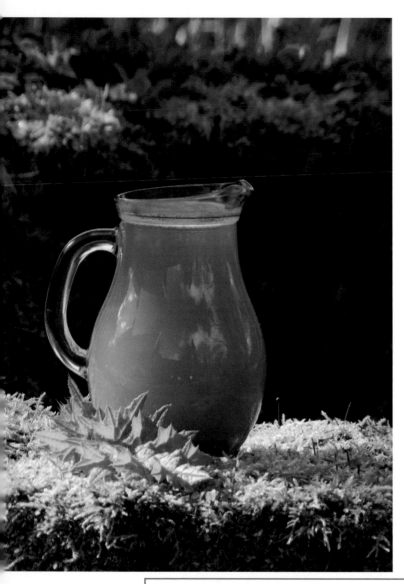

(100 proof vodka, ie 50% alcohol in UK terms), of first-year basal leaves, extracting for two to three weeks. The dosage was 6–10 drops per 20 lb of body weight, two to three times a day. Symptom relief and structural improvement were rapid, and were confirmed by medical doctors.

The mechanism appears to be bull thistle's action as a powerful anti-inflammatory, based on Native American oral traditions. The presence in bull thistle of the flavonoid genkwanin-4'O-glucoside (the only thistle to have it) may help the body's immune system identify and eliminate dormant bacteria.

The reports are promising for sufferers of juvenile SpA and some forms of arthritis caused by micro-organisms (hence not osteoarthritis, which is the result of joint overuse). Further trials will hopefully be undertaken.

Julie finds in her practice that a spear thistle tincture is helping patients who have Lyme disease with joint symptoms.

Green thistle energiser
- arthritis
- acidity
- liver health
- vitality

With thanks to Katrina Blair for inspiring this recipe

Green thistle energiser

We use spear thistle in this recipe, as it is the thistle we are fortunate (yes!) to have in our garden. It is biennial, so this drink is best made from the first-year rosette of leaves, before the thistle flowers in its second year. Cut at the base of the leaves where there are no spines.

Put in a blender: about 8 **thistle leaves** (or a whole thistle including roots if you are weeding), half an **unpeeled lemon**, and a 750ml bottle of **apple juice**. Blend until bright green. Strain the pulp out (gets rid of any spines), and drink the bright green liquid. This lemonade is delicious!

Valerian *Valeriana officinalis*

Valerian has been a useful food, perfume and medicine for over two thousand years, but with unexpected twists in its story. It has well-attested sedative and relaxant effects, but in some 'hot' patients can over-stimulate instead. Despite modern reservations on its root odour it is a valuable and effective herbal ally.

Wild valerian is a beautiful marsh and dryland plant, but its reputation is inseparable from its smell. The white-pink flowers have a vanilla-like odour that is delicate in single flowers and heady in colonies, while the smell of the roots is often dismissed in terms approaching disgust.

It would surprise our ancestors to read modern herbal accounts that describe dried valerian root as smelling like tom cats or old socks, as nauseating and unpleasant. An old Greek term *phu*, still applied in the name of some varieties of valerian, is sometimes said to be onomatopoeic, describing the sound of rejection (*phew!*) when encountering the roots.

This claim tells us much about a modern Western sensibility. In the past, valerian was thought to be sweet-smelling enough to place the roots among bedlinen, and a Japanese form of *Valeriana officinalis*, called kesso root, is a popular perfume, as is the related Indian valerian (*V. jatamansi*).

In modern commerce the oil of valerian is used in blended

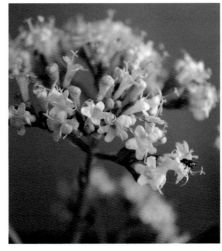

perfume oils, for 'mossy' and 'leathery' tones. Valerian essential oil in aromatherapy provides indications that its odour alone can have a sedative effect.

In addition to various medicinal uses, valerian leaves were a salad herb of the Anglo-Saxons. Gerard in 1597 related that valerian (or setwall, in another older name) was indispensable in *broths, pottage or physicall meats*.

A close relative is common cornsalad or lamb's lettuce (*Valerianella locusta*), a salad crop in our garden; it is locally wild in southern Britain and the US.

Caprifoliaceae
Honeysuckle family

Description: Tall, perennial, to 2m (6ft), with sparse, erect stems and Apiaceae-like umbels of white-pink small, scented flowers; leaflets opposite; roots, rhizomes and stolons, highly scented when dried.

Habitat: Widespread in marshy land in Britain but also in limestone grassland (it was once grown commercially in Derbyshire).

Distribution: Widespread in Britain and Ireland. Introduced in Canada and northern US.

Related species: Marsh valerian (*V. dioica*) is rare and non-medicinal; red valerian (*Centranthus ruber*) is common in southern Britain, but also non-medicinal. Common cornsalad (*Valerianella locusta*) is another relative, which grows wild on thin poor soils, and makes a garden salad vegetable. Over 150 species worldwide; native in temperate Western Europe, West-ern Asia, USA.

Parts used: Roots, above-ground parts.

Valerian roots: this dense mat is the usual source of medicinals, though we like to use the flowers.

Cats find the smell of valerian hard to resist, with old stories of them breaking into apothecary shops to get to it. Valerian was once a rat bait, and some say the Pied Piper of Hamelin attracted the town's rodents more by hidden valerian root in his pockets than his hypnotic flute-playing!

Away from the smell and taste of valerian, its history reveals an interesting case of one individual adapting a classic use of a plant for his personal health, thereby moving valerian to modern status.

Fabius Columna, or Fabio Colonna (1567–1650), was an early Italian plantsman, now largely forgotten. Born in Naples, he trained as a lawyer and linguist, but became interested in plants because from birth he had suffered from epilepsy and could not find a cure.

Contemporary physicians failing him, Columna went back fifteen hundred years to the source of European herbalism, Dioscorides. His *De Materia Medica* proposed valerian for similar purposes.

Columna dried valerian roots and swallowed the powder in various combinations of wine, water and milk. It was successful for him (though he may have relapsed later) and relieved symptoms in other people he treated too. Columna's *Phytobasanos* of 1592 publicised his experiences with valerian – and incidentally gave the world the flower term 'petal'.

The book made little impact in England, with the leading herbalists Gerard and Parkinson ignoring the epilepsy finding. John Pechey (1707), however, reported that Columna's use of valerian for epilepsy was *more effectual in this Case than the Roots of Male-Peony* [Paeonia mascula].

Columna's rediscovery of an ancient use for valerian opened

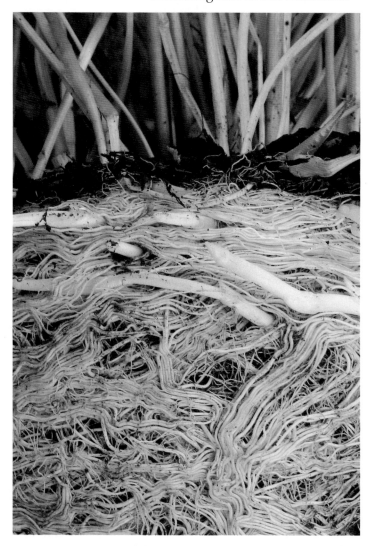

out its applications in treating nervous disorders more generally. By 1772 John Hill had published the 12th edition of his own book *The Virtue of Wild Valerian in Nervous Disorders*.

American herbalists of the 18th and 19th centuries helped bring valerian into mainstream medicine. It was included in the *U.S. Pharmacopoeia* as an anti-spasmodic and sleep aid from 1820 to 1936. Valerian remains 'official' as a sedative in the latest *British Herbal Pharmacopoeia* (1996).

But the smell issue was always there. The notorious tincture of valerian, Tincturea Valerianae ammoniata, mixing valerian root oil with oil of nutmeg and lemon, and ammonia, was described by Mrs Grieve (1931) as *an extremely nauseous and offensive preparation.*

Nonetheless it was a widely prescribed Victorian medicine. One example is Gustave Flaubert's novel, *Madame Bovary* (1856), where the country doctor Charles Bovary administers valerian to his fretful wife, Emma, for her nerves, along with camphor baths.

The tincture was used for shell-shock (now called post-traumatic stress disorder) in World War I and for treating civilians.

Finally, a word about **Red valerian** (*Centranthus ruber*), also known by a variety of attractive names like drunken sailor, bouncing Bess, pretty Betsy, kiss me quick, red money and scarlet lightning.

This member of the wider Valerian family was first recorded in Gerard's London garden in 1597. A fashionable introduction from Italy, he called it a 'great ornament' in his garden. It later spread around the west and south of England, and blows bright red in the wind from its haunts on city buildings. It has no medicinal uses, though the fleshy leaves are tender enough for spring salads.

... whereupon it hath been had (and is to this day among the poore people of our Northerne parts) in such veneration amongst them, that no broths, pottage or physicall meats are worth any thing, if Setwall [valerian] were not at an end.
– Gerard (1597)

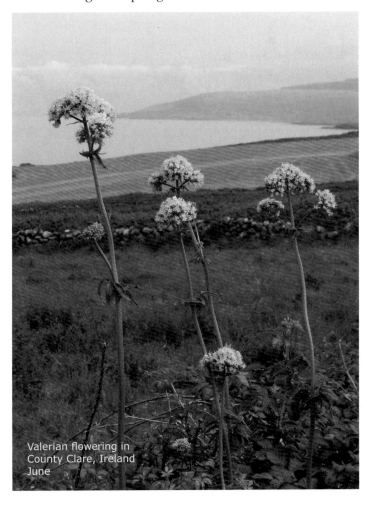

Valerian flowering in County Clare, Ireland June

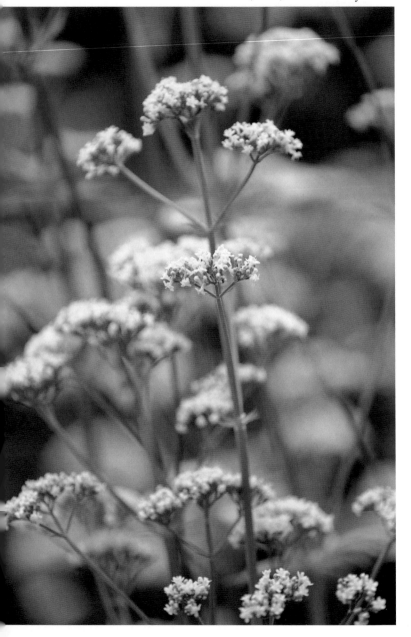
Above-ground parts of valerian: an under-used resource

Use valerian for...

The medieval accolade 'all-heal' was conferred on valerian, and this name could be an English version of Latin *valere*, to be well. Indeed, the plant was known to Parkinson (1640) as a standby for headaches, colds and coughs, eye problems, colic and modest wound-healing (another old name for it was 'cut finger').

It is worth remembering these more mundane properties of valerian, which remain useful alongside its proven value as a sedative and relaxant for stress and tensions, whether musculoskeletal or nervous.

The American herbalist 7Song makes a pertinent point on people's reactions to the plant as a sedative. He finds, and others have confirmed, that about one in nine or ten people become agitated, 'wired' rather than calmed by it. Indeed he says this reaction is the most common contrary effect of any herb he uses.

He has adopted a conservative protocol for valerian. He will see a new insomnia patient around the middle of the day, in his office, and give them a small amount of fresh root valerian tincture as an initial test for their reaction. Dosage and treatment details are adjusted in light of the patient's response.

Julie finds valerian well indicated when stress or headache is accompanied by digestive problems; the tincture, tea or capsules can help reduce anxiety and panic attacks, palpitations and high blood pressure. Valerian has proven efficacy for insomnia accompanied by worries, fears and high emotion.

As an antispasmodic valerian eases muscles of the stomach, shoulders and neck; the tightness of period pain and irritable bowel syndrome are also relieved.

Valerian combines well with other sedative and hypnotic remedies, like passionflower, hops, lemon balm and chamomile. It is best avoided when a patient is taking hypotensive medication, which can lead some to next-morning drowsiness, in which case drivers and users of heavy machinery should avoid the plant or the drug.

We think the above-ground parts should be used more, with milder but similar results for the patient. Baths, steam distillation and home flower essences are routes for further exploration. There are also commercial flower essences, including one for the nervous system and one for delight and joy.

Modern research

The pharmacology of valerian is complex, with over 150 compounds named already. Previous research efforts to identify specific compounds as causative, eg valepotriates or valeric acid, have latterly been displaced by emphasis on the synergistic positive actions of the plant as a whole. Or, use the herb!

Responses to valerian, as we have seen, can be paradoxical, and moreover its actions can vary, by locality (compare taller marshy plants with shorter limestone ones), seasonality, dosage, length of treatment (in case of cumulative effect) and preparation.

Such variations aside, valerian is in general safe, non-addictive (an important factor in sedatives) and effective as a dose-dependent herb for sleep-promotion.

Half a Spoonful of the Powder of the Root, before the Stalk springs, taken once or twice, in Wine, Water or Milk, relieves those that are seiz'd with the Falling-sickness [epilepsy].
– Pechey (1707)

Providing the dose is appropriate and the preparation is properly made and conserved from good quality plant material, Valerian is unquestionably the supreme remedy in all cases of nervous trouble either on its own or combined with other plants.
– Barker (2001)

Harvesting valerian

Traditionally, the roots of valerian are used, but we have found that the flowers also give good results. The flowers have a vanilla scent, but the tincture or glycerite has the same smell as the roots, which cats and some people love and others dislike. Our friend Glennie Kindred gave us a good tip for harvesting valerian root – grow it in a large pot sunk into the ground, then at the end of the summer lift the plant and harvest the roots that have been going round the inside of the pot. These can easily be trimmed, and the plant replanted with no ill effects.

Valerian flower glycerite

Pick enough **valerian flowers** to fill a jar. Add 4 parts **vegetable glycerine** and 1 part **vodka** to cover the flowers. Leave in a warm sunny place for 2 to 4 weeks, strain out and bottle the liquid.

Dosage: Take a teaspoonful before bed for help with sleep, or ½ teaspoon several times daily for anxiety.

Valerian flower glycerite
• insomnia
• anxiety
• digestive tension
• tension headache
• neck & shoulder tension

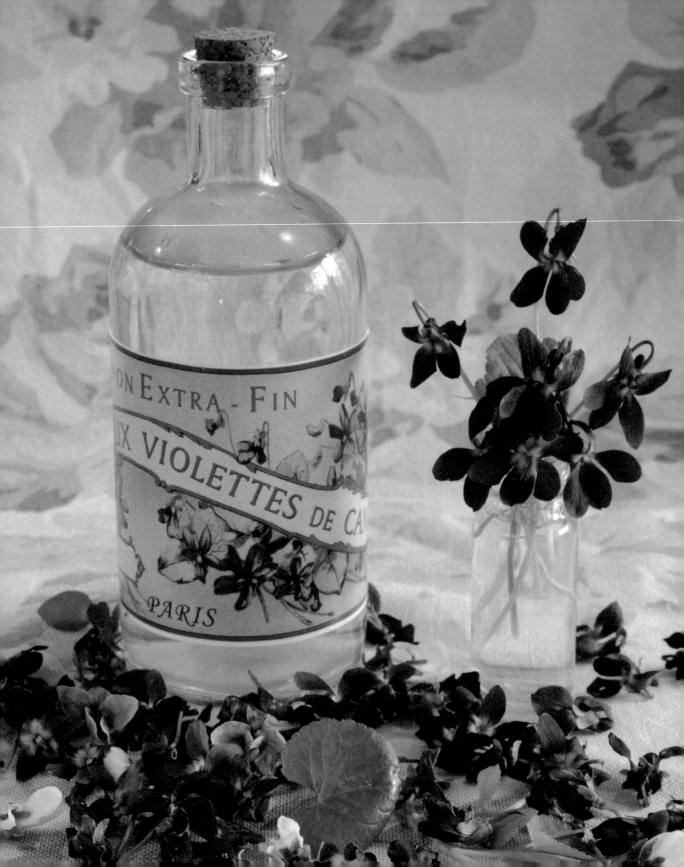

Violet *Viola odorata*

Sweet violets have always been valued for their beauty and scent, and as a syrup, crystallised sweet or a tea they are on the pleasant and child-friendly side of medicinal. They nonetheless act powerfully as expectorants for the respiratory tract, as cooling for hot and inflammatory conditions, particularly of the skin, and as an ally in some forms of cancer treatment.

Violaceae
Violet family

Description: Sweet violet (*Viola odorata*), named for its scent, spreads largely by runners; has early spring flowers, usually purple but can be white or pink-red, and heart-shaped leaves.

Habitat: Usually lowlands in British Isles (except mountain pansy, *V. lutea*), woods with light shade, roadsides, hedgebanks; prefer lime-rich soils (except marsh violet, *V. palustris*); pansies favour arable fields with disturbed ground.

Distribution: Europe, North America, India and China; also many garden species, which hybridise with wild violets or are escapes.

Related species: About 20 British Violas, notably common dog violet (*V. riviniana*); of the pansies field pansy (*V. arvensis*) is more abundant than heartsease, wild pansy (*V. tricolor*); in North America Canada violet (*V. canadensis*) is widespread, as is common blue violet (*V. sororia*). All Viola species can be used medicinally.

Parts used: Flowers, leaves, root.

Sweet violets have long been celebrated for their perfume and springtime beauty, peeping up in shady woods when the snowdrops finish. Dog violet species are later-flowering but equally beautiful, the rather disparaging 'dog' in their name referring to their lack of scent (in the same way as the unscented wild rose is a dog rose).

An early Western herbal, written by Macer in the 12th century, sets out the conventional valuation of violets: *Neither the rose colour ne the lylie may over-passe the violet, neither in beaute, neither in strengthe or vertue, neither in odour.*

Among the many poets who couldn't get enough of them was the Romantic Leigh Hunt, who in 1820 coined the phrase 'shrinking violet', for the plant's apparent modesty. He clearly wasn't aware that the carpet of purple violets he admired was the result of its vigorous and competitive runners.

A much earlier poet, Horace (65–8 BC), lamented that his fellow Romans spent more time growing violets to flavour their wine than growing olives. As the ancients knew, violets lend their colour and scent to liquids – wine, water (teas), syrup, vinegar or honey.

Violet flowers are cooling and demulcent, and had a reputation among the Greeks and Romans as a remedy for easing drunkenness and headaches, when applied to the head as a garland. Richard Surflet, in 1600, repeated the formula: *The flowers of March violets applied unto the brows, doe assuage the headach, which commeth of too much drinking and procure sleepe.*

Violets were also much used for the complexion – think of the Victorian obsession with violet water. Earlier, the Rev John Lightfoot, writing in 1777 of Scottish customs, advised his female readers irresistibly: *Anoint thy face with goat's milk in which violets have been infused and there is not a young prince on earth who would not be charmed with thy beauty.*

Etching of sweet violet and associated insects by Maria Sibylla Merian (1717), John Innes Historical Collections, courtesy of the John Innes Foundation

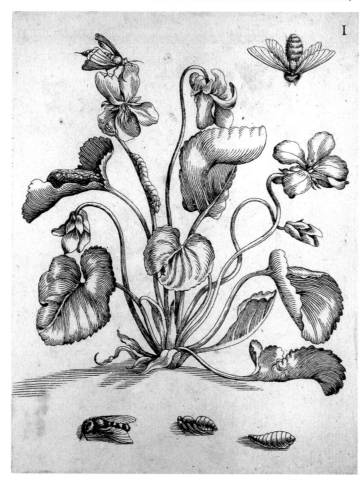

One 'young prince' we know well is Shakespeare's Hamlet. In an early scene of the play Laertes warns his sister Ophelia about Hamlet's volatile temperament. Sweet violet's smell is the chosen apt metaphor: *A violet in the youth of primy nature, / Forward, not permanent, sweet, not lasting, / The perfume and suppliance of a minute. / No more.*

What perfumiers (and dramatists) long knew pharmacologists confirm: compounds from violets called ionones have been isolated, which temporarily block our sense of smell, then release it. This means violets smell good to us over and over again – perhaps the secret of their enduring appeal?

It is not only the flowers that go into perfume. The famous Vera Violetta perfume (1892) used sweet violet leaves. Most violet perfume today, regrettably, is synthetic.

Use violets for...

The violet group (Violas) broadly consists of violets and pansies, including heartsease, but we are focused on true violets here. Heartsease is useful for heart concerns, skin problems such as eczema, lymphatic congestion, bladder irritation and cancer.

Behind violet's idealised image lies a coarser truth: it makes you spit. That is, violets are technically expectorants, and are still 'official' in Britain for this use. One area of their action is described as pectoral, for relieving chest issues such as harsh coughs, asthma, whooping cough and bronchitis.

The plant also contains mucilage, contributing to a demulcent effect of soothing an irritated respiratory tract, stomach or intestines. Violet is also used by herbalists for its anti-tumour action, especially for breast, lung and gastrointestinal cancers.

Violet syrup is a traditional and still-used remedy for children suffering from coughs and croup, with the additional benefit of lowering cough-related fevers. The syrup acts as a gentle juvenile laxative and was also used as a mouthwash for inflamed gums and a gargle for sore throats.

Violet's cooling properties as a tea or syrup come into play where there is excess heat or inflammation, including migraines with feelings of heat, and for arthritis and rheumatism. Externally, violet poultices will reduce the pain of swellings or cracked nipples, and ease inflammatory skin issues, such as eczema, psoriasis and acne, and cradle cap in babies.

The root of violet was once used as a purgative – much more 'medicinal' than the syrup, and stretching Culpeper's view of violet to its limit: … *a fine pleasing*

plant of Venus, of a mild nature and no way hurtful.

In cases when sickness prevents sleep, Askham's herbal (1550) recommended boiling violet plants in water and soaking the feet 'to the ancles'; when the patient goes to bed, the herb should be bound to his temples, *and he shall slepe wel, by the grace of God.*

American herb scientist James Duke suggests eating violet flowers can help treat varicose and spider veins. He reasons that the flowers contain generous amounts of rutin, which supports capillary wall integrity and strength.

An infusion made of violet leaves eases tension headaches and was a reputable cancer remedy from medieval times. Among South Africa's black population in the 1980s violet leaves were chewed

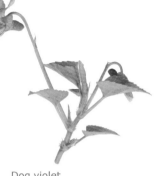

Dog violet

To dispel drunkenness and repel migraine/ The violet is sovereign;/ From heavy head it takes the pain,/ And from feverish cold delivers the brain.
– Regimen Sanitatis Salernitanum (The Salernitan Rule of Health), c. 12thc.

The decoction of Violets is good against all hote Fevers, and all inward inflammations, … The syrupe is good against the inflammations of the lungs and breast, the pleurisie and cough, and also against fevers, especially in children.
– Langham (1583)

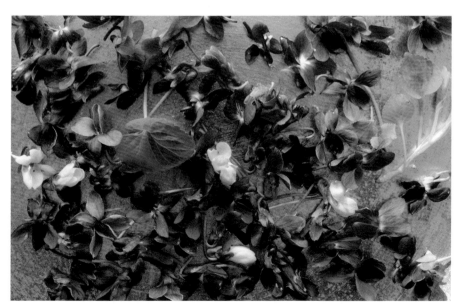

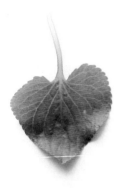

and also crushed to make a poultice applied to skin cancers and abnormal skin growths. This 'neoplastic' quality of violet now attracts clinical research, as does its potential value in breast and stomach cancer treatment, HIV and immune disorders.

Modern research
The Viola family is rich in novel plant-protective peptides called cyclotides, and 1995 research identified cycloviolacin O1.

A study into cycloviolacins in *Viola odorata* (2010a) found them to be promising chemosensitising agents against drug-resistant breast cancer; a similar study of the same compounds in *V. tricolor* (2010b) showed them to be cytotoxic in cancer cell lines.

The same cyclotides were isolated in Chinese medicinal herb *V. yedoensis* (*zi hua di ding*) (2008), and showed anti-HIV activity through disrupting HIV cell membranes. Another Chinese study (2011) found the same plant antibacterial to various forms of *Streptococcus* and to *E. coli* and *Salmonella* through its coumarin content.

Confirming traditional uses, Iranian research (2014) found an essential oil from *Viola odorata* (two drops taken nasally before sleep) offered relief to 50 patients with chronic insomnia.

A study (2015) of sweet violet, via a flower syrup was used in a double-blind randomised controlled trial to treat 182 children with intermittent asthma.

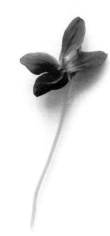

Sweet violet

Violet leaf tea
- sore throats
- coughs
- inflammation
- mild constipation

Violet glycerite
- mild asthma
- sore throats
- coughs
- inflammation
- mild constipation

Harvesting violets
Because sweet violet spreads mainly by runners rather than seed in spring (if there is a second flowering in autumn, the reverse is true), your picking of the flowers will not affect its viability. It also grows in colonies, but only pick what you need.

The leaves can be picked year round in milder areas, but are at their best in spring and summer. They can readily be dried for use thoughout the year.

Violet leaf tea
Use 2 or 3 fresh **leaves** or a rounded teaspoon of crumbled dried leaves per mug of **boiling water**. Leave to infuse for at least 5 minutes, then strain and drink.

Violet flower glycerite
Fill a small jar with **sweet violet flowers**, then pour in **vegetable glycerine** to fill. Shake and keep the jar in a warm place until the violets lose their colour, then strain and bottle.

Crystallised violets

The crystallising liquid used in this vegan recipe is best prepared ahead of time, as the gum arabic can take some time to dissolve.

Put in a small jar: 1 tablespoon **gum arabic powder** (also called Acacia gum) with 3 tablespoons **water or rosewater**. Shake well and leave overnight for the powder to dissolve. This mixture will keep in the fridge for months.

Pick about 20 **violets**, leaving some stalk on each flower. Dip a flower into the liquid, holding it by the stem. Shake off as much excess liquid as you can, then sprinkle the flower with **caster (superfine) sugar** and hang it on the edge of a cup or glass to dry – the stem has a handy bend that makes this easy. Once the cup rim is full, you can put it in an airing cupboard to speed drying, or the violets can be laid gently on a dehydrator tray to finish drying.

When the violets are dry, keep them in an airtight jar until you want to use them. Unlike violets that have been crystallised with egg white, these will keep for a year or more as long as they are stored airtight.

Sweet violets

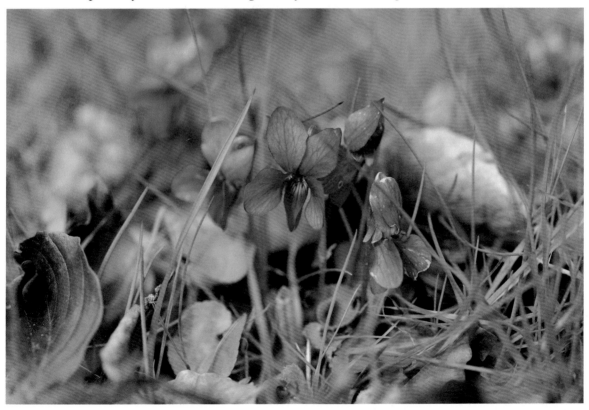

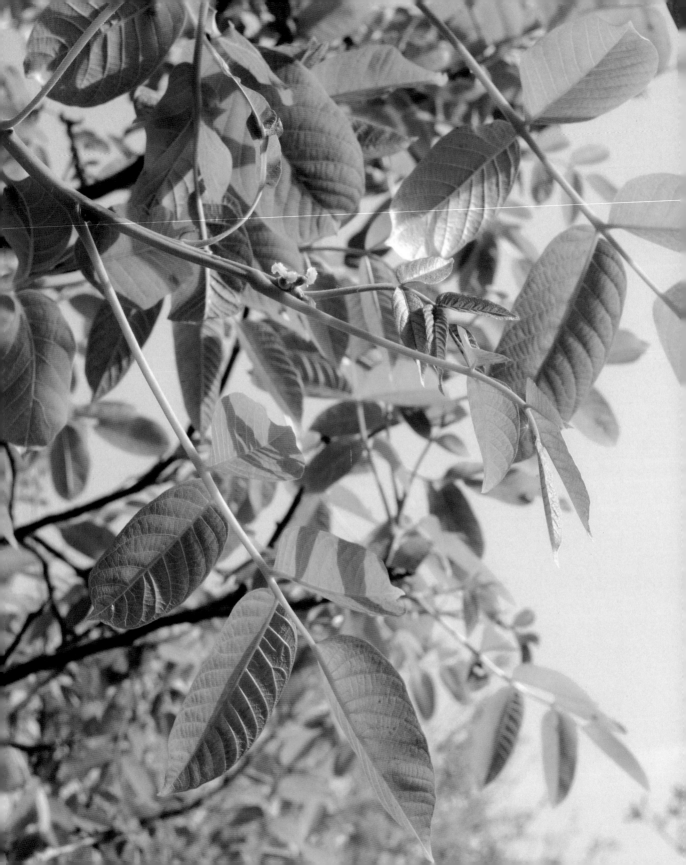

Walnut *Juglans regia*

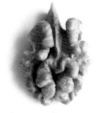

Walnut was thought by the Romans and Greeks to be native to Persia (Iran), from where it spread by trade both to the west and east in ancient times. Central Asia is now regarded as the likely origin. The nut, both green and brown, and leaves are the main parts used, and the tree enjoys an enviable reputation as a food, aphrodisiac, wood, oil, dye and medicine.

The scientific names of the common walnut recall an elite, even a divine past: *Juglans* meant 'nuts of Jupiter' and *regia* was royal. A 'food of the gods' to the Romans meant that walnuts conferred sexual vigour, and who was more vigorous than the god Jupiter? Among common mortals walnuts were symbolically thrown at Roman weddings.

We now know that walnuts contain plentiful arginine and zinc, both of which support the human sexual response. In more general terms eating walnuts regularly has long been known as good practice for maintaining vigorous health, especially in older age.

Walnuts have been a **food** from prehistoric times and across every culture where the tree grows. The nuts are light in weight and a handy size to gather and carry, and are highly nutritious.

In current terminology walnuts are a superfood that can reduce cholesterol levels and have a positive effect on heart health.

Walnuts have high levels of polyunsaturates, especially omega-3 fatty acids, which is good news for health but unfortunately not for the nut's storage. Even with modern freezing methods walnuts remain prone to rancidity.

The green, unripe rinds are edible, if sour, as well as being good for pickling. John Parkinson (1640) wrote that preserved green nuts in sugar made a 'dainty junket', and also good for 'weake stomackes'.

As a **wood**, walnut was the English cabinet-maker's timber of choice until imported mahogany largely supplanted it in the 18th century, though it remains popular. It proved unsuitable for house- or ship-building, however.

Walnut oil is used for salads and for cooking in southern Europe, but is costly, partly because it does not keep well. It also has too low a boiling point for good frying.

American black walnut in particular yields an excellent fast **dye**. A black stain emerges

Juglandaceae
Walnut family

Description: A graceful tree growing to 25m (80ft); lime-green oval leaves with 3 to 9 leaflets, aromatic but with a smell coarsening as leaves mature and dry; soft green husks harden into a shell, turning the familar beige brown; flesh is in two 'brain-like', nutritious halves.

Habitat: Likes temperate conditions but grows to 2,000m (7,000ft) altitude; sensitive to late frosts.

Distribution: Native to central Asia, introduced across Northern Hemisphere.

Related species: Black walnut (*Juglans nigra*) and butternut (white walnut) (*J. cinerea*) in North America, and paper-shell walnut (*J. mandschurica*) in China. Pecans and hickories are closely related North American nuts.

Parts used: Bark, leaves, husks, green and ripe nuts.

Why Wall-Nuts, having no affinity with a wall [should be so called]. *The truth is, Gual or Wall to the Old Dutch signifieth 'strange' or 'exotick' (whence Welsh, that is foreigners); these nuts being no natives of England or Europe, and probably first fetch'd from Persia.*
– Fuller (1682)

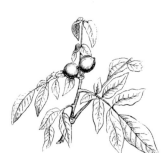

Walnut, etching by JC Loudon (1838)

easily from the nuts, both in green and ripe stages, and handling is inevitably messy – users beware!

The mature nut, as everybody knows, resembles the **human brain** in miniature (in Afghanistan the nut is called *charmarghz*, or 'four brains'). Herbalist William Coles, writing in 1657, said the nuts had 'the perfect Signature of the Head', meaning that walnuts resembled a brain so must be useful for brain treatment. And he just might be proved right.

Use walnut for...
Walnut species in the temperate world have similar medicinal actions, with common astringent, tonic and anti-inflammatory properties, among others.

Native Americans, for example, had a range of uses for black walnut (and later the settler-introduced common walnut): as an expectorant and purgative; to treat toothache, headache and greying hair; for colic, diarrhoea and skin complaints; as an insecticide and antifungal.

In early modern Europe walnut was a pestilence or plague herb. Culpeper, for one, stated of the green unripe nuts: *you shall find them exceeding comfortable to the stomach, they resist poison, and are a most excellent preservative against the Plague, inferior to none.*

In London's plague year of 1666, the eminent doctor Thomas

Willis offered *For the Poorer Sort, that Recipe of the Ancients*. This was two handfuls of rue, fig and walnut kernels (24 each), and half an ounce of salt, all beaten in a mortar. Parkinson in 1640 had attributed a similar plague recipe to Mithridates, king of Pontus (135–63 BC).

The action the apothecaries and physicians were looking for here was in the expectorant, emetic and purgative spectrum. Dried and powdered walnut bark taken as a tea could produce any of these responses, depending on dosage.

The green, unripe shell and the early green leaves have high astringency, utilised widely as a gargle for mouth and throat ulcers. In mild doses an infusion of green walnuts would soothe coughs, asthma and stomach ulcers, while stronger doses were for dissolving stones and cancerous tumours.

Other well-established uses included walnut as a blackening hair dye, though the Roman naturalist Pliny's two thousand-year-old recipe will be less popular now: boil green walnut husks with lead, ashes, oil and earthworms, and paste on the head.

Externally, cooled walnut tea was applied to inflammatory skin conditions such as eczema and herpes simplex via rubbing, compresses or in hand, foot or body baths. American herbalist Susun Weed suggests a black walnut tea soak for fungal toenails or a spritz of tincture for the skin.

A revived Appalachian use, led by Alabama herbalist Phyllis Light, is using the black husks to treat hypothyroidism or goitre. Matthew Wood has confirmed this in hundreds of cases, and calls black walnut *a superlative remedy for hypothyroid.*

While most former uses are now forgotten, walnut's value as an anti-diarrhoeal, insecticide and a dye remains current. Two of the many older virtues, those for skin inflammations and sweating, remain in the 'official' European pharmacopoeia for walnut today.

Modern research

Walnut is often known as 'brain food', and modern research shows why: it increases seratonin levels in the brain (2011). Walnuts as a nutritious food source improved learning and memory function (in rats using maze tests), but also prove a satisfying food in weight-reduction diets. Walnuts in a controlled diet reduced the effects of metabolic syndrome, which is a precursor of diabetes and cardiovascular disease (2012).

A sample of 200 people in a US study (2002) established a positive link between walnut intake and reduced levels of coronary heart disease, with the walnut sample showing lowered blood cholesterol and weight.

Forced-swimming tests in mice (2013) with and without walnut in the diet found that the walnut sample had an anti-fatigue action. This reinforces folk usage of walnuts as a sustaining, easily carried or gathered walking food.

Walnuts are linked to prevention of neurodegenerative disease by maintaining brain health through increasing age (2014a). Another study (2014b) demonstrated improvement in memory deficits and learning skills in mice with induced Alzheimer's disease.

It can be concluded that the benefit/ risk assessment for Juglans regia *leaves preparations is positive for use in therapeutical dosages in specific conditions of the mild superficial inflammatory conditions of skin and in excessive perspiration of hands and feet.*
– European Medicines Agency (2013)

Harvesting walnuts
The green nuts are harvested while the shells inside the husks are still soft for pickling or for making tincture or nocino, a green walnut liqueur. The leaves can be picked any time while they are green, and the ripe nuts are harvested in the autumn.

Muhammara
This Middle eastern walnut spread is traditionally served with pita bread. Mix in a food processor to make a coarse paste: 1 cup **walnuts**, ½ cup **breadcrumbs**, 3 large **roasted red peppers**, 1 teaspoon **cumin**, 2 tablespoons **pomegranate molasses** (or honey), 2 tablespoons **lemon juice**, ½ teaspoon **salt** and 3 tablespoons **extra virgin olive oil**.

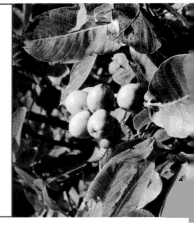

Wild carrot *Daucus carota,* ssp. *carota*

Wild carrot is a tough and beautiful umbellifer that has made the amazing transition from central Asian weed to worldwide food crop. Common on our roadsides, wild carrot can readily be distinguished from its poisonous cousin the hemlock and used medicinally, for urinary tract, reproductive and skincare benefit.

Apiaceae (Umbelliferae) Carrot family

Description: Biennial, to 1m (3ft); fine-leaved, delicate; central florets often red-purple within white umbel; long, fine-cut bracts, which turn upwards, forming a distinctive ball ('bird's nest'); short hairs; stem ridged, unmarked; seeds small, bristly.

Habitat: Grassland, roadsides, wasteland, especially with dry soils.

Distribution: Common in east and south of British Isles, less so upland areas of central Wales and Scotland; naturalised in North America, where it is usually named Queen Anne's lace.

Related species: Cultivated carrot (*D. carota* ssp. *sativus*) is the familiar orange vegetable, with dense green leaves, sometimes seen wild as an escape; sea carrot (*D. carota* ssp. *gummifer*) is local to southern British coasts.

Parts used: Roots, leaves, seeds.

In midsummer the massed white umbels of wild carrot lining the wayside look delicate and 'lacy'. But why the plant should be called Queen Anne's lace – the old British name and now the most frequently used North American name – is something of a mystery.

There are at least three contending Queen Annes and one Saint Anne, and in each case there is a drop or more of blood involved (especially in the case of Anne Boleyn, whose head was cut off). But the elusive historical truth is less important than the visual mnemonic: 'wild carrot' has lacy flowers with pink or purple florets in the centre.

The name and symbol no doubt helped countryfolk of old to distinguish the medicinal and nutritious wild carrot from its deadly poisonous cousin the hemlock (*Conium maculatum*). The two plants have an overlapping wayside habitat and similar British and American distribution; indeed, they can grow alongside and flower at much the same time. Fortunately, hemlock stems have purple or reddish blotches (the *maculatum* of its scientific name) on the stems, while wild carrot has none. These warning blotches are present even when hemlock is a small seedling.

Use wild carrot for…

The seeds of wild carrot are gathered for medicine-making. These are covered with small bristly hairs, which helps them stick to passing animals or humans. Certainly gardeners know that planting the seeds is fiddly because they adhere in a clump, which is why the seeds are often mixed with sand to separate them out and give control over the sowing distance.

The seeds can be eaten, in teaspoonful doses, but they are easier to digest if taken with a little oil, say hemp seed or olive oil (American herbalist Robin Rose Bennett favours almond butter). The oil helps activate the seeds; indeed, if you are taking carrot roots for their vitamin A or beta-carotene, an oil improves absorbtion. Commercial carrot seed oil is an essential oil distilled from wild carrot seed.

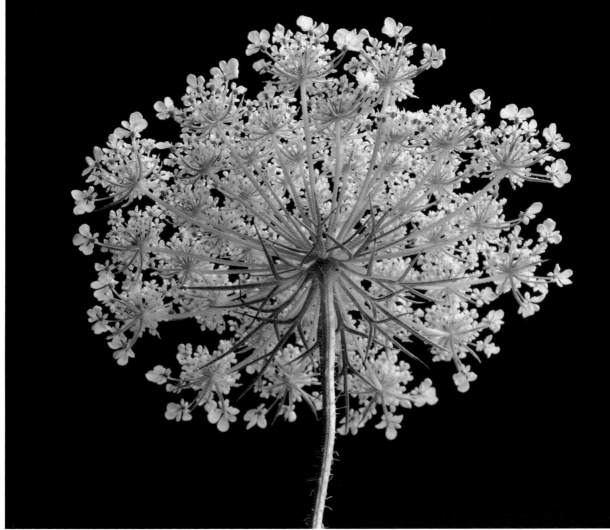

Carrot roots are also macerated in oil for use in skincare products and suntan lotions. Some people may be allergic to these products.

Carrot seeds and roots made into a tea (infusion or decoction respectively) are a traditional diuretic, with a specific action in eliminating urinary stones, and offering relief in urinary tract infections and cystitis. American herbalist Jim Mcdonald likes to combine carrot and goldenrod for urinary issues.

Herbalist Ryan Drum uses chopped carrot leaves or the juice in his gout remedy; he also found that men taking carrot for urinary discomfort had the inadvertent benefit of relief in the initial stages of BPH (benign prostate enlargement) and persistent prostatitis.

Carrot was used to treat worms: Julie's grandmother used grated carrot as a one-day mono-diet for pinworm. This also treats children's threadworms.

Wild carrot flower head, showing the finely divided bracts and hairy stem beneath

Wild carrot seed's double action of relaxing and stimulating unfolds almost entirely on urinary and reproductive functions.
– Holmes (2006)

I like to say that it [carrot] 'helps thread the urine through the kidneys'.
– Wood (1997)

Carrot ID: seedhead curls inwards as it matures (right), giving the characteristic 'bird's nest' effect; with the fine bracts still showing below; the leaf (below) is finely divided, and the whole plant is hairy, with no spots or blotches on the stems. Stems are solid, not hollow.

I regularly prescribe wild and/or domestic carrot greens for my gout patients. … This treatment is long-term (lifetime) to tolerance, especially for high-protein diet-induced gout. The best results are from finely chopped leaves in salads or soups, or leaves juiced in a wheatgrass juicer.
– Drum (nd)

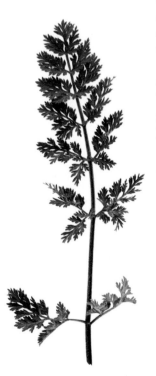

The seed has another familiar use as a 'morning-after' contraceptive. The mechanism seems to be that taking seed extracts prevents implantation of a recently fertilised egg, although stopping the extracts after a period of use may make the woman more fertile. This would explain why carrot seed is variously said to be both abortifacient and reproductive.

Herbalists have a spectrum of views on using carrot seed as a natural birth control, or as a possible strategy (ie taking the seeds and then stopping) for fertilisation. Endocrinal-level research into carrot's action is continuing, and for the time being no firm conclusions can be offered. Accordingly we'd suggest avoiding herbal use of carrot seed during pregnancy (as opposed to eating carrots normally).

Other uses for wild carrot include benefits for asthma sufferers – in ancient Greece carrots were known to calm wheezy horses; as a poultice for cancer sores – a remedy used in Suffolk until about 1920; for help with sugar and tobacco addictions – carry carrots with you and munch when the craving grows; and for a child or infant with diarrhoea a purée of the leaves or root is soothing and replaces lost nutrients. Finally, a carrot flower essence is good for organisation and creativity – it helped us organise our time while writing this book.

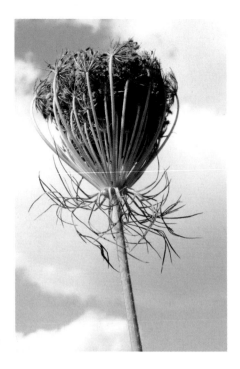

Modern research

Carrot consumption by laboratory rats (2003) modified normal cholesterol absorption and bile acids excretion, and increased antioxidant status. The study found: *these effects could be interesting for* [human] *cardiovascular protection.*

Human subjects drank fresh-squeezed carrot juice (16fl oz daily) for three months (2011a). The finding was that this may protect the cardiovascular system by increasing total antioxidant status and by decreasing lipid peroxidation independent of cardiovascular risk markers.

In a Chinese meta-study in 2014 carrot intake was inversely associated with prostate cancer risk, while the findings of a 2015 meta-study showed an inverse relationship between the consumption of carrots and the risk of gastric cancer.

Carrot juice containing β-carotene or purified β-carotene had antioxidative potential in preventing damage to lymphocyte DNA in smokers (2011b).

If cigarettes are cancer sticks, carrots are anti-*cancer sticks. ... So even if you don't quit smoking, you should still be munching on carrots.*
– Duke (1997)

[Carrot] *essence is for organisation, bringing a feeling of having enough time and support to be more relaxed, creative and spontaneous so that you can reach your goals.*
– Marjoram (nd)

Carrot top pesto

Put a couple of handfuls of **young carrot tops** in a saucepan with water to cover and boil for a few minutes, just until they start to wilt. Rinse them under cold water and squeeze dry.

Put in a food processor with 1 clove chopped **garlic**, ½ cup **whole almonds**, with enough **extra virgin olive oil** to blend into a paste (about ½ cup). Add **salt** and **pepper** to taste.

Grated pecorino or other cheese can also be added, as can dill tops and young ground elder leaves.

Carrot seed lozenges

Carrot seeds are covered in small bristles, so are more palatable ground to a powder. Grind 2 tablespoons **carrot seed** in an electric coffee mill or spice grinder. They take longer to grind than you might expect. Strain through a fine sieve to remove any larger bits. You'll end up with just under a tablespoon of powder. Add 1 tablespoon thick **tahini** (sesame paste) and 1 teaspoon of **set honey** (or to taste). Mix until smooth, then roll out with your hands into a thick pencil shape and refrigerate. Cut into a dozen small lozenges, which can be kept in the fridge or freezer, and eat one or two a day.

Carrot top pesto

- gout
- urinary discomfort
- high in potassium
- low libido

Carrot seed lozenges

- sluggish digestion
- tiredness
- convalescence
- low libido

Caution: Be certain of identifying wild carrot before using it. Avoid carrot seeds during pregnancy.

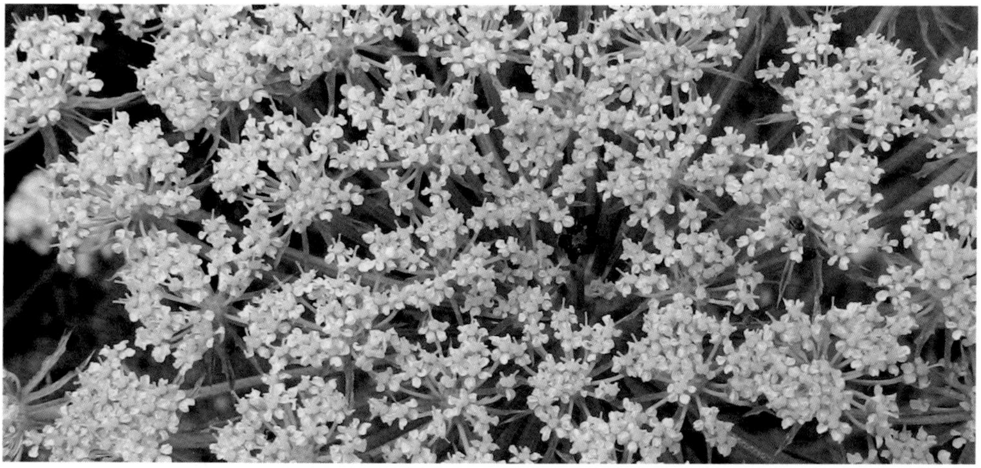

Wild carrot flowers usually have a pink or purple flower in the centre of the umbel

Wild strawberry *Fragaria vesca*

Rosaceae
Rose family

Description: Creeping, 5 to 30cm (3 to 10in) tall, with rooting runners and white flowers, which have rounded edges and no gaps between petals; veined, shiny and pointed trifoliate leaves; fruit resembles a miniature garden strawberry, with pips protruding, sepals turned down.

Habitat: Common on roadsides, hedgebanks, in coppiced woodland or rocky terrain; likes dry, often lime-based soils, eg quarries, railway embankments.

Distribution: Widespread across British Isles, Europe; an introduced alien in North American woods.

Related species: Barren strawberry (*Potentilla sterilis*) is also common, but its fruit is unstrawberry-like. Garden strawberry (*Fragaria* x *ananassa*) is larger, and may escape to waste ground; Virginia strawberry (*Fragaria virginiana*) is the wild American species, and *F. chiloensis* is the Chilean, once abundant from Chile to Alaska.

Parts used: Berries, leaves, root.

There is nothing quite like the sweet burst of flavour of a tiny wild strawberry, but medicinally the leaves are used to treat digestive and urinary disorders. Modern research is examining strawberry's phytochemical content, with powerful antioxidant potential for treating chronic conditions.

As one of the most recognisable and familiar fruits in the world, the strawberry has been enjoyed for its delicious taste, juiciness and sweet fragrance from Roman times – pips were found in an excavated latrine along Hadrian's Wall – and, from a time before writing, strawberry pips have been dug up at many Mesolithic and Neolithic archaeological sites across Europe.

An early enthusiast and one of the first to mention liking wild strawberries with cream was Cardinal Wolsey (1475–1530). A little later, the physician to James I and VI, Dr William Butler (1535–1618), summarised best the many gustatory tributes paid to this exquisite plant: *Doubtless God could have made a better berry, but doubtless God never did.*

Sugar, to our mind, is optional, and so indeed is cream, if the berries are picked in the sun and eaten. Adding vanilla to the cream will tempt us, while some people soak their berries first in orange juice or kirsch. Matthew's mother sprinkled hers with black pepper.

The origin of the name 'strawberry' is much debated, but one theory can be discounted, namely that it is a berry grown amid straw. This practice arrived centuries after the plant had already been named. More likely its common name is adapted from an Anglo-Saxon term for the berry that 'strews' or spreads itself. The Latin name leaves no doubt: *Fragaria* means sweet-smelling and *vesca* refers to something small.

Unusually, this native wild species did not develop into the strawberry of commerce, but has remained distinct. The strawberry we buy arose from the cross-breeding in the mid-18th century of two introduced species, one from North America and one from South America. Until then garden strawberries were essentially wild strawberries, uprooted and taken into the garden. John Parkinson explained in 1629: *I must also enforme you, that the wilde Strawberry that groweth in the Woods is our Garden Strawberry, but bettered by the soyle and transplanting.*

This was always a limit on strawberry production, with the wild species yielding small-sized fruit in relatively meagre quantities; it tasted wonderful and commanded high prices, but was easily bruised and had a short shelf life. Meeting impatient demand for cheap strawberries was a horticultural holy grail. It needed botanical exploration in the Americas to achieve it.

One notable consumer to make the most of strawberry's availability was the Napoleonic-era *grande dame* Madame Tallien (1773–1836), who reputedly poured 10kg (22lb) of strawberry juice at a time into her bath – but she did not bathe daily.

Meanwhile the wild strawberry has long had its own cultivar, the delicious Alpine strawberry (*F. vesca semperflorens*), or *Fraise des bois* in French.

Use strawberries for…
Eating strawberries is wonderful and indulgent, but is it also good for you? The answer, happily, is yes, whether wild strawberries or cultivated varieties.

Strawberry is alkalising, with high quantities of vitamins and phytochemicals that give it strong antioxidant properties. Its actions are traditionally described as diuretic, laxative and nutritive, and it has been used historically to treat urinary and kidney stones, gout, rheumatism and dysentery, among other conditions.

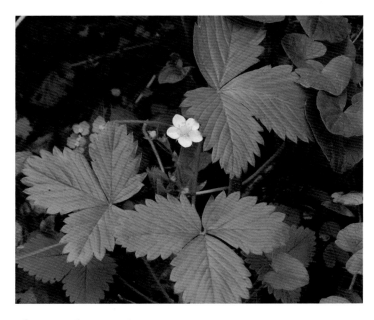

The great botanical systematiser Carl Linnaeus (1707–78) had success with a strawberry fast for his gout, and popularised the cure. Gout is a painful condition caused by excess uric acid, a by-product of purine breakdown, accumulating in the joints and forming crystals. Purines are compounds found in most foods, but particularly in meats and yeast products, including alcohol.

Recent research suggests it is the vitamin C of strawberries that keeps uric acid levels low, thus minimising the risk of gout.

Some researchers, on the other hand, say that strawberries also contain oxalates, which in some people contribute to conditions like stones, urinary tract infections, and indeed gout! The evidence is conflicting, and if you suffer from such conditions

… Mrs Elton, in all her apparatus of happiness, her large bonnet and her basket, was very ready to lead her way in gathering, accepting, or talking. Strawberries, and only strawberries, could now be thought or spoken of. 'The best fruit in England – every body's favourite – always wholesome. … delicious fruit – only too rich to be eaten much of … only objections to gathering strawberries the stooping – glaring sun – tired to death – could bear it no longer – must go and sit in the shade.'
– Jane Austen (1816)

The many valuable uses of strawberry have not been entirely understood and utilized.
– Wood (2008)

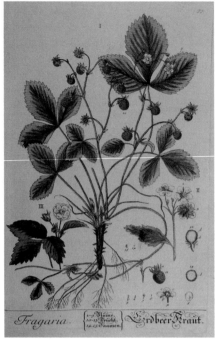

Wild strawberry, painting by Elizabeth Blackwell (1750), courtesy of the Wellcome Library

Fragaria. *Erdbeer Kraut.*

Eccentric esculent

Something to munch on when you next eat a strawberry: what we call its fruit or flesh is actually a swollen receptacle, also termed a false or accessory fruit. The real fruit is the achenes, the tiny pips, each containing a single seed, which are dotted on the *outside* of the fleshy receptacle. The cashew shares this quality of the true 'nut' (or pip) being actually the fruit.

Strawberries mislead us: we gobble down the false fruit while obliviously ingesting the real fruit and seeds: it is a brilliant plant trick for spreading itself far and wide! That is, along with the aggressive runners (properly stolons) that enable strawberries to colonise and make a dense ground cover.

and want to treat them through diet and herbs, you are advised to seek practitioner help. If you feel like emulating Linnaeus, taking strawberries as a gout fast should be part of a longer-term controlled diet, including avoiding high-purine foods and alcohol.

The alkalising effect of strawberry underlies its former use in treating tartar (mineralised tooth plaque).

The colour pigments in strawberries (anthocyanins) once served as a rouge to redden light-skinned faces and as medicine for sunburn, burns and minor skin ailments.

Thomas Green's *Universal Herbal* of 1820 says: *It would be unpardonable not to inform our fair readers of these attributes.* At the

same time, it should be noted that some people can suffer an allergic reaction to strawberry on the skin, including urticaria.

The best-known herbal use of strawberry is making an infusion of the leaves, whether using wild-gathered or cultivated forms. Similar to the leaf tea made from its rose family cousins, raspberries or blackberries, strawberry tea is mildly astringent. This astringency underlies its traditional use in relieving diarrhoea and dysentery and settling an over-acid stomach.

The roots as a decoction or tincture are stronger and more 'binding', but are less used than the leaves.

An early English reference to strawberry use is found in The *Old English Herbarium*, written around the year 1000, which recommends the juice of the wild plant, mixed with honey and pepper, for sufferers from asthma or abdominal pain.

The French herbalist Jean Palaiseul (1973) suggests that chilblains in winter can be prevented by rubbing the affected parts in summer with crushed strawberries, and using poultices of pulped strawberries overnight. A messy, if fragrant remedy!

Modern research
There has been much research into strawberries as functional foods, ie valuing it for its nutrients but also as a source of phytochemicals with

antioxidant power. For example, an influential paper by Hannum (2004) suggests that strawberry phytochemicals like ellagic acid and various flavonoids inhibit LDL-cholesterol oxidation and plaque stability and decrease tendency to thrombosis (ie reducing cardiovascular risk).

The same research also found that strawberry phytochemicals attack COX enzymes (ie reduce inflammatory processes), and have anti-cancer effects on tumours and carcinogenesis, with marked benefits for the ageing brain.

Research in 2014 suggests frozen strawberries have greater antioxidant potential than fresh or dried ones, while organically grown berries inhibited colon and breast cancer cells (2006), and Vitamin C had a synergistic action with the other compounds.

Other work (2015) indicates how polyphenols in strawberries are effective in treating 'oxidative stress-driven pathologies', which includes cancers, cardiovascular diseases, type II diabetes, obesity, neurodegenerative diseases and inflammation.

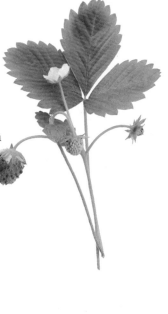

Harvesting wild strawberries is hard work, with lots of bending and scrambling, for what are often tiny fruits, but it is well worth the effort. When you find a precious patch of the ripe red fruit, take a shallow basket and line it with a tea towel, so that the collected berries are not crushing each other too much.

Distilled strawberry water
Set up a saucepan as described on page 233, placing the strawberries around your central bowl in a large saucepan and adding enough water to cover them. Place the lid on upside down, with ice on top, and heat gently. When most of the water containing the strawberries has evaporated and been collected in the bowl, remove the lid and bottle your strawberry water.
Dose: 1 dessertspoon internally as needed to calm the heart.

Strawberry leaf tea
This is best made with the fresh leaves, which being evergreen are available most of the year. For maximum flavour, crush the leaves gently with your hands or with a rolling pin before making the tea.

Use 3 or 4 **strawberry leaves** per mug of **boiling water**, steeped in a teapot for about 5 minutes. Strain as you pour into cups. It will be a pretty light yellow colour, with a delicate and refreshing taste. Try it with lemon added.

Of all the many astringents available I find small doses of this one [strawberry leaf] almost irreplaceable in the treatment of peptic, especially gastric ulcers.
– Barker (2001)

Distilled strawberry water
• eyewash for infections or grit in the eyes
• heart palpitations
• cleaning wounds and ulcers

Strawberry leaf tea
• peptic ulcers
• stomach over-acidity
• diarrhoea

Woundwort

Marsh woundwort, *Stachys palustris;* Hedge woundwort, *S. sylvatica*

**Lamiaceae
Deadnettle family**

Description: Both main species are perennials of up to a metre tall. Marsh woundwort (*Stachys palustris*) has spear-shaped leaves and pinkish-purple flowers. Hedge woundwort (*S. sylvatica*) has nettle-shaped leaves and dark reddish-purple flowers, and smells unpleasant when crushed.

Habitat: Marsh wound-wort grows in damp places; hedge wound-wort prefers woodland and shade, and is often a garden weed.

Distribution: Both are widely distributed in Britain and Ireland, and in much of Europe and Asia. Marsh woundwort is also found in parts of the US and Canada, where it is considered a weed.

Related species: Over 300 species in the genus worldwide. Field woundwort, *S. arvensis*, is a near-threatened annual weed on arable land. Betony, *S. officinalis*, is a well-known medicinal plant, common in England and Wales. The woolly white *S. byzantina*, lamb's ear, is often grown in gardens.

Parts used: Above-ground parts. The tuber of *S. palustris* is edible.

Marsh woundwort and hedge woundwort are, unsurprisingly, useful for treating wounds. They are also an effective remedy for insect bites and stings, an antispasmodic and show promise as cardioprotective and being useful in diabetes.

Also called hedgenettles, woundworts are closely related to the medicinal herb betony (or wood betony), *S. officinalis* syn. *Betonica officinalis*. The Chinese artichoke, *S. affinis*, is similar but is grown for its edible white tubers.

The edible swollen white roots of marsh woundwort are also very tasty as a vegetable, and are smoother and easier to clean. They can be eaten raw, being sweet and crunchy, and are delicious fried in a little butter or oil, having a flavour much like skirret.

John Gerard, writing in 1597, reports how he learnt the use of this herb from a labourer he met in Kent. Gerard was a barber-surgeon of some repute in London, and named the plant Clown's woundwort, because the man in question had 'clownishly' turned down Gerard's expert help and preferred to treat his scythe wound with his own home-made woundwort poultice.

Gerard's plant was almost certainly marsh woundwort, as his woodcut shows the small tubers that form among the roots.

Gerard found in his practice that woundwort worked much faster to heal wounds than the balm he had previously used.

He gives two examples of cases where it rapidly healed otherwise mortal wounds. One gentleman, Mr Edward Cartwright, had been stabbed through the base of the sternum into his lungs, and was dangerously feverish. *With this Clownes experiment and some of my*

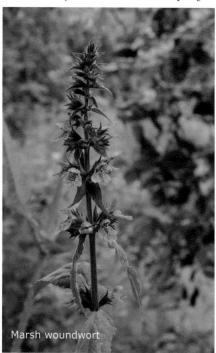
Marsh woundwort

foreknown helpes, Gerard mashed the woundwort with hog's grease and applied it. *By God's permission I perfectly cured* [him] *in a very short time.*

The second case was of a shoemaker's apprentice who had tried to kill himself by stabbing himself through the trachea, in the chest and twice in the abdomen.

Gerard says: *the which mortall wounds, by Gods permission, and the vertues of this herbe, I perfectly cured within twenty daies: for which the name of God be praised.*

Use woundwort for...

On a less dramatic scale, woundwort is a great first aid remedy for minor injuries. Simply crush the leaf in your hands or chew it, then apply. Drinking the tea as well will increase the healing effects. You can also use the tea to soak some gauze and apply it as a fomentation.

A fresh leaf also works well for insect bites and stings, crushed or chewed and rubbed on the bite. Marsh woundwort is more effective than hedge woundwort, but if the latter is all you have to hand it will still help.

Woundwort tea can be beneficial for hay fever and other allergies, as well as for headache and neuralgia. It has similar relaxing effects to betony, well known for being relaxing and protective for the nervous system.

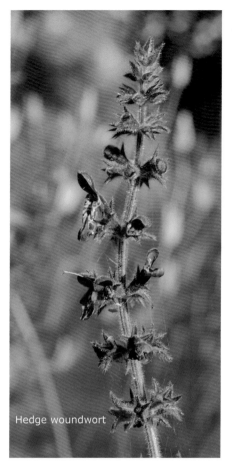

Hedge woundwort

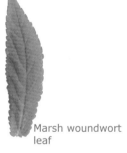

Marsh woundwort leaf

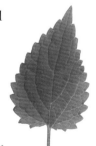

Hedge woundwort leaf

The leaves heerof stamped with Axungia or Hogs grease, and applied unto green wounds in manner of a pultis, doth heale them in such short time & in such absolute maner, that it is hard for any that hath not had the experience thereof to beleeve:
– Gerard (1597)

The stincking Dead Nettles, any of the kinds of them, boyled in wine and drunke, doth wonderfully helpe all inward wounds and hurts, bruises, falls or the like, and are singular good also for the spleene, and the diseases thereof: but especially for the hemorrhoides or piles.
– Parkinson (1640)

Try it for sleep – have a cup of the tea in the evening. It has been used for cramps (both externally and internally), and also used for gout and pains in the joints. Hand and foot baths using the warm tea are a good way to administer external treatments.

The astringency of both types of woundwort can be used to treat diarrhoea and dysentery. They can be combined with avens, tormentil, silverweed, cinquefoil, agrimony, oak, blackberry leaf and other astringent plants for gum problems, as a mouthwash.

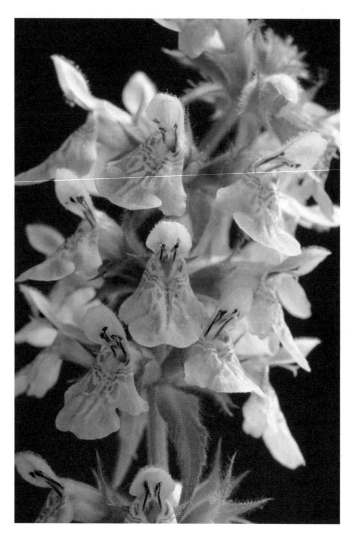

Marsh woundwort can help relax menstrual cramps, and can be combined with black horehound's antispasmodic effects. Woundwort also combines well with the same plant for anxiety and insomnia.

Parkinson mentions woundwort for cancers, a finding that is supported by results of modern research on the essential oil of marsh woundwort.

Modern research
A study of the essential oils of six Mediterranean species of *Stachys* (2009) found that the essential oil of *S. palustris* consisted mainly of carbonylic compounds, showed an anti-free radical effect and a 77% anti-proliferative effect on ACHN cell line (cancer).

Another study (2011) looked at the antibacterial and antifungal properties of the essential oils of 22 different species of *Stachys*. Most of them demonstrated moderate activity against the organisms tested.

Marsh woundwort flowers are beautiful in close-up

Woundwort fresh poultice
- pimples
- cuts & grazes
- insect bites & stings

Woundwort fresh poultice
Crush or chew a leaf or two and apply to insect bites and stings, cuts, grazes and spots. Marsh woundwort is the most effective.

Marsh woundwort roots
The white fleshy roots and tubers are easiest to harvest if you grow your marsh woundwort in a pot sunk into damp ground. In autumn, lift the plant from the pot and harvest the roots/tubers, then replant.

The fresh roots have a raw peanut flavour. When boiled gently so they still have a little crunch, they taste like starchy bean sprouts, very mild and pleasant. Serve with garlic butter, or add to stir fries.

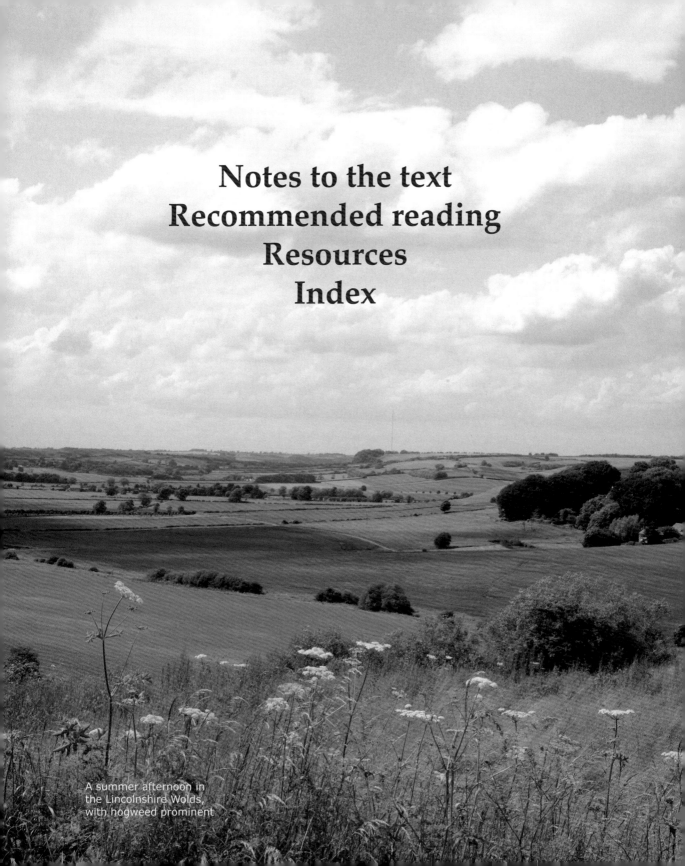

Notes to the text
Recommended reading
Resources
Index

A summer afternoon in
the Lincolnshire Wolds,
with hogweed prominent

Notes to the text

Full citation given in first reference only, thereafter author and page number (or short title if more than one work by that author). Original year of publication is in square brackets; place of publication London unless otherwise stated. For PubMed citations, we give date and reference number (or short title) for follow-up on a search engine. Scientific names of the plants are as given in The Plant List, www.theplantlist.org

Motto [222]: William Coles, *Adam in Eden: Nature's Paradise* (London, 1657) 54; Gabrielle Hatfield, *Memory, Wisdom and Healing* (Stroud, Glos, 1999) 14.

Preface [223]: Charles Dickens, *Nicholas Nickleby* (1839) ch 8; 'undiscovered country': see Robert Macfarlane, *The Wild Places* (2008 [2007] 225; Christopher Hedley, seminar (6 Dec 2014); David Winston, 'The American Extra Pharmacopoeia', www.herbalstudies.net [accessed 21 Sep 2016]; John Ruskin, qtd ES Rohde, *A Garden of Herbs* (Boston MA, 1931) 1.

Introduction [225]: Plantlife, *The Good Verge Guide* (2016).

Harvesting from the wayside [226]: James Green, *The Herbal Medicine-Maker's Handbook: A Home Manual* (Berkeley CA, 2000) 10; Nicholas Culpeper, *Pharmacopoeia Londinensis, Or, The London Dispensatory Further Adorned* (1653) 1–2; anon, *Stiches in Time: The Wayside Flowers & Country Remedies* (Brockhampton, Heref, 2008) 12; Dr John R Christopher, *School of Natural Healing* (Springville UT, 1996 [1976]) viii.

Using your wayside harvest [229]: Christopher Hedley & Non Shaw, *A Herbal Book of Making & Taking* (2016 [1993]) 2.

ALEXANDERS [236]: Geoffrey Grigson, *The Englishman's Flora* (1958) 229; John Parkinson, *Theatrum Botanicum* (1640) 929; William Salmon, *Botanalogica* I (1710) 10; John Aubrey, in *Wiltshire Collections*, ed JE Jackson (1862) 12, cited by Katie Peebles, in *Studies in Medievalism XXVI* (forthcoming, Cambridge, 2017); Columella: www.seedaholic.com [accessed 8 Dec 2015]; RE Randall, *J*

Ecology 91 (2) (2003) 325–40; Culpeper, *Pharm Lon* 19; Covent Garden: Gabrielle Hatfield, *Hatfield's Herbal* (2007) 7; PubMed: (2014) 24924290; (2012) 21902563; (2008) PMC2731181; Anne Pratt, *Haunts of the Wild Flowers* (1866) 310; John Parkinson, *Paradisi in Sole* (1629) 492; *The Syon Abbey Herbal, AD 1517*, ed J Adams & S Forbes (2015) 227.

ASH [240]: overview: Forestry Commission, www.forestrygov.uk [accessed 21 Sep 2016]; 'Betty': *The Guardian*, 22 Apr 2016; biochar: www.carbongold.com [accessed 21 Sep 2016]; John Wesley, *Primitive Physick* (Bristol, 1765 [1747]) 102; Robert Penn, *The Man who Made Things out of Trees* (2015) 7; Oliver Rackham, *The Ash Tree* (Toller Fratrum, Dors, 2014) 8; French herbalist: Jean Palaiseul, *Grandmother's Secrets* (1973 [1972]) 38; William Langham, *The Garden of Health* (1578) 39; Maurice Mességué, *Health Secrets of Plants and Herbs* (1979 [1975]) 40; PubMed: (2014) 24877717; (2015) 24562238; (2010) 20035854; (2004) 15120454; EMA Monograph 239271 (2011).

AVENS [244]: 'antidote': *Hatfield's Herbal* 184; eugenol research: (2011) 1627964; *Ortus Sanitatis*, quoting Platearius of Salerno: James T Shipley, *Dictionary of Early English* (Lanham MD, 2014 [1955]) 92; Parkinson, *Theatrum* 138; Henriette Kress, *Practical Herbs* 1 (Helsinki, 2011) 96; David Hoffmann, *Medical Herbalism* (Rochester VT, 2003) 114–17; Sir John Hill, *The Family Herbal* (Bungay, Suff, 1812 [1755]) 19; Edward Baylis, *A New and Compleat Body of Practical Botanic Physic* (1791) 66; www.wildplantforager.com/blog [accessed 22 Sep 2016]; PubMed: (2013) 23738465; (2015) PMC4461949; (2016)

27353564; Palaiseul 39; Julian Barker, *The Medicinal Flora of Britain and Northwestern Europe* (West Wickham, Kent, 2001) 178.

BISTORT [248]: Mrs M Grieve, *The Modern Herbal* (1931) 105; root, snake names: eg Lesley Gordon, *A Country Herbal* (Exeter, 1980) 23; Grigson 247; Turner: Grigson 248; David Blackwell, pers comm, 2014; bistort competitions: eg Stephen Barstow, *Around the World in 80 Plants* (East Meon, Hamp, 2014) 263; Lord Haw Haw, Amundsen: Barstow 260; tanning: Thomas Green, *The Universal Herbal* II (Liverpool, 1820) 376; PubMed: (2014) 24742754; (2016) 26929003; (2008) 18067063; (2015) 26360047; (2011) 21413092; Barker 93.

BLACK HOREHOUND [252]: cattle rejection: Gordon 93; Turner: Grigson 349; Cape use: Ben-Erik Van Wyk et al, *Medicinal Plants of South Africa* (Pretoria, 1997) 54; Richard Lawrence Hool, *Health from British Wild Herbs* (Southport, 1924 [1918]) 5–6; Hoffmann 533; Matthew Wood, *The Earthwise Herbal: Old World Medicinal Plants* (Berkeley CA, 2008) 126–7; Dioscorides: Andrew Chevallier, *Encyclopedia of Herbal Medicine* (2016 [1996]) 176; PubMed: (2010) 20645243; (2008) 18817140; (2003) 15138012; (2014) PMC4099109; John Gerard, *Herball* (1597).

BLACKTHORN [256]: Ötzi: James H Dickson et al, 'The Iceman Reconsidered' (2005), www.scientificamerican.com [accessed 22 Sep 2016]; 'thorn in the flesh': II Cor 12.7; Maj Thomas Weir: Susan Lavender & Anna Franklin, *Herbcraft* (Chieveley, Berks, 1996) 114; 'lady of pearls': *Hatfield's Herbal* 27; Parkinson, *Theatrum* 1034; Palaiseul 286; anon, qtd Hatfield, *Memory* 56; Hill, *Family Herbal* 314; Brooks & Hellier, wine merchants, qtd Roger Phillips, *Wild Food* (1983) 132; *umeboshi*: *The Oxford Companion to Food*, ed Alan Davidson (Oxford, 1999) 726; PubMed: (2009) 20120103; (2014) 24243401; (2013) 23815554; Abbé Kneipp, qtd Palaiseul 286.

BUGLE [260]: Gerard: qtd *Hatfield's Herbal* 46; surgeons: eg Parkinson, *Theatrum* 528; Culpeper, *Pharm Lon* 15; Grigson 354; Langham 99; Parkinson, Theatrum 526; Baylis 223–34; William Kemsey, *The British Herbal* (1838), cited in *Hatfield's Herbal* 46–7; harpagide: *Potter's Herbal Cyclopaedia*, ed EM Williamson (Saffron Walden, Ess, 2003) 75; Thomas Green I, 70; PubMed: (2011) 22015320; (2008a) 19478420; (2008b) 18520054.

BUTCHER'S BROOM [264]: Chevallier, *Encyclopedia* (2016) 265; 'knee holly': Langham 111; Parkinson, *Theatrum* 253; rodents: Richard Mabey, *Flora Britannica* (1996) 433; meat trade: *The Encyclopedia of Herbs and Herbalism*, ed Malcolm Stuart (1979) 256; Devon: *Hatfield's Herbal* 52; Christine Herbert, pers comm, 31 Oct 2016; Elizabeth Blackwell, *A Curious Herbal* (1750 German edn of 1739 edn) pl 155; PubMed: (2009) 19620698; (2000) 11152059.

CHICORY [266]: Passover/seder, leaf recipe: Maida Silverman, *A City Herbal* (Woodstock NY, 1997 [1977]) 34–5; Pliny: Lisa Manniche, *An Ancient Egyptian Herbal* (1989) 88; Linnaeus: Silverman 33; names: *Ox Comp Food* 167; Peter Holmes, *The Energetics of Western Herbs*, 2 vols (Boulder CO, 2006 [1989]) I, 449; Camp, poster: Paul Chrystal, *Coffee: A Drink for the Devil* (Stroud, 2016); names: *Ox Comp Food* 167; recurring wartime coffee substitute: Silverman 35; oligofructose: 'Food Unwrapped', Channel 4 TV, 3 Jan 2016, and www.nutriline.org [accessed 4 Jan 2016]; eye issues: HK Bakhru, *Herbs that Heal* (New Delhi, 1990) 66; James Duke, *The Green Pharmacy* (Emmaus PA, 1997) 247; PubMed: (2002) 12860315; (2012)

PMC3372077; (2010) 21694986; (2015) 26151029; Parkinson, *Theatrum* 776.

CRANESBILL [270]: Mrs Grieve 233; Thomas Bartram, *Bartram's Encyclopedia of Herbal Medicine* (1998 [1995]) 134; Culpeper, *Pharm Lon* 18; Salmon I, 229; species numbers: Clive Stace, *Field Flora of the British Isles* (Cambridge, 1999) 316–21; Jim Mcdonald, wild geranium video, 13 Feb 2011; Deni Bown, *Encyclopedia of Herbs & Their Uses* (1995) 288; Holmes II, 797; Michael Moore, *Medicinal Plants of the Mountain West* (Santa Fe NM, 1979) 69; *vrouebossie*, rose geranium: Van Wyk et al, 134; Matthew Wood, *The Earthwise Herbal: New World Medicinal Plants* (Berkeley CA, 2009) 164; PubMed: (2007) 18173115; (2015) 4491959; (2012) 23413565.

CREEPING JENNY & YELLOW LOOSESTRIFE [274]: Parkinson, *Theatrum* 544; Mrs Grieve 549; Turner: Grigson 289; *herbe aux cent maux*: Barker 317; Culpeper, *Pharm Lon* 22; Parkinson, *Theatrum* 555; Hill, *Family Herbal* 204; Dan Bensky & Andrew Gamble, *Chinese Herbal Medicine: Materia Medica* (Seattle WA, 1993 [1986]) 144–5; PubMed: (2002) 12776538; (2013) 263665578.

DAISY [278]: Mrs Pratt, *Haunts* 111; Chaucer, 'The Legend of Good Women' (1385); day's eye: Grigson 400; Milton, 'L'Allegro', l. 75; Shelley, 'The Question', ll. 10–11; Clare, 'The Village Minstrel', ll. 811–12; Hill, *Family Herbal* 107–8; Barker: quote, *bellis* meaning 450; Roman use, soup: Anne McIntyre, *The Complete Floral Healer* (1996) 73; Parkinson, *Theatrum* 532; modern uses: Rachel Corby, *The Medicine Garden* (Preston, 2009) 44; bruisewort: *Hatfield's Herbal* 92; Wesley 67; Elizabeth Blackwell pl 200; Nikki Darrell, pers comm, 27 Jun 2015; Chris Gambatese, pers comm, 17 Jun 2016; PubMed: (2012) 22775421; (2013) 24346069; (1997) 9434600; (2014) 24617777; (2016) 27178360; (2005) 16036165.

FLEABANE [284]: genera: Stace 487–9; Linnaeus: Mrs Grieve 321; Egypt: Manniche 109–10; Parkinson, *Theatrum* 128; Salmon I, 372; Rudolf Koch & Fritz Kredel, *Das Blumenbuchje Zeichungen*, 3 vols (Mainz, 1929–30) III, 215; PubMed: (2012) 02014782; (1992) *Field Mus Nat Hist* 1442; (2014a) 25532299; (2014b) *J Pure App Microbio* 8 (4): 267985.

FORGET-ME-NOT [288]: naming: eg Jack Sanders, *The Secrets of Wildflowers* (Guilford CT, 2014) 121; Gerard: *Hatfield's Herbal* 138; Coleridge, 'The Keepsake', ll. 10–13; DH Lawrence, *Lady Chatterley's Lover* (1928) ch 15; Mrs Grieve 322; Parkinson, *Theatrum* 692; PubMed: (2014) *Acta Phys Plant* 36 (8): 2283–6; (2011) 22462056; (2008) *Chem Nat Comp* 44 (5): 632–3; Parkinson, *Theatrum* 692.

FUMITORY [292]: 'official' (1618): Culpeper, *Pharm Lon* 18; (1996): *British Herbal Pharmacopoeia 1996* (Exeter, 1996) 84; names: Grigson 60; Shakespeare, *King Lear* 4.4.2–6; Mrs Pratt, *Haunts* 74; *Hatfield's Herbal* 142; EMA/HMPC/576232/2010; Mességué 129; Christophe Barnard, seminar, Avignon, 26 Apr 2015; Mrs CF Leyel, *Herbal Delights* (1987 [1937]) 280; Holmes II, 692; Palaiseul 123; India: Elizabeth M Williamson, *Major Herbs of Ayurveda* (Edinburgh, 2002) 150; PubMed: (2012) 23569991; (2014) *J Intercult Ethnopharm* 3 (4): 173–8; (2011) 3371888; Anne Pratt, *Flowering Plants, Grasses, Sedges, and Ferns of Great Britain* 1 (1873) pl 14.

GOLDENROD [296]: Aaron's rod: Grigson 398; *S. odora*, Liberty Tea: Silverman 63; Parkinson, *Theatrum* 543; Gerard: Grigson 399; William Cobbett (1818), qtd Gordon 87; John Muir (1905), qtd Silverman 63; Palaiseul (1973) 131; Culpeper, *Pharm Lon* 17; German treatments: Aviva Romm, *Botanical Medicine for Women's Health* (St Louis MO, 2010) 296; tea: Maria Treben, *Health through God's Pharmacy* (Steyr, Austria, 1982) 24; cf green tea: www.herbalremediesadvice.org [accessed 15 Jul 2016]; *BHP 1996* 91; ragweed: Steven Foster & James Duke, *Eastern/Central Medicinal*

Plants and Herbs (New York, 2000) 139; PubMed: (2004) 15638071; (2014) 23872883; (2002) 12467138; (2008) 18380925; (2009) 19827029; (2012) 23137724.

GREATER CELANDINE [300]:
Holmes I, 410; Barker 129; Mességué 86; Anne van Arsdall, *Medieval Herbal Remedies* (New York, 2002) 127; Treben 25–6; *Hatfield's Herbal* 155; Langham 128; Pechey 46; Mrs Pratt, *Haunts* 214; PubMed: (1995) 7757387; EMA/HMPC/369801/2009.

GROUND ELDER [303]: Barstow 232; Hill, *Family Herbal* 157; Grelda: Richard Mabey, *Weeds* (2010) 198; Gerard: qtd Pamela Michael, *Edible Plants & Herbs* (2007 [1980]) 107; St Gerard: Bown 229; bishopweed: Grigson 232–3; 'Wildman' Steve Brill & Evelyn Dean, *Identifying and Harvesting Edible and Medicinal Plants* (New York, 2002 [1994]) 260; Mabey, *Weeds* 197; Parkinson, *Theatrum* 944; Tabernaemontanus 1588, qtd in (2009) 19063957; 'all the tastier': John Wright, *Hedgerow* (2010) 101; PubMed: Olga Tovchiga et al, papers, 2012–16; (1987) 24225783; (2007) 17574359.

GROUND IVY [308]: alehoof, gill: Mrs Grieve 442; 'poor name': Grigson 352; Bartram 207–8; *BHP 1996* 95; Hildegard: www.whisperingearth.co.uk [accessed 28 Sep 2016]; Langham 8; 'recent survey': Henriette Kress, *Practical Herbs 2* (Helsinki, 2013) 76–9; Parkinson, *Theatrum* 677; PubMed: (2011) 3218471; (2006) 16530364; (2013) 24477256; (2014) 24850617.

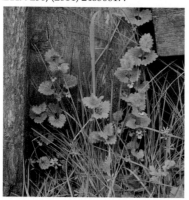

GYPSYWORT [312]: Lyte: qtd Grigson 342–3; Barker 383; Constantine Samuel Rafinesque, *Medical Flora* (1828): see www.henriettes-herb.com [accessed 28 Sep 2016]; Holmes II, 555; Hoffmann 463; PubMed: (2006) 16150466; (1994) 8135877; (2013) 3719484; (2008) 18083068.

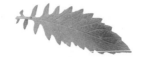

HEATHERS [315]: genera: Stace 193–4; George Buchanan, qtd in DC Watts, *Dictionary of Plant Lore* (Burlington MA, 2007) 188; Mrs Pratt, *Haunts* 249–50; Scottish uses: Tess Darwin, *The Scots Herbal* (Edinburgh, 1996) 106–9, and William Milliken & Sam Bridgewater, *Flora Celtica* (Edinburgh, 2013) passim; honey: Milliken & Bridgewater 72–3; Leyden: qtd anon [Elizabeth Kent], *Flora Domestica* (1831) 200; ale/wine: ibid. 58–60; moorland tea: Darwin 108; Koch & Kredel, III, 210; Matthiolus, Clusius: Parkinson, *Theatrum* 1486; PubMed: (2014) 25550074; (2013) 24383325; (2010) 19827032; (2011) 22181981; Dr R Spittal, 'The Heather Bell' (nd), qtd GP Morris & NP Willis, *The Prose and Poetry of England and America* (New York, 1845) 540, www.electricscotland.com [accessed 21 Oct 2016].

HERB ROBERT [320]: redness: Palaiseul 96; Rupert: Barker 212; Robert, Robin Goodfellow: Grigson 114–17, and Katherine Kear, *Flower Wisdom* (2000) 153, 155–6; South Africa: Van Wyk et al, 134; Pechey 118–19; red-water fever, Ireland: David E Allen & Gabrielle Hatfield, *Medicinal Plants in Folk Tradtion* (Portland OR, 2004) 175–6; PubMed: (2010) 21046015; (2004) 15165415; (2012) *Med. Chem. Res.* 21 (5): 601–15; (2014) 3274083; Mrs Pratt, *Haunts* 41; Chevallier 216.

HOGWEED [324]: 'commonest': M Blamey, R & A Fitter, *The Wild Flora of Britain and Ireland* (1977) 180; Heracles/Hercules: Stuart 201; giant hogweed: eg Mabey, *Weeds* (2010) 228–33; French uses: Cathy Skipper, pers comm, 10 Nov 2015; Wood, *Earthwise:*

New World 188; PubMed: (2008) *Planta Med* 74 – PF18; (2013) 23541934; (2014) 24697288; (2010) 20657619; (2006) 16504434; Roger Phillips, *Wild Food* (1983) 50; buds: Mina Said-Allsopp, pers comm, 9 Jan 2016.

LESSER CELANDINE [328]: Wordsworth: Miranda Seymour, *A Brief History of Thyme* (2002) 18; DH Lawrence, *Sons and Lovers* (1913) ch 6; names: Grigson 50; 'broom handle': Seymour 18; Parkinson, *Theatrum* 618–19; Pechey 47; Hoffmann 289–90; Culpeper, *Pharm Lon* 17; 'as in other cases': Allen & Hatfield 83; causes: Barker 119; PubMed: (2015) 25729484.

MOUSE-EAR HAWKWEED [332]: Hill, *Family Herbal* 236; William Curtis, *Flora Londinensis* 2 (1835 [1778]) 274; Parkinson, *Theatrum* 790; *BHP 1983*: Bartram 298; Leo Hartley Grindon, *The Manchester Flora* (1859) 304; expectorant: Hoffmann 512; Pechey 162; Barker 498; New South Wales: www.weeds.dpi.nsw.au [accessed 4 Oct 2016]; PubMed: EMA/HMPC/68034/2013; (2011) *Open Life Sci* 6 (3): 397–404; (2010) 21054887; (2009) 3274148; Chevallier 220.

NAVELWORT [336]: Parkinson, *Theatrum* 741–2; Mrs Grieve 455; names: Grigson 200; Gerard: Mrs Pratt, *Haunts* 192; Culpeper, *Pharm Lon* 25; Sarah Raven, *Wild Flowers* (2011) 100; Miles Irving, *The Forager Handbook* (2009) 294; Barker 16; Bach: www.bachessenceproducers.com [accessed 30 Sep 2016]; Pechey 168; PubMed: (2012) 22672636; Van Arsdall 170.

OX-EYE DAISY [340]: Grigson 405–6; gools: www.hikersnotebook.net [accessed 26 Sep 2016]; dermatitis: PubMed (1999) 10439521; www.extension.colostate.edu [accessed 26 Sep 2016]; Pechey 69; Salmon I, 289; Thomas Green I, 294; Hill, *Family Herbal* 107; Mabey, *Flora Britannica* 373; PubMed: (2015) 26121329.

PINE [344]: John Evelyn, *Sylva* (1664) I, 242; Pechey 188; Julia Lawless, *The Encyclopaedia of Essential Oils* (Shaftesbury, 1992) 157; drovers:

Hatfield's Herbal 268; Matthiolus: Parkinson, *Paradisi* 608; Linnaeus, flour: Laura Mason, *Pine* (2013) 153, 156; sanitoria, asthma: Nikki Darrell, *Conversations with Plants* (Cork, 2014) I, 176; 'truism': Parkinson, *Theatrum* 1538; Peter Conway, *Tree Medicine* (2001) 234–5; Keats, 'Ode to Psyche' (1819) l. 53; Charlotte du Cann, *52 Flowers that Changed My World* (Uig, Isle of Lewis, 2012) 172; Michael Moore, *Medicinal Plants of the Desert and Canyon West* (Santa Fe NM, 1989) 89; Euell Gibbons, *Stalking the Healthful Herbs* (New York, 1966) 122, qtd Mason 156; Wood, *Earthwise: New World* 269; Crispin Van de Pas, *Hortus Floridus* (Arnhem, 1614) pl 78; PubMed: (2009a) 2794845; (2005a) 15752644; (2000) 10857921; (2002) 11996210; (2005b) 16028975; (2009b) *Food & Bio Proc* 88 (2–3): 247–52.

PRIMROSE & COWSLIP [350]: Chevallier 256; Plantlife survey, 9 Jun 2015, www.plantlife.org [accessed 3 Aug 2016]; St Peter's keys: Philippa Back, *The Illustrated Herbal* (1987) 48; Freya, overpicking: McIntyre 181; W Strehlow & G Hertzka, *Hildegard of Bingen's Medicine* (Santa Fe NM, 1988) 82; Treben 22; Parkinson, *Paradisi* 247; George Eliot, *Mill on the Floss* (1860), bk 1, ch 7; Pechey 60; Milton: Colonial Dames of America, *Herbs and Herb Lore of Colonial America* (New York, 1995 [1970]) 48; Germany, 'official': NG Bisset & M Wichtl, *Herbal Drugs and Phytopharmaceuticals* (Stuttgart & Boca Raton FL, 2001 [1994]) 389, 391; Wesley 123; Saskia Marjoram: www.saskiasfloweressences.com [accessed 26 Sep 2016]; PubMed: (2012) PMC 3318187; (1994) 23195935.

PURPLE LOOSESTRIFE [355]: 'reliable drama': Raven 316; 'long purples': Grigson 209; 'iron hard': Sybil Marshall, *Fenland Chronicle* (Cambridge, 1980 [1967]) 196; 'purple plague': Timothy Lee Scott, *Invasive Plant Medicine* (Rochester VT, 2010) 255–60; Salmon 650, 652; '2.7 million seeds': www.seagrant.umn.edu [accessed 4 Oct 2016]; '$45m': www.refugeassociation.org [accessed 4 Oct 2016]; Mcdonald: www.herbcraft.

org [accessed 4 Oct 2016]; Parkinson, *Theatrum* 547; Anna Parkinson, pers comm, 28 May 2013; Mrs Grieve 497; PubMed: (2010) 20554008; (2012) 22829057; (2015) 25985768; (2005) 15975734.

ROWAN [360]: names: Grigson 186–7; 'rowan': *Hatfield's Herbal* 296; James VI & I, *Demonologie* (Edinburgh, 1598) IV, 3; tanning, dyeing: Mrs Grieve 69; parasorbic acid: Irving 285; PubMed: (2008) 18819524; (2010) 21195756; 'The Laidly Worm', qtd Wright 77; Rev J Evans, *Letters Written through a Tour of North Wales* (1798) 112; Alys Fowler, *The Thrifty Forager* (2011) 172.

SANICLE [364]: 'molecular': Raven, 25; ancient woodland: Oliver Rackham, *Woodlands* (2006) 325; 'Celui qui…': qtd WT Fernie, *Herbal Simples* (Philadelphia, 1895) 508; Grigson 224; Parkinson, *Theatrum* 534; Elizabeth Blackwell pl 63; Hool 28; PubMed: (1999) 10441789; (1996) 8769089; (2013) 23770053; Jethro Kloss, *Back to Eden* (New York, 1939) 309; Wood, *Earthwise: Old World* 461, attrib to Peter Holmes.

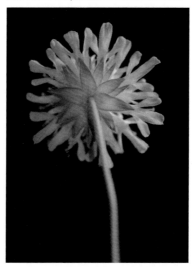

SCABIOUS [368]: genera: www.theplantlist.org [accessed 23 Sep 2015]; Knaut: Mrs Grieve 721; 'rough stalks': Mabey, *Flora Britannica* 363; devil's bit name: Grigson 386–7, Barker 385; devil's 'envy': *Grete Herball* (1526), in Grigson 387; plague: Marcus Harrison,

Plants and the Plague (Lostwithiel, Corn, 2015) 197–201; Parkinson, *Theatrum* 490; Culpeper: Mrs Grieve 722; Hill, *Family Herbal* 306; Stuart 268; Holmes I, 233; PubMed: (2015) 25841374; (2012) 22492499; (2010) 2984435.

SEA BUCKTHORN [373]: migrant birds: Mabey, *Flora Britannica* 233; HCA Vogel, *The Nature Doctor* (1989 [1952]) 387; Parkinson, *Theatrum* 1008; elder health: eg Barker 246; 'New Nordic': www.washingtonpost.com, 25 Jul 2016 [accessed 10 Oct 2016]; 'Siberian pineapple': *Sea Buckthorn*, ed V Singh & H Kallio (New Delhi, 2003) 486; John Wilkes, ed, *Encylopaedia Londinensis* 10 (1811) 192; PubMed: (2012) 3317027; (2006) 16968106; (2011) 21960663; (2009) 19425187; (2003) 12854177; (2013) 23096237; (2016) *Afr J Biotech* 15 (5): 118–24; Wright 156; harvesting: eg Irving 290; ice cream sauce: noted Davidson 708.

SILVERWEED, TORMENTIL & CINQUEFOIL [378]: tormentil names: Grigson 161; 'austere': Hill, *Family Herbal* 342; silverweed names: Grigson 159; argentina, goosewort: Stuart 245; prince's feathers: Zöe Hawes, *Wild Drugs* (2010) 70; Alexander Carmichael: radix4roots.blogspot (2011) [accessed 7 Oct 2016]; Ray: Grigson 160; Wright 78; cinquefoil: Mrs Grieve 316; cinquefoil names: Grigson 162–3; crampwort: Holmes II, 795; Vogel 218; Mrs Leyel, *Cinquefoil: Herbs to Quicken the Five Senses* (1957) 9; Parkinson, *Theatrum* 399; 'sisters': Palaiseul 257; Pechey 236; PubMed: (2009) 19857087; (2014a) 4202341; (2003) 12913771; (2014b) 25483225; (2008) 18664379; (2011) 20677176; Barker 180.

SOWTHISTLE [382]: genera: Stace 452–3, 475; Margaret Roberts, *Margaret Roberts' Book of Herbs* (Johannesburg, 1983) 120; Barstow 167; Arthur Lee Jacobson: www.arthurleej.com [accessed 2 Oct 2016]; Pliny: Mabey, *Flora Britannica* 365; Popeye, worldwide uses: Irving 158; passover, Five Boro: Brill & Dean 201–2; Ray: qtd Grigson 322; warts, latex: Allen

& Hatfield 282; Parkinson, *Theatrum* 807; opium: Brill & Dean 202; Nepal: Narayan P Manandhar, *Plants and People of Nepal* (Portland OR, 2002) 433; elder medicine in China: Silverman 151; PubMed: (2002) 12716920; (2012) 3292812; (2011) 3305921.

SPHAGNUM MOSS [392]: Mrs Grieve 554; British/Irish species: British Bryological Society, *Mosses and Liverworts of Britain and Ireland: A Field Guide* (2010) 276–310; Cathcart, poem: Peter Ayres, *Field Bryology* 110 (2013): www.rbg-web2.rbge.org.uk [accessed 1 Oct 2016]; Nelson Coon, *Using Wild and Wayside Plants* (New York, 1980 [1957]) 84–5.

SPEEDWELL [386]: Mrs Grieve 831; species: Stace 414–18; 'victory': Grieve 831; Roberts 62; Parkinson, *Theatrum* 552; Francke: Bown 368; Pechey 222; *thé d'Europe*: Barker 408; Leclerc, poor man's tea, eyebright, whooping cough: *Hatfield's Herbal* 326; cholesterol, Roman compliment, priest: Treben 40–1; brooklime like scurvy grass: Raven 292; Wright 128; PubMed: (2013) 23142555; (1985) 4021513; (2014) 24892270.

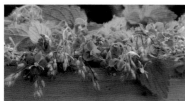

SWEET CHESTNUT [394]: Evelyn I, ch 8; Bartram 109; Pechey 53; Bach remedy: Conway 153; bud: Joe Rozencwajg, *Dynamic Gemmotherapy* (New Plymouth NZ, 2008) 39–40; *The Times* (London) 22 Aug 2015; PubMed: Quave et al (2015) 4546677.

THISTLE [398]: 'Scotch thistle': Mabey, *Flora Britannica* 455; Scott: www.nrscotland.gov.uk [accessed 9 Oct 2016]; Irving 147; Hill, *Family Herbal* 337; silymarin: Holmes I, 196; Barker 483; Katrina Blair, *The Wild Wisdom of Weeds* (White River Junction VT, 2014) 311–31; Wesley 80, 117; Blair 321–2; Matthew Alfs (2014), *Medical Herbalism* 17 (2): 8–15.

VALERIAN [403]: odour: Antony Dweck, in Peter J Houghton (ed), *Valerian: The Genus Valeriana* (Amsterdam, 1997) 2; 'phu', kesso root, jatamansi: Mrs Grieve 824, 828–9; Gerard, *Herball* (1636 edn) 1078; Robert Thornton, *A New Family Herbal* (1810) 35; Pied Piper, eg Doug Elliott, *Wild Roots: A Forager's Guide* (Rochester VT, 1995) 87; Fabius Columna: Seymour 119; Pechey 240; John Hill, *The Virtues of Wild Valerian in Nervous Disorders* (1772 [1758]); *U.S. Pharmacopoeia*: Roy Upton et al, *Valerian Root* (American Herbal Pharmacopoeia, Santa Cruz CA, 1999) 2; *BHP 1996* 176; 'nauseous': Grieve 827; Gustave Flaubert, *Madame Bovary* (1857): qtd Seymour 119; Parkinson, *Theatrum* 124–5; 7Song, seminar, Avignon, 28 Apr 2015; 150 compounds: Upton 8; Barker 431.

VIOLETS [408]: 'dog': Grigson 79; Macer: qtd *Hatfield's Herbal* 336; Leigh Hunt, *The Indicator* (1820); Horace: qtd Bown 370; Romans: Barker 251; Richard Surflet, *A Countrie Farme* (1600); Lightfoot: qtd *Hatfield's Herbal* 336; Hill, *Family Herbal* 362; Maria Sybilla Merian, *Erucam ortus…* (Amstelaedami, 1718) pt 2, pl 1; *Hamlet* 1.3.7–10; ionones: www.boisdejasmin.com [accessed 29 Sep 2016]; Violetta: Bown 370; 'pectoral': Palaiseul 306; 'official': *BHP 1996* 178; Nicholas Culpeper, *The English Physician Enlarged* (1814 [1652]) 337; Askham: qtd Mrs Grieve 835; Duke, *Green Pharmacy* 446; South Africa: Roberts 45; Salerno: qtd Palaiseul 306; Langham 663; PubMed: (1995) 7703226; (2010a) 20564026; (2010b) 20580652; (2008) 18081258; (2011) 22242426; (2014) 25763239; (2015) 25954025.

WALNUT [414]: Jupiter: Stuart 208; Parkinson, *Theatrum* 1413–14; Thomas Fuller, *The History of the Worthies of England* (1682 [1662]) 76; Evelyn I, ch 9; JC Loudon, *Arboretum et Fruticetum Britannicum* (1838); Roger Deakin, *Wildwood: A Journey through Trees* (2007) 317; brain/charmarghz: Davidson 833; Coles: Mrs Grieve 844; Culpeper, *Pharm Lon* 11–12; Willis: Harrison 223; Langham 666; Pliny, hair recipe: Stuart 208; Susun Weed, video

[last accessed 30 Oct 2016]; Wood, *Earthwise: New World* 208; PubMed: (2011) 22048906; (2012) 23756586; (2002) 11983340; (2013) 24396383; (2014a) 24500933; (2014b) 25024344; EMA/HMPC/346740/2011, 26.

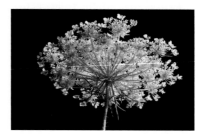

WILD CARROT [418]: Forgotten Herbs blog, July 2016; Robin Rose Bennett: blog, 1 July 2012; Holmes II, 574; Matthew Wood, *The Book of Herbal Wisdom* (Berkeley CA, 1997) 230; Ryan Drum: blog, nd; Jim Mcdonald: blog, 13 Feb 2006; bird's nest: Elliott 75; Suffolk: Gabrielle Hatfield, *Country Remedies* (Woodbridge, Suffolk, 1994) 24; PubMed: (2003) 14569406; (2011a) 3192732; (2014) 24519559; (2015) 26819805; (2011b) 3259297; Duke, *Green Pharmacy* 400; Saskia Marjoram: www.saskiasfloweressences.com [accessed 26 Sep 2016].

WILD STRAWBERRY [422]: Hadrian's Wall: *Hatfield's Herbal* 331; Wolsey, Mme Tallien: Ernest Small, *Top 100 Food Plants* (Ottawa, 2009) 493; Dr Butler: Izaak Walton, *Compleat Angler* (1653) pt I, ch 5; Parkinson, *Paradisi* 526; Linnaeus: Richard Pulteney, *A General View of the Writings of Linnaeus* (1805) 478–80; Jane Austen, *Emma* (1816) ch 36; Wood, *Earthwise: Old World* 261; Elizabeth Blackwell pl 77; Thomas Green I, 574; Van Arsdall 168; Parkinson, *Theatrum* 758–9; Hill, *Family Herbal* 329; Palaiseul 294; PubMed: (2004) 15077879; (2014) 24345049; (2006) 16478244; (2015) 25803191; Barker 180.

WOUNDWORT [426]: Gerard: Wood, *Earthwise: Old World* 471; Parkinson, *Theatrum* 609; blog: monica.wilde.com, 16 Aug 2015 [accessed 5 Oct 2016]; PubMed: (2009) 22339365; (2011) *Phytochem Lett* 4 (4): 448–53.

Recommended reading

Barker, Julian. *The Medicinal Flora of Britain & Northwestern Europe: A Field Guide.* West Wickham, Kent, 2001

Barstow, Stephen. *Around the World in 80 Plants.* East Meon, Hampshire, 2014.

Bartram, Thomas. *Bartram's Encyclopedia of Herbal Medicine.* London, 1998 [1995]

Blair, Katrina. *The Wild Wisdom of Weeds: 13 Essential Plants for Human Survival.* White River Junction, VT, 2014

Blamey, Marjorie, Richard Fitter and Alastair Fitter. *Wild Flowers of Britain & Ireland.* London, 2003

Brill, "Wildman" Steve, with Evelyn Dean. *Identifying and Harvesting Edible and Medicinal Plants in Wild (and Not so Wild) Places.* New York, 1994

Bruton-Seal, Julie & Matthew Seal. *Hedgerow Medicine.* Ludlow, Shropshire, 2008
_____ *The Herbalist's Bible.* Ludlow, Shropshire, 2014

Campbell, Ffyona. *The Hunter-Gatherer Way: Putting Back the Apple.* South Hams, Dorset, 2014 [2012]

Cech, Richo. *Making Plant Medicine,* 4th edn. Williams, OR, 2016 [2000]

Chevallier, Andrew. *The Encyclopedia of Herbal Medicine,* 2nd edn. London, 2016 [1996]
_____ *Herbal Remedies.* London, 2007

Coon, Nelson. *Using Wild and Wayside Plants.* New York, 1980 [1957]

de la Forêt, Rosalee. *Alchemy of Herbs.* New York, 2017

Duke, James A. *The Green Pharmacy.* Emmaus, PA, 1997

Easley, Thomas & Steven Horne. *The Modern Herbal Dispensatory: A Medicine-Making Guide.* Berkeley, CA, 2016

Furnell, Dennis. *Health from the Hedgerow: A Naturalist's Encyclopaedia of Medicinal Plants.* London, 1985

Gordon, Lesley. *A Country Herbal.* London, 1980

Green, James. *The Herbal Medicine-Maker's Handbook: A Home Manual.* Berkeley, CA, 2002

Grieve, Mrs M, ed. and introd. Mrs CF Leyel. *A Modern Herbal.* London, 1998 [1931]; online at www.botanical.com

Grigson, Geoffrey. *The Englishman's Flora.* London, 1975 [1958]

Harrap, Simon. *Harrap's Wild Flowers: A Field Guide to the Wild Flowers of Britain & Ireland.* London, 2013

Harrison, Marcus. *Plants and The Plague: The Herbal Frontline.* Lostwithiel, Cornwall, 2015

Hatfield, Gabrielle. *Country Remedies: Traditional East Anglian Plant Remedies in the Twentieth Century.* Woodbridge, Suffolk, 1994
_____ *Memory, Wisdom and Healing: The History of Domestic Plant Medicine.* Stroud, Gloucestershire, 1999
_____ *Hatfield's Herbal.* London, 2007

Hedley, Christopher & Non Shaw. *Herbal Remedies: A Practical Beginner's Guide to Making Effective Remedies in the Kitchen.* Bath, 2002 (1996)
_____ *A Herbal Book of Making & Taking.* London, 2016 [1993]

Hoffmann, David. *The New Holistic Herbal: A Herbal Celebrating the Wholeness of Life,* Shaftesbury, Dorset, 1986 [1983]

Hughes, Nathaniel & Fiona Owen. *Weeds in the Heart.* Privately published, 2016

Kress, Henriette. *Practical Herbs.* Helsinki, Finland: vol. 1, 2011; vol. 2, 2013

Mabey, Richard. *Flora Britannica.* London, 1996

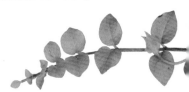

_____ *Weeds: How Vagabond Plants Gatecrashed Civilisation and Changed the Way We Think About Nature.* London, 2010

Masé, Guido. *The Wild Medicine Solution: Healing with Aromatic, Bitter, and Tonic Plants.* Rochester, VT, 2013

McIntyre, Anne. *The Complete Floral Healer.* London, 1996

Milliken, William & Sam Bridgewater. *Flora Celtica: Plants and People in Scotland.* Edinburgh, 2013

O'Ceirin, Cyril & Kit. *Wild and Free: Cooking from Nature.* Dublin, 1978

Palaiseul, Jean. *Grandmother's Secrets: Her Green Guide to Health from Plants.* London, 1973 [1972]

Phillips, Roger. *Wild Food.* London, 1983

Pienaar, Antoinette. *The Griqua's Apprentice: Ancient Healing Arts of the Karoo.* Trans. Catherine Knox. Cape Town, 2009

Plantlife. *The Good Verge Guide: A Different Approach to Managing Our Waysides and Verges.* London, 2016

Pole, Sebastian. *Cleanse, Nurture, Restore with Herbal Tea.* London, 2016

Rackham, Oliver. *The Illustrated History of the Countryside.* London, 2003 [1986]

Roberts, Margaret. *Healing Foods.* Pretoria, South Africa, 2011

Rohde, Eleanour Sinclair. *A Garden of Herbs.* Boston, MA, 1921; online at archive.org

Scott, Timothy Lee. *Invasive Plant Medicine: The Ecological Benefits and Healing Abilities of Invasives.* Rochester, VT, 2010

Silverman, Maida. *A City Herbal: Lore, Legend, & Uses of Common Weeds*, 3rd edn. Woodstock, NY, 1997 [1977]

Tobyn, Graeme, Alison Denham & Margaret Whitelegg. *The Western Herbal Tradition: 2000 Years of Medicinal Plant Knowledge.* Edinburgh, 2011

Treben, Maria. *Health through God's Pharmacy: Advice and Experiences with Medicinal Herbs.* Steyr, Austria, 1983 [1982]

Waller, Pip. *The Domestic Alchemist: 501 Herbal Recipes for Home, Health & Happiness.* Lewes, East Sussex, 2015

Wood, Matthew. *The Book of Herbal Wisdom.* Berkeley, CA, 1997

_____ *The Earthwise Herbal: A Complete Guide to New World Medicinal Plants.* Berkeley, CA, 2009

—— *The Practice of Traditional Western Herbalism.* Berkeley, CA, 2004

Wright, John. *Hedgerow.* River Cottage Handbook No. 7. London, 2010

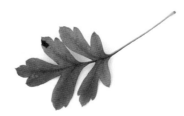

Resources

Finding an herbal practitioner
Word of mouth is often the best way to find a good herbalist. Ask friends or your local health food store to see who they can recommend.

You can also contact the professional associations below for a list of practicing members:

American Herbalists Guild (AHG)
PO Box 3076
Asheville, NC 28802
Tel. (617) 520-4372
www.americanherbalistsguild.com

Canadian Herbalist Association of BC (CHAofBC)
www.chaofbc.ca

The Ontario Herbalists Association
www.herbalists.on.ca

Workshops
Hedgerow Medicine
www.hedgerowmedicine.com
The authors' website, offering workshops, short courses; see also closed Facebook group *Forgotten Herbs*, which we moderate.

Suppliers
You can find most of what you need in grocery, health, kitchen and hardware stores. Here are a few suppliers who carry some of the harder-to-source supplies you might want.

Al-Ambiq
www.al-ambiq.com
Beautiful hand-made copper stills from Portugal.

Frontier Co-op
PO Box 299
3021 78th St
Norway, IA 52318
Tel. 1-844-550-6200
www.frontiercoop.com
Beeswax, empty capsules, etc.; also herbs, spices, body care

G Baldwin & Co
www.baldwins.co.uk
Mail order and shop: brown glass bottles, lanolin, beeswax; also dried herbs, essential oils.

Lakeland Ltd
www.lakeland.co.uk
Mail order and shops: jam- and jelly-making supplies, kitchen equipment.

Just Botanics
www.justbotanics.co.uk
Mail order for tinctures, oils, dried herbs, gums, resins, powders and empty capsules.

The London Teapot Company
www.chatsford.com
Mail order, manufacturer: Chatsford teapots with basket strainers for loose teas.

Neals Yard Remedies
www.nealsyardremedies.com
Beeswax, lanolin, brown glass bottles; also herbs, body care

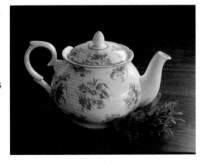

Plant information
American Botanical Council
http://abc.herbalgram.org
Information on medicinal plants; publishes *Herbalgram*

American Herb Association
www.ahaherb.com

Hedgerow Medicine
www.hedgerowmedicine.com
The authors' website, for workshops, courses, seasonal recipes

Henriette Kress
www.henriettes-herb.com
Herbal information website, with texts of many older herbals

Michael Moore
www.swsbm.com
Inspirational website of the late American herbalist (1941–2009), featuring distance learning.

The Herb Society of America
www.herbsociety.org
Publishes *The Herbarist* magazine

The Herb Society
www.herbsociety.org.uk
Promotes interest in all aspects of herbal use, publishes *Herbs* magazine.

Plantlife International
www.plantlife.org.uk
Wild-plant conservation charity

Plants for a Future
www.pfaf.org
Database and related book

State of the World's Plants
sotwp_2016
Pioneering report by Kew Royal Botanic Gardens.

United Plant Savers
PO Box 147
Rutland, OH 45775
http://unitedplantsavers.org
Charity protecting native medicinal plants of North America

USDA Plants Database
http://plants.usda.gov
Distribution maps for wild plants in the US and Canada   (including all those in this book)

The Wildlife Trusts
www.wildlifetrusts.org
Local groups, nature reserves.

Herbal medicine-making
For more detailed information on making your own herbal medicines, we recommed starting with these two books:

Making Plant Medicine by Richo Cech (Williams, OR, 2016)

The Herbal Medicine-Maker's Handbook: A Home Manual by James Green (Berkeley, CA, 2002)

Seeds and plants
Many plant nurseries sell wildflower seeds and plants. Two of our favourites are:

Poyntzfield Herb Nursery
www.poyntzfieldherbs.co.uk
For beautifully packed seeds and plants.

British Wild Flower Plants
www.wildflowers.co.uk
Largest supplier of British native plants.

Strictly Medicinal Seeds
PO Box 299
Williams, OR 97544
Tel. (541) 846-6704
www.strictly medicinal seeds.com
Run by herbalist Richo Cech, author of *Making Plant Medicine*; excellent selection of medicinal plants and seeds; comprehensive annual catalog

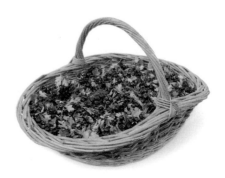

Index

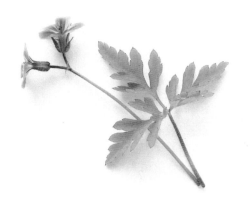

The authors

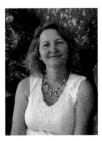

JULIE BRUTON-SEAL is a practising medical herbalist, iridologist and cranio-sacral therapist. A Fellow of the Association of Master Herbalists (AMH), she is also a writer, photographer, artist and graphic designer. Julie co-authored the vegetarian cookbook *Vegetarian Masterpieces* (1988).

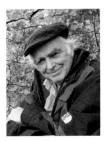

MATTHEW SEAL has worked as an editor and writer in books, magazines and newspapers for over forty years, in both the UK and South Africa. He is author of *Survive and Thrive in the New South Africa* (2000), and was the founder of the Professional Editors' Group there in 1993. He has served as the publications director of the Society for Editors and Proofreaders (SfEP).

Julie and Matthew teach courses and workshops in herbal medicine. For more information, visit the Facebook pages for their books and see their website: www.hedgerowmedicine.com

Other books by Julie and Matthew:

Hedgerow Medicine

Harvest wild plants and weeds and make your own remedies from the hedgerow. A practical guide to 50 common plants, telling you exactly what to do with them and how to use them, with recipes for each plant.

Published in North America as *Backyard Medicine.*

My absolute herbal inspiration nowadays being Julie and Matthew's wonderful book Hedgerow Medicine, *which to my mind is the best home-use British herbal that has ever been written - such a beautiful, inspiring and empowering book!*

Rose Titchiner, flower essence maker and author

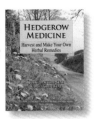

Kitchen Medicine

You have a pharmacy at your fingertips in your own pantry, and this practical book shows you how to use herbs, spices, fruits, vegetables, oils, vinegars and other familiar kitchen items to treat common ailments.

This is the best book I have ever seen on this subject and I just want to buy it for everyone I know! It is a great resource, an inspiration, a thing of great beauty and healing. Everyone should have a copy in their kitchens!

Permaculture Magazine

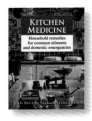

Make Your Own Aphrodisiacs

This attractive book is full of delicious recipes for romance, and is sumptuously illustrated. From ashwagandha to yohimbe via chocolate, roses, horny goat weed and more, this is a guide to herbs that really work as aphrodisiacs. Many of these herbs are also rejuvenating tonics.

It was published in North America as *Aphrodisia: homemade potions to make love more likely, more pleasurable and more possible.*

This would make a lovely Christmas present or indeed a fun, but informative, gift for lovers of both plants and people at any time of the year. I liked its small size – handy for the bedroom – and the rich, colourful pictures lend themselves very well to romance and the love of life in general.

The Herbalist

The Herbalist's Bible
John Parkinson's Lost Classic Rediscovered

A selection from and commentary on the biggest and best herbal ever written in English, John Parkinson's magnum opus, the largely forgotten *Theatrum Botanicum* or *Theater of Plants* (1640). Herbalist to Charles I, Parkinson took 50 years to write this book, and his experience comes through clearly in the Vertues (medicinal uses) for the chosen plants. Julie and Matthew add their own comments and illustrations.

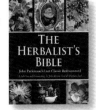

... a fascinating fusion of old and new.

The English Gardener

Skyhorse Publishing books may be purchased in bulk at special discounts for
sales promotion, corporate gifts, fund-raising, or educational purposes. Special
editions can also be created to specifications. For details, contact the Special
Sales Department, Skyhorse Publishing, 307 West 36th Street, 11th Floor, New
York, NY 10018 or info@skyhorsepublishing.com.

Skyhorse® and Skyhorse Publishing® are registered trademarks of Skyhorse
Publishing, Inc.®, a Delaware corporation.

Visit our website at www.skyhorsepublishing.com.

10 9 8 7 6 5

Library of Congress Cataloging-in-Publication Data is available on file.

Cover design by Mona Lin

Print ISBN: 978-1-5107-5382-2
Ebook ISBN: 978-1-5107-5462-1

Printed in China

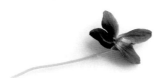

Please note: The information in *The Big Book of Backyard Medicine* is compiled from a
blend of historical and modern sources, from folklore and personal experience.
It is not intended to replace the professional advice and care of a qualified
herbal or medical practitioner. Do not attempt to self-diagnose or self-prescribe
for serious long-term problems without first consulting a qualified professional.
Heed the cautions given, and if already taking prescribed medicines or if you
are pregnant, seek professional advice before using herbal remedies.